Geography of Health

About the Author

Swati Rajput is a Professor at the Department of Geography, Shaheed Bhagat Singh College, University of Delhi. She holds her M.Phil. and Ph.D. degree from the Department of Geography of Delhi School of Economics, University of Delhi, India. She has been recognized as a National Resource Person in the Social Sciences by UNFPA and MHRD. She received Delhi University Gold Medal and the NS Pradhan Award. In 2020, she received the Venus International Women's Award for her commend able research in the field of gender studies.

She is an expert in the fields of Health and Well-being Geography, Food and Nutrition Security, Agricultural Geography and Urban Ecology. She has published numerous research papers in national and international journals, as well as chapters in renowned books. She has two books in her credit "Urban Green Space, Health Economics and Air Pollution in Delhi" (2021) and "Sustainable Smart Cities of India: Challenges and Future Perspectives (2017)".

GEOGRAPHY OF HEALTH

Swati Rajput

CONCEPT PUBLISHING COMPANY PVT. LTD.
NEW DELHI - 110059

ISBN: 978-93-5594-851-9 (HB)
ISBN: 978-93-5594-734-5 (PB)

First Published 2024

Published and Printed by

Concept Since 1974 **Concept Publishing Company Pvt. Ltd.**
A/15-16, Commercial Block, Mohan Garden
New Delhi-110059 (India)
T: +91-11-41101460
E: publishing@conceptpub.com, *W*: www.conceptpub.com

Cataloging in Publication--Courtesy: D.K. Agencies (P) Ltd. <docinfo@dkagencies.com>

Rajput, Swati, author.
Geography of health / Swati Rajput.
pages cm
Includes bibliographical references and index.
ISBN 9789355947345 (PB)
ISBN 9789355948519 (HB)

1. Medical geography. 2. Medical geography--India. 3. Public health. 4. Public health--India. 5. Medical policy. 6. Medical policy--India. 7. Medical statistics. 8. India--Statistics, Medical. I. Title.

LCC RA792.R35 2024 | DDC 614.42 23

Preface

Health and Well-being is the ultimate goal to attain. As the world is passing through the biggest uncertainty of COVID-19, the relevance of health studies has become increasingly significant. The world is witnessing significant changes in the landscape of health, diseases, and health systems. These changes are driven by various factors, including globalization, demographic shifts, urbanization, climate change, and advancements in technology. Geographers play a critical role in understanding various health parameters. It is widely recognized that health is not simply a personal attribute, but is also influenced by social, economic, and environmental factors, and it is these factors which vary considerably across space. The geography of health, therefore, raises important questions about health equity and highlights the impact that place has on the spatial variation of diseases, health resources and outcomes. This book aims on exploring the subject matter of geography of health, focusing on how geography affects health outcomes, the distribution of health resources, the factors that contribute to health disparities and health related policies and programmes at national and international level.

This book will hopefully be a meaningful addition to literature and content in this sub-field of Geography. The book is devoted to the students and researchers who want to explore this discipline and develop basic understanding of various aspects of health geography.

The book begins with examining the definition and concept of health and health geography. It develops the idea for a reader to understand the basics of health and well-being. It focuses upon approaches and scope of geography of health. Health outcomes are influenced by a complex range of factors that are related to each other and vary across regions, including geographical, demographic, socio-economic status, environmental conditions, lifestyle factors, and cultural practices. These determinants of health build up basic understanding about the disparities that exist between different regions. The book further examines these factors in detail, highlighting their unique roles in shaping health outcomes and identifying regions with high or low health conditions. It also contributes by explaining the impact of geography on health outcomes. The social determinants of health have a significant impact on health outcomes and account for a large proportion of health disparities between regions. Economic conditions are also a crucial factor influencing health outcomes and access to healthcare services, as people living in poverty are more likely to experience poor health outcomes. Access to healthy environments is equally important, as environmental pollution and unsafe living conditions can contribute to a range of health problems.

The book also discusses various communicable and non-communicable diseases and their affect on huge population of the earth. Communicable diseases spurt at a place and spread to other places. This spread can be well explained from a geographical perspective. The geographical conditions and location of a place are majorly responsible for the existence of the disease. Later, the movement of population and goods lead to its spread beyond administrative and political boundaries. The book highlights the spread of communicable diseases over space and time. Non-communicable diseases, also known as lifestyle diseases are prevalent in the modern world. Non-communicable diseases are influenced by the food habits, excessive use of chemicals, sedentary lifestyle etc. The book reinstates the epidemiological shift and its relevant reasons. Mental health is yet another significant area of discussion. The book talks about the concept of mental health and its significance. It also discusses the type of mental and psychological disorders that human beings are facing in the contemporary world. Finally, the book highlights the national and international policies, programmes and institutions for improving access to healthcare services and reducing health disparities between regions. It is an undeniable truth that health is one of the most valuable assets humans possess. It encompasses physical, mental, and social well-being, enabling individuals to lead fulfilling lives. Therefore, there exists a need to prioritize investments in healthcare systems, social infrastructure, and policies that promote equitable access to resources, quality healthcare, and opportunities for personal development.

The book relies upon well published data and maps from the sites and documents of recognized official international and national agencies like World Health Organization (WHO), United Nations Children's Fund (UNICEF), American Psychiatric Association (APA), Ministry of Health and Family Welfare, Indian Council of Medical Research (ICMR) etc.

The purpose of the book is to make readers aware about the holistic concept of health, physical health and mental health. The purpose is also to understand the role of geography in understanding the occurrence and spread of various diseases. The book is very relevant to the undergraduate and post-graduate students of Geography and health studies. The book covers all important topics of "Geography of Health" and "Geography of Health and Well-being" for BA Hons, Generic Elective and BSc. Hons. students studying in CBCS, LOCF and NEP: UGCF mode.

Swati Rajput

Acknowledgements

Writing a book is an enormous job but extremely rewarding. It gives the pleasure of doing something valuable for the community one belongs to. Teaching has always been my passion and writing a meaningful text has been my fervent desire. I am fortunate to have a family who has always encouraged me and given me an environment to thrive. I am indebted to my husband and family members for their continuous support. Heartfelt thanks to my teachers and colleagues who were involved in the curriculum design and discussions on improvement of the subject. The phases of discussions with them during examination and evaluation helped to understand diverse perspectives on many subtopics. The thought of writing a book on "Geography of Health" was conceived while teaching this paper for the last few years. The dire need for a textbook, in this field, that caters to the entire syllabus fostered my thought of giving shape to my valuable notes. So I am grateful to my students and their immense love that encouraged me to pen down this work. I hope the readers benefit from it. My heart felt thank to Shaheed Bhagat Singh College and its principal, Prof. Arun Kumar Attree, for providing a conducive environment for professional and academic growth. I am thankful to Mr. Sanjeev Kumar for applying his cartographic skills and helping with illustrations. I am grateful to Prof. Pascal Geldsetzer for permitting to use the maps and data from his studies. The medicine practitioners were also consulted to build-up basic understanding of various aspects. The book is written in a geographical context so any shortcomings or contradiction to knowledge of medicine or epidemiology is regretted.

Swati Rajput

Contents

List of Tables and Figures

TABLES

FIGURES

Chapter

1

Health

Definition, Concept and Approaches

1.1 Definitions and Concept

Mahatma Gandhi wrote a book entitled "*Key to Health*" while he was confined in the Aga Khan Palace at Poona during 1942-1944. He wrote "it is necessary to understand the meaning of the word 'health', before entering upon a description of the human body. Health, means body ease. He is a healthy man whose body is free from all diseases; he carries on his normal activities without fatigue. Such a man should be able with ease to walk ten to twelve miles a day, and perform ordinary physical labour without getting tired. He can digest ordinary simple food. His mind and his senses are in a state of harmony and poise. This definition does not include prize fighters and such like. A man with extraordinary physical strength is not necessarily healthy. He has merely developed his musculature, possibly at the expense of something else" (Gandhi, 1948).

Health has become an important term of discussion in the contemporary world. The word "Health" has been derived from the word "Hoelth". In 1973, Dolfman, a Professor in Health Administration in Philadelphia, wrote that Health is a word which has been used to express a certain thought or concept, such as a state or condition of well-being" (Dolfman, 1973). World Health Organization considers health "as a state of complete physical, mental and social well-being and not merely the absence of disease or infirmity" (WHO, 1948: 100). Health geography thus looks into the spatiotemporal aspect of human health.

Long before the germ theory paradigm shift in the late 1800s, relationships between geography and health were recognised throughout human history, predating current health delivery systems and offering insights into the transmission of infectious agents. There have been numerous instances throughout history where geography and place have had a significant impact on how people perceive risk and health. Hippocrates first acknowledged the links between geographic factors and health outcomes in his work "*On Airs, Waters, and Places*" (about 400 BC), which effectively serves as the foundation for modern medical geography. Due to the fast urbanisation and poor sanitation that accompanied the industrial revolution in the 1700s, a wide professionals, researchers, and other interested persons can gather data about the distribution of the world's diseases in an attempt to find patterns of transmission and possibly cures to some of the more deadly illnesses such as HIV/AIDS and various cancers" (Briney, 2020).

Although there are medical geographers who still usefully employ more positivistic approaches to problems, health geography in this sense is predicated on place processes and does not focus on generalizability. It employs a wide range of theoretical frameworks and deals with nuanced concepts with which to approach and to interpret its subject matter (Cutchin, 2007).

Social epidemiology emerged as a distinct field during the last few decades. Major motivators were stress research, a return to ecological thinking in epidemiology, and the emergence of the "population health" movement of the 1990s (Berkman & Kawachi, 2000). The concerns of social epidemiology, as its name and background suggest, are social phenomena that influence health inequalities in populations. The social phenomena of interest vary, but socio-economic stratification, social capital, social networks, discrimination, and segregation are commonly investigated; but the conceptual and methodological approaches remain those of epidemiology. As Berkman and Kawachi (2000) suggest, the boundaries between social epidemiology and other types, such as environmental epidemiology, are often fuzzy. Social epidemiologists have drawn on concepts and techniques that implicate the geographic concepts of space and place, and they have begun to use geographic information systems (GIS) in earnest. Moreover, the increasing importance of the concept of neighbourhoods in social epidemiology (Kawachi & Berkman, 2002) implies that its subject matter is thoroughly geographic in nature even if it is not overtly conceptualized as such.

Wil Gesler's important book, *"The Cultural Geography of Health Care"* (1991), suggested the use of cultural ecology as one of the several frameworks for thinking about health and healthcare problems. To explain the utility of cultural ecology, Gesler drew on traditional cultural geography's notions of culture and environment interaction. He stressed that the interaction was bidirectional in that humans shaped their environments in order to survive and flourish, but they also needed to adapt and adjust to environmental changes in order to try and establish a balance in the relationship. Although Gesler was writing about healthcare, his ideas may be applied to environmental health and well-being (Cutchin, 2007).

Medical geography had a crux of illness and disease while health geography talks about holistic approach to health challenges. Medical geography laid emphasis on body and health geography equates body, mind and environment together. According to Curtis, the framework for understanding and explaining health includes:

1. The idea of health as "balance" and illness as "imbalance".
2. The notion of the body as a machine and of illness as malfunction of the machine.
3. The idea of locus of control (the perception of the degree of control the individual has over his or her own health).
4. Health or illness seen as the outcome of faith or divine will.
5. Ideas about health providing freedom or release to do as one pleases or as functional ability to carry out key roles such as work as an employee or a homemaker.
6. The concept of health as resilience against threats of infection or hazards.
7. Ideas about access to the means for good health such as healthcare and a reasonable standard of living.

Chapter 1

Health

Definition, Concept and Approaches

1.1 Definitions and Concept

Mahatma Gandhi wrote a book entitled "*Key to Health*" while he was confined in the Aga Khan Palace at Poona during 1942-1944. He wrote "it is necessary to understand the meaning of the word 'health', before entering upon a description of the human body. Health, means body ease. He is a healthy man whose body is free from all diseases; he carries on his normal activities without fatigue. Such a man should be able with ease to walk ten to twelve miles a day, and perform ordinary physical labour without getting tired. He can digest ordinary simple food. His mind and his senses are in a state of harmony and poise. This definition does not include prize fighters and such like. A man with extraordinary physical strength is not necessarily healthy. He has merely developed his musculature, possibly at the expense of something else" (Gandhi, 1948).

Health has become an important term of discussion in the contemporary world. The word "Health" has been derived from the word "Hoelth". In 1973, Dolfman, a Professor in Health Administration in Philadelphia, wrote that Health is a word which has been used to express a certain thought or concept, such as a state or condition of well-being" (Dolfman, 1973). World Health Organization considers health "as a state of complete physical, mental and social well-being and not merely the absence of disease or infirmity" (WHO, 1948: 100). Health geography thus looks into the spatiotemporal aspect of human health.

Long before the germ theory paradigm shift in the late 1800s, relationships between geography and health were recognised throughout human history, predating current health delivery systems and offering insights into the transmission of infectious agents. There have been numerous instances throughout history where geography and place have had a significant impact on how people perceive risk and health. Hippocrates first acknowledged the links between geographic factors and health outcomes in his work "*On Airs, Waters, and Places*" (about 400 BC), which effectively serves as the foundation for modern medical geography. Due to the fast urbanisation and poor sanitation that accompanied the industrial revolution in the 1700s, a wide range of novel public health challenges were created. The pioneer work of John Snow, a doctor, correctly determined the exposure point during the Broad Street cholera outbreak in 1854. Snow's well-known cholera outbreak map from 1854 illustrates visually how cases were concentrated near the Broad Street pump, the source of tainted water that sparked the epidemic. Given that bacteria were still unknown to science at the time, it is amazing that Snow was able to use this map to locate the infected pump and comes to the conclusion that cholera was a watery disease.

According to *International Encyclopedia of Human Geography*, Medical geography uses the concepts and paradigms of the discipline of geography to investigate human-environmental relationships of disease, nutrition, and medical care systems, of which maps and geographic information science (GI Science) are arguably most prominent today….Medical geographers are also, foremost, problem solvers who deal with both environmentally based problems and those of anthropogenic origin. Their workplaces include academia, private and public organizations (Earickson, 2009).

Medical Geography concentrated on effect of location on human health. It tries to answer questions as to why people living in dry areas have different health problems than in humid areas. Do diseases vary across different latitudes and altitudes? It was only after 1800 when cholera gripped London, the researchers and scholars got curious. As more and more people became ill, they believed they were becoming infected by vapours escaping the ground. John Snow, a doctor in London, believed that if he could isolate the source of the toxins infecting the population then only cholera could be contained. As part of his study, Snow plotted the distribution of deaths throughout London on a map. After examining these locations, he found a cluster of unusually high deaths near a water pump on Broad Street. He then concluded that the water coming from this pump was the reason people were becoming sick and he had authorities remove the handle to the pump. Once people then stopped drinking the water, the number of cholera deaths dramatically decreased (Briney, 2020).

The Commission on "International Geographical Union" defined Medical Geography in the year 1952 as "the study of Geographical factors concerned with the cause and effect of health and diseases." Realizing the narrowness of such a definition, in 1976, the IGU (International Geographical Union) in Moscow, abolished the 24 years of old term of Medical Geography and adopted a much broader perspective of Geography of Health and Health Care (Hyma *et al.*, 1986).

Table 1.1: Evolution of Definition of Health and Medical Geography and Health Geography

Year	Agency	Definition
1948	World Health Organization	Health as "a state of complete physical, mental, and social well-being and not merely the absence of disease or infirmity.
1958	René Dubos, a French-American microbiologist	Health as "a quality possessed by all living organisms, which enables them to survive and flourish in their environment.

(*Contd.*)

Year	Agency	Definition
1974	Lalonde Report	Health as "a resource for everyday living and not the objective of living. Health is a positive concept emphasizing social and personal resources as well as physical capacities."
1981	John Woods	Medical geography is a sub-field of geography defined as "the systematic study of the spatial dimensions of health, disease, and healthcare".
1986	World Health Organization	Medical geography to include "the application of geographical methods and perspectives to aspects of health and healthcare."
1991	Joint Committee on Health Education and Promotion Terminology	Health as a "complex and multifaceted concept encompassing the physical, mental, emotional, and social dimensions of life."
1998	Susan Hanson and Patricia Lawn	Medical geography has "progressed to a new perspective, which emphasizes environmental factors, social and psychological phenomena and human behaviour."
2000	World Health Organization	A pragmatic concept of health—the ability to conduct a socially and economically productive life—was accepted indirectly, which was an essential goal of this strategy.
2004	Ward *et al.*	Health geography as "the application of geographical information, perspectives, and methods to the study of health, disease, and healthcare delivery", recognizing the multidisciplinary nature of the field.
2007	Kearns and Moonen	Health geography should be defined as "the study of the distribution of health-related phenomena and the processes that shape them over space and time."
2014	WHO	Health geography as "the science and art of applying geographic information, perspectives, and methods to the study of the health of populations, communities, and individuals."

Source: Compiled by Author.

The "web of causation" remains a generally accepted but inadequately developed model that was first introduced in a 1960 U.S. Epidemiology textbook, reflecting in part the emphasis placed today on epidemiologic procedures rather than epidemiologic theories of disease causation. It is a conceptual model that recognises that diseases or health outcomes are complex and are influenced by multiple factors. *The Atlas of United States Mortality*, developed by the Centres for Disease Control and Prevention (CDC) in the United States, is still used today to examine a variety of health-related variables across the country. The spatial distribution of persons of all ages and the locations with the best and worst air quality are just a few examples of the data. These kinds of topics are crucial since they affect the spread of diseases like lung cancer and asthma as well as the population growth of a region. Along with the United States, "Here, the public, medical professionals, researchers, and other interested persons can gather data about the distribution of the world's diseases in an attempt to find patterns of transmission and possibly cures to some of the more deadly illnesses such as HIV/AIDS and various cancers" (Briney, 2020).

Although there are medical geographers who still usefully employ more positivistic approaches to problems, health geography in this sense is predicated on place processes and does not focus on generalizability. It employs a wide range of theoretical frameworks and deals with nuanced concepts with which to approach and to interpret its subject matter (Cutchin, 2007).

Social epidemiology emerged as a distinct field during the last few decades. Major motivators were stress research, a return to ecological thinking in epidemiology, and the emergence of the "population health" movement of the 1990s (Berkman & Kawachi, 2000). The concerns of social epidemiology, as its name and background suggest, are social phenomena that influence health inequalities in populations. The social phenomena of interest vary, but socio-economic stratification, social capital, social networks, discrimination, and segregation are commonly investigated; but the conceptual and methodological approaches remain those of epidemiology. As Berkman and Kawachi (2000) suggest, the boundaries between social epidemiology and other types, such as environmental epidemiology, are often fuzzy. Social epidemiologists have drawn on concepts and techniques that implicate the geographic concepts of space and place, and they have begun to use geographic information systems (GIS) in earnest. Moreover, the increasing importance of the concept of neighbourhoods in social epidemiology (Kawachi & Berkman, 2002) implies that its subject matter is thoroughly geographic in nature even if it is not overtly conceptualized as such.

Wil Gesler's important book, *"The Cultural Geography of Health Care"* (1991), suggested the use of cultural ecology as one of the several frameworks for thinking about health and healthcare problems. To explain the utility of cultural ecology, Gesler drew on traditional cultural geography's notions of culture and environment interaction. He stressed that the interaction was bidirectional in that humans shaped their environments in order to survive and flourish, but they also needed to adapt and adjust to environmental changes in order to try and establish a balance in the relationship. Although Gesler was writing about healthcare, his ideas may be applied to environmental health and well-being (Cutchin, 2007).

Medical geography had a crux of illness and disease while health geography talks about holistic approach to health challenges. Medical geography laid emphasis on body and health geography equates body, mind and environment together. According to Curtis, the framework for understanding and explaining health includes:

1. The idea of health as "balance" and illness as "imbalance".
2. The notion of the body as a machine and of illness as malfunction of the machine.
3. The idea of locus of control (the perception of the degree of control the individual has over his or her own health).
4. Health or illness seen as the outcome of faith or divine will.
5. Ideas about health providing freedom or release to do as one pleases or as functional ability to carry out key roles such as work as an employee or a homemaker.
6. The concept of health as resilience against threats of infection or hazards.
7. Ideas about access to the means for good health such as healthcare and a reasonable standard of living.

In their book entitled "*Health Disease and Society: A Critical Medical Geography*", Jones and Moon pinpointed that there is an urgent need for medical geographers to go outside the body to develop an alternative social and environmental perspective on health in which geography can play an important part with other social sciences. In terms of content, two distinct areas of study, or 'traditions', can be recognized:

- *First*, there is the disease ecology tradition with the geographer attempting to elucidate the social and environmental causes of ill-health; such work is closely allied to epidemiology, which itself is trying to discover the patterns and determinants of disease.
- The *second*, and more recent, area of study is the geography of medical care which is concerned with the consumption of care in respect of such matters as distribution and accessibility (Jones and Moon, 1987).

One mark of novelty in health geography is its emerging connection with a critical human geography defined by Painter (2000: 126) as: . . . a rapidly changing set of ideas and practices within human geography linked by a shared commitment to emancipatory politics within and beyond the discipline, to the promotion of progressive social change and to the development of a broad range of critical theories and their application in geographical research and political practice (Kearns and Moon, 2002).

1.2 Approaches to Geography of Health

According to Pyle (1979) and Phillips (1981), there are 5 approaches to health geography. Below are the elaboration and application of the approaches suggested by them:

1.2.1 *The Cartographic Approach*

This approach deals with mapping of related spatial data and their variations, modelling and quantifying relationship between them. The works of Aiken, Mcclleland, and Hopps have established the importance of this technique to Health Studies. Hopps in his work of 1969 has stressed on the significance of computerized mapping in Geographical studies on Health (Hyma *et al.*, 1986). The cartographic approach in health geography, researchers and policymakers can visually communicate complex health data and patterns, identify spatial trends and disparities, and inform evidence-based decision-making. Cartographic techniques are widely used for mapping disease distributions like the mapping of infectious diseases, like malaria, dengue fever, or COVID-19 to visually identify areas of high prevalence and track the spread of these diseases over time. Disease mapping allows researchers and policymakers to identify hot spots, understand geographic patterns, and allocate resources more effectively. Maps can be utilized to highlight disparities in health outcomes across different geographic areas. For instance, researchers may map mortality rates, disease prevalence, or access to healthcare services at the regional or neighbourhood level. Such maps can reveal spatial patterns of health inequalities, allowing policymakers to identify areas that require targeted interventions.

The cartographic approach is valuable for mapping the distribution of healthcare facilities and services. By plotting the locations of hospitals, clinics, or specialized health centres on maps, researchers can identify gaps in healthcare accessibility, explore spatial variations in service provision, and evaluate the geographical distribution of resources. This information aids in healthcare planning, resource allocation, and addressing issues related to healthcare access. The cartographic approach is applied in mapping environmental health risks and exposures. For instance, maps can be created to display the distribution of air pollution levels, toxic waste sites, or areas prone to natural disasters. These maps help identify areas with higher environmental health risks and inform policies to mitigate or prevent exposure to such risks.

Cartographic approach can also be utilized to spatially represent health behaviours and lifestyles. For example, mapping physical activity levels, smoking prevalence, or dietary habits can provide valuable insights into patterns of health behaviours and their spatial variations. This information can support targeted health promotion strategies and interventions.

1.2.2 *The Positivist Approach*

Positivism is an approach in social science research that emphasizes the use of objective and quantitative methods to study phenomena. It originated in the natural sciences and was subsequently applied to social sciences, including health geography. In health geography, positivism is often used to understand the spatial distribution of health-related phenomena and their relationships with various environmental factors. This approach deals with natural science methods and accurate measurement. The approach uses quantitative methods to do enquity. It views the body as a machine and examines from a bio-medical perspective. Such an approach ignores socio-cultural or political processes. The application of positivism in health geography involves the collection and analysis of statistical data on health outcomes, disease prevalence, and environmental factors at different geographical scales. These data can be used to identify patterns, correlations, and trends, leading to a better understanding of health issues and their spatial variations. Criticisms of this approach highlight concerns over objectivity, reductionism, and the potential exclusion of qualitative and subjective aspects of health experiences. Many scholors have applied positivist approach to do quantification like John Snow also known as one of the founders of modern epidemiology. His work during the 19th century involved mapping the distribution of cholera cases in London and linking them to contaminated water sources. Snow's use of data collection, spatial analysis, and statistical methods to understand disease transmission laid the foundation for the positivist approach within epidemiology and health geography. Another scholor is Alan Lopez in the Global Burden of Disease Study conducted extensive research on global health metrics using the positivist approach. She and her team applied rigorous data collection and statistical analysis to estimate disease burdens, mortality rates, and risk factors across different populations and regions. Their work provides valuable insights into the global distribution of health conditions, allowing policymakers to prioritize interventions and allocate resources effectively.

1.2.3 *The Behavioural Approach*

This approach analyses human perception and behaviour and it seeks to understand the decision making process. The behavioural approach emphasizes the scientific study of observable behavioural responses and their environmental determinants. In other words, it is the study of the connection between our minds and behaviour. In health geography such an approach helps in understanding psychological and social, cultural factors that determine health and illness variations over space. In *Ichiro Kawachi and the Social Capital Theory*, Ichiro Kawachi explores the impact of social capital on health outcomes and behaviours. Social capital refers to the networks, norms, and trust that exist within social relationships. Scholars adopting this perspective would analyze how social networks and social cohesion influence health behaviours, access to healthcare, and health outcomes at different geographical scales, such as neighbourhoods or communities. Mark Rosenberg developed an applied social ecological framework that highlights the multiple levels of influence on health behaviours. This framework considers individual, interpersonal, community, and societal factors that shape health behaviour. By adopting this approach, geographers can study how social and physical environments affect health behaviours and the utilization of healthcare services, aiming to develop interventions that address these multiple levels of influence.

1.2.4 *The Structuralist Approach*

It focuses upon social, political and economic structures. It considers health as a commodity and, therefore, healthcare as preventive rather than curative. The approach believes that poverty is the underlying factor for illness and diseases. For example, Vicente Navarro has extensively studied the political economy of health, focusing on the influence of political and economic structures on health outcomes. His work highlights how power relations, social class, and economic policies shape health inequalities. He examines the impact of neoliberalism, globalization, and welfare state structures on health and proposes policies that address social determinants to improve population health. Another example is Clare Bambra in her study "*Geographies of Health Inequalities*" explores the geographical distribution of health inequalities and their underlying structural causes. She examines how regional, national, and international policies, as well as socio-economic structures, interact to shape health disparities across different geographic areas. Her research sheds light on the role of place-based factors, such as access to resources, social cohesion, and governance, in influencing health outcomes.

1.2.5 *Ecological Approach*

According to Helen and Peter, ecological approaches focus on human as biological entity, recognizing them as part of interdependent ecological systems. In other words, it builds up the understanding that health outcomes are influenced by the interplay of multiple factors at different scales, including the physical environment, social conditions, and individual behaviours. This approach recognizes the dynamic relationship between people and their environment, emphasizing the importance of studying health within the context of broader ecological systems. Health Geography has several studies based on the ecological approach, like the Health and Place Study (Fullilove, 1996) which examined the impact of physical and social environments on health outcomes in urban neighbourhoods. It highlighted how aspects such as dilapidated housing, crime rates, and lack of access to resources can contribute to poor health outcomes. The study emphasized the importance of considering both the physical and social dimensions of place in understanding health disparities.

A study by Hay *et al.* in 2002, *Socio-Ecological Determinants of Malaria,* employed an ecological approach to understand the determinants of malaria transmission in Africa. It explored the interactions between the physical environment (i.e., climate, water bodies), mosquito vectors, human behaviour, and socio-economic conditions. The study highlighted the need for multi-level interventions that address both environmental and social factors to effectively control malaria.

Similarly, a study on *Neighbourhood Walkability and Diabetes* by Creatore *et al.*, in 2016, analyzed the association between neighbourhood walkability and the risk of diabetes. It found that individuals residing in highly walkable neighbourhoods had a lower risk of developing diabetes compared to those in less walkable areas. The study highlighted the role of the built environment in influencing physical activity and subsequent health outcomes. Disease ecology and disease geogenes are the two terms associated with this approach.

The Ecological Associative studies concentrated on spatial context of Epidemiological studies, the influences of topographic, climatic, biotic and socio-economic cycles and their influences on health of people, environmental repercussion and associated health hazards (Mcclleland, 1859; Adams, 1889; Hesterlow, Scomer, Man, Sergent, Fonarff and Justaz, 1900 to 1983; Ashley and Dixit, 1983).

1.2.6 *The Welfare Approach*

The approach attempts to answer the questions of who gets what and where. It also highlights on the fact that how improvement in the quality of life can be achieved by the gradual reform of existing society.

According to the *Dictionary of Human Geography* edited by R.J. Johnston, D. Gregory and David M. Smith (1994), "in a spatially disaggregated society, the general level of welfare may be written as:

$$W = f(S1 \ldots\ldots Sn),$$

where, S is the level of living or social well-being in a set of n territorial subdivisions". In other words, welfare is some function of the distribution of good and bad among groups of the population defined by area of residence.

Another book "*Health and Inequality: A Geographical Perspective*", (2004) explains the importance of geographies and inequality in health services and health conditions of people. Health geography is primarily concerned with the spatial understanding of health, healthcare and health challenges among people. Variation in diseases, types of disease, mortality and life expectancy are all referred to as areas of research in health geography. Geographical research concerns processes operating in time as well as space, linking health over the life course with processes of human migration, environmental change, and duration of exposures to different environmental risk factors. Geography considers "health" broadly defined as physical or mental health, well-being, and health-related practices, and addresses a range of different substantive issues (Curtis, 2016). One of the remarkable works is of Sir Michael Marmot who worked on the social determinants of health and health inequalities. He emphasizes the importance of addressing the disparities in health outcomes and access to healthcare services among different socio-economic groups. His research examines the role of social and economic factors, such as income, education, and employment, in shaping health inequities and advocates for policies that address these social determinants to achieve better health outcomes for all.

1.3 Epidemiology

Parkin in 1873 considered "epidemiology" as the branch of medical sciences dealing with epidemics. According to Lilienfeld, epidemiology is the study of distribution of a disease or a physiological condition in human populations and of the factors that influence the distribution (Lilienfeld, 1980). Later, International Epidemiological Association (IEA) considered it to be the study of frequency, distribution and determinants of diseases. Last in the *Dictionary of Epidemiology* wrote, "Epidemiology is the distribution and determinants of health related states and events in population and the application of this study to control health problems" (Last, 1983). In other words, Epidemiology is the "study of distribution and determinants of health-related states among specified populations and the application of that study to the control of health problems."— *A Dictionary of Epidemiology.*

It is to understand that occurrence of communicable disease (spread from one person to another through a variety of ways that include: contact with blood and bodily fluids; breathing in an airborne virus; or by being bitten by an insect) or non-communicable (diseases that do not spread through infection or through other people, but are typically caused by unhealthy behaviours) are due to interaction between host, agent and environment. Host is the human body, agent is any organism or substance that may initiate the disease and environment is natural and social surroundings around us. In fact in broader sense epidemiology considers environment as internal and external environment. Internal environment consists of human organs, tissues, cells and genes. The external environment is all that which surrounds us. According to International Epidemiological Association, epidemiology aims to describe the magnitude and distribution of health and disease; identifies risk factors in pathogenesis of disease; and helps to provide the data essential to planning, implementation and evaluation of services for prevention, control and treatment of disease.

1.4 Well-being: Concept and Definition

The definition given by WHO in 1984 citing health as a complete physical, mental and social well-being and not merely absence of disease; not only redefined health but also gave a very important term " well-being". The term explicitly shifts discussion away from being limited to biomedicine and healthcare sectors towards holism and inter-sectorality in which the settings of health experiences are central. Geographers of health have done much to emphasize the importance of relationships between health, and the places and spaces which produce and reproduce experiences of health or are constructed through policy to respond to ill-health (Jones & Moon, 1993; Litva & Eyles, 1995; Kearns & Moon, 2002). Contemporary research includes identification of determinants of spatial inequalities in health (Graham, 2000; Curtis *et al.*, 2002, 2004; Boyle *et al.*, 2004; Fagg *et al.*, 2006), the importance of particular spaces and places such as neighbourhoods (Cummins & MacIntyre, 2002; Diez-Roux, 2003; Wilson *et al.*, 2004) or therapeutic landscapes (Andrew, 2004; Gesler *et al.*, 2004; Milligan *et al.*, 2004; Conradson, 2005; Smyth, 2005); impacts of different health experiences on the construction of places (Bush *et al.*, 2001; Smith & Easterlow, 2005; Wakefield & McMullan, 2005) and contextualized analyses of policy responses (Moon & Brown, 2001; Atkinson, 2002; Fleuret & Séchet, 2002, 2006; Kearns & Barnett, 2000). The broader lens that well-being brings to considerations of health opens up further arenas for geographers of health to explore in terms of the processes that promote, remedy or regenerate health and ill-health (Fleuret and Atkinson, 2007).

The *Merriam-Webster Dictionary* defined well-being as "The state of being happy, healthy, or prosperous". Well-being is also known as wellness, prudential value or quality of life, refers to what is intrinsically valuable relative to someone. So the well-being of a person is linked to what is ultimately good for this person, what is in the self-interest of this person (Roger, 2017). The World Health Organisation (WHO) states that "well-being exists in two dimensions, subjective and objective. It comprises an individual's experience of their life as well as a comparison of life circumstances with social norms and values."

Well-being from a geographical perspective, includes:

1. A socio-economic focus on spatial and social injustice in which inequalities in consumption, access to services and standards of living are studied. This refers back to the notion of satisfying needs (e.g. Benzeval *et al.*, 1995; Acheson, 1998; Graham, 2000). The socio-economic well-being strives towards education, health and income of all sections of society.
2. An environmental approach in which the quality of air and water, pollution levels, exposure to nuisance (e.g. noise) and risk, the sensorial experience of places and the therapeutic virtues of the landscape are studied. This refers back to primary needs of human beings (senses) as well as to representations, standards, attitudes and values depending on the human— environment—culture triplet (Tuan, 1974).
3. A social welfare approach in which the consequences of vulnerability in terms of health and quality of life are studied. Welfare geography reveals what gets where and how.

1.5 Relationship between Health and Well-being

Well-being and health co-exists. Health depends upon well-being and well-being gets influenced by both physical and mental health. The concept of well-being has evolved over time and has been shaped by various philosophical, cultural, and scientific beliefs.

The ancient Greeks, including philosophers like Aristotle, emphasized the importance of a balanced life, where well-being was seen as a state of flourishing or eudaimonia. This concept emphasized the pursuit of virtues and fulfilling one's potential. Eudaimonia is a combination of well-being, happiness and flourishing. It is the ultimate goal of human beings. McIntyre, who describes human life as a whole with a history which links our birth, life and death in a continuous narrative, describes the virtues as dispositions, which will enable us to live through this narrative sustaining us in the relevant kind of quest for the good, by helping us to "overcome the harms, dangers, temptations and distractions which we encounter, and which will furnish us with increasing self-knowledge and increasing knowledge of the good." Aristotle's definition of eudaimonia focuses on the "pursuit of virtue, excellence, and the best within us" (Huta & Waterman, 2014: 1426). Aristotle believed that happiness came from living a life aligned with virtues (Hursthouse, 1999). He presented these ideas in Nichomachean Ethics, where he describes how to achieve eudaimonia:

> "A life of eudaimonia is a life of striving. It is a life of pushing yourself to your limits, and finding success. A eudaimonistic life will be full of the happiness that comes from achieving

something really difficult, rather than just having it handed to you." (*Eudaimonia: Definition, Meaning, & Examples*—The Berkeley Well-Being Institute (*berkeleywell-being.com*))

Another philosophy linked to well-being that prevailed in the 4th century BC by Socrates was philosophy of hedonism. The Cyrenaics, a Greek School of this Philosophy, taught that the only intrinsic good is pleasure, which meant not just the absence of pain, but positively enjoyable momentary sensations. Of these, physical ones are stronger than those of anticipation or memory. They did, however, recognize the value of social obligation, and that pleasure could be gained from altruism (Tim, 2019). Hedonism focuses on the 'feeling good' aspect of happiness. When taken to the extreme, it can translate into the pursuit of pleasure and simply doing whatever you want that helps you attain this. Let's say, for example eating junk food gives us pleasure. This act of eating junk food can give hedonic pleasure but can give displeasure in future.

> According to our point of view, 'positive' psychological well-being could be defined as the cognitive and affective reactions to the perception of adequate personal characteristics and achievements, efficient interaction with the world and social integration, and positive progress in time. 'Negative' well-being could be defined as the cognitive and affective response to perceived deficit(s) in the aforementioned areas. Accordingly, positive well-being includes component, such as life satisfaction, positive mood and energy (Argyle and Crossland, 1987; Diener, 2000; Watson and Tellegen, 1985), whereas negative well-being includes components such as distress and negative mood, symptoms and hyperarousal (Clark and Watson, 1991; Diener, 2000; Karademas, 2007).

Throughout history, various religious and spiritual traditions have emphasized the connection between well-being and one's relationship with the divine. Concepts like salvation, enlightenment, or *nirvana* were central to achieving well-being in such traditions.

> Religion may benefit psychological well-being because it encourages supernatural beliefs that can help people deal with stress (Koenig, Harold, King, and Carson, 2012). Social psychologists identify "stress buffering" mechanisms, such as a perceived connection with the divine, as key ways people may deal with difficult life events (Schieman, Scott, Bierman, and Ellison, 2013). And religious meaning may help people manage suffering, both in their lives and in the lives of those around them (Crystal, 2005). This appears to be particularly important for older people, who tend to experience suffering on a more regular basis (Krause, Neal, 2003).

1.5.1 *Objective and Subjective Well-being*

There are two broad conceptual approaches of well-being for research, i.e., Objective and Subjective well-being. Well-being when observed from economic and social perspective, it is objective well-being. The subjective well-being deals with well-being of each individual.

The objective approach defines well-being in terms of quality of life indicators such as material resources (e.g. income, food, housing) and social attributes (education, health, political voice, social networks and connections). The subjective approach emphasises subjective well-being, that is people's own evaluations of their lives, especially their life satisfaction (a cognitive evaluation), happiness (a positive emotional state) and unhappiness (a negative emotional state) (Diener and Suh, 1997).

Where origin of subjective philosophy of well-being can be traced to the time of Aristotle, the objective philosophy of well-being is not very old. Its origin comes from Amartya Sen's work of Welfare Economics. The main differences between subjective and objective well-being is as below:

Table 1.2: Difference between Objective and Subjective Well-being

	Objective Well-being	Subjective Well-being
Focus	It focuses on external indicators of well-being and is often assessed by certain standards or criteria.	It focuses on internal indicators of well-being and is often assessed by individual personal criteria.
Assessment and Observation	Objective well-being refers to the assessment of well-being based on observable and measurable factors.	Subjective well-being, also known as psychological well-being or happiness, refers to an individual's self-perceived quality of life, satisfaction, and emotional experiences.
Factors	Objective well-being can include factors such as income, education level, employment status, physical health, and life expectancy.	It focuses on an individual's personal factors of well-being, reflecting their thoughts, feelings, and overall happiness or life satisfaction.
Quantification or Evaluation	These factors are often quantifiable and can be measured objectively using reliable data and indicators.	Subjective well-being is typically assessed through self-report measures, such as questionnaires or surveys that ask individuals to rate their level of happiness, life satisfaction, or overall well-being. It considers factors such as positive emotions, negative emotions, and cognitive evaluations of one's life circumstances.
Example	For example, objective well-being might involve measuring the average income levels or life expectancy in a specific population. These measures provide a tangible understanding of people's material and physical well-being and can be compared across different individuals or groups.	For example, subjective well-being might involve asking individuals to rate their level of happiness on a scale from 1 to 10 or to report their overall life satisfaction. These self-reported measures provide insights into an individual's own perception of their well-being, regardless of external circumstances.

Source: Author.

1.5.2 *Relationship between Aspects of Health and Well-being*

From the above discussion, it is quite clear that Health and Well-being are two separate concepts, where health talks about physical and mental fitness, well-being is a broader concept where health becomes part of it. According to WHO "well-being exists in two dimensions, subjective and objective. It comprises an individual's experience of their life as well as a comparison of life circumstances with social norms and values."

1.5.3 *Health Impacts Well-being*

Health has a significant impact on overall well-being. When individuals are in good health, it often leads to higher levels of well-being in various aspects of life. Health can impact well-being in following ways:

1. **Physical Health and Functioning:** Physically healthy person happens to enjoy a higher level of comfort and functioning in his daily life. For example, being free from chronic pain, having good mobility, and having the energy to engage in activities they enjoy can contribute to a greater sense of well-being. Many studies show that physical health issues from cancer to obesity impacts mental health and well-being of people. According to The American Heart Association, "Physical activity boosts mental wellness. Regular physical activity can relieve tension, anxiety, depression and anger."
2. **Mental Health and Well-being:** Physical conditions such as chronic illnesses or disabilities can have a significant impact on mental health and overall well-being. Conversely, when individuals are in good physical health, they are more likely to experience positive emotions, higher self-esteem, and better life satisfaction, all of which contribute to overall mental well-being. According to World Humanitarian Movement, mental health problems can have a significant impact on children's lives. They can affect a child's ability to form and maintain relationships, perform well in school, and enjoy activities they once loved. In some cases, untreated mental health issues can also lead to more serious problems such as substance abuse, school dropout, and homelessness. According to World Health Organisation (WHO), the self-harm rates in the adolescent age group are found in the highest numbers at a global level. Emotional stress and other concerns are a major contributing factor for most of the physical illnesses. Further research findings suggest that factors like physical illness, limited basic resources, inability to provide for self and family as well as unfulfilled desires in life are major factors that impact mental health and well-being (https://manodarpan.education.gov.in/assets/img/pdf/CBSE_MH_Manual).
3. **Health, Social Connections and Well-being:** Physical health can influence social interactions and relationships, which are crucial for well-being. When individuals have good health, they are more likely to participate in social activities, maintain friendships, and form meaningful connections. Having strong social support networks is associated with higher well-being, and physical health can significantly impact a person's ability to engage in these social connections. People with good mental health are mostly part of social groups. They not only remain positive but also make other think positive. This way individuals, physical and mental condition help to build good social environment around him/her.
4. **Health, Individual Achievement and Well-being:** Physical and mental health can contribute to personal fulfilment and a sense of achievement. When individuals are healthy, they are more likely to pursue and accomplish their goals, whether it is in their personal or professional life. Attaining goals and feeling successful can add to a person's overall well-being and life satisfaction.
5. **Health and Emotional Stability:** Physical and mental health plays a role in emotional stability and resilience. Certain physical conditions, such as hormonal imbalances or

chronic pain, can affect emotional well-being and increase the risk of mood disorders. Good physical health, on the other hand, contributes to emotional stability and resilience, allowing individuals to better cope with stress and life challenges.

6. **Health and Quality of Life:** Overall, good health significantly contributes to an improved quality of life, which is a crucial aspect of well-being. When individuals are in good health, they can engage in activities they enjoy, maintain independence, and have a higher overall satisfaction with life. This, in turn, enhances their overall well-being. Healthy and active person also performs well in their jobs and can tend to earn more. The increased earnings can help them to improve their and family's quality of life and standard of living.
7. **Healthy Environment and Well-being:** Environmental factors, such as access to clean air, water, and safe living conditions, can directly influence health and well-being. For example, living in a polluted and unsafe environment may lead to respiratory problems, stress, and reduced overall well-being. On the other hand, being in a clean and safe environment promotes physical health, mental peace, and overall well-being.

1.5.4 *Well-being Impacts Health*

Well-being can have a significant impact on overall health. When a person's well-being is high, it often leads to positive health outcomes in various ways. Well-being can impact health in following ways:

1. **Stress Reduction:** High levels of stress can have detrimental effects on physical and mental health. On the other hand, individuals with high well-being often have effective stress management strategies, such as regular exercise, mindfulness, or engaging in hobbies they enjoy. By reducing stress levels, they experience improved cardiovascular health, immune system function, and better mental health.
2. **Immune System Function:** Well-being can play a role in bolstering the immune system. Positive emotions and a sense of fulfilment release hormones that stimulate the immune system, thus enhancing body's ability to fight off illnesses and infections. Conversely, chronic stress and negative emotional states can weaken the immune response, making individuals more susceptible to illnesses.
3. **Better Mental Health:** Well-being is closely linked to mental health. Engaging in activities that promote well-being, such as socializing, pursuing hobbies, or practicing self-care, can contribute to better mental health. This includes reduced rates of anxiety, depression, and improved overall psychological well-being. Conversely, poor mental well-being can lead to various mental health disorders, affecting a person's overall health.
4. **Improved Physical Health:** When individuals have higher levels of well-being, they are more likely to engage in behaviours that promote good health. For example, they are likely to maintain a balanced diet, exercise regularly, and get enough sleep. These behaviours can prevent chronic diseases, improve cardiovascular health, and lead to a higher overall level of physical well-being.
5. **Increased Resilience:** Well-being equips individuals with greater resilience, the ability to bounce back from challenging situations and adversity. Resilience can protect against the negative health effects of stress and other life difficulties. Those with higher well-being

can more effectively cope with setbacks, maintaining their physical and mental health in the face of adversity.

6. **Higher Life Expectancy or Longevity:** Research suggests that individuals with higher levels of well-being tend to live longer. Positive emotions, contentment, and life satisfaction have been found to be associated with a reduced risk of mortality and a longer lifespan. This connection between well-being and longevity underscores the impact well-being can have on overall health.

The relationship between health and well-being is not just one-way—health influences well-being and well-being itself influences health. There are a number of correlations between well-being and physical health outcomes, improved immune system response, higher pain tolerance, increased longevity, cardiovascular health, slower disease progression and reproductive health (Fig. 1.1).

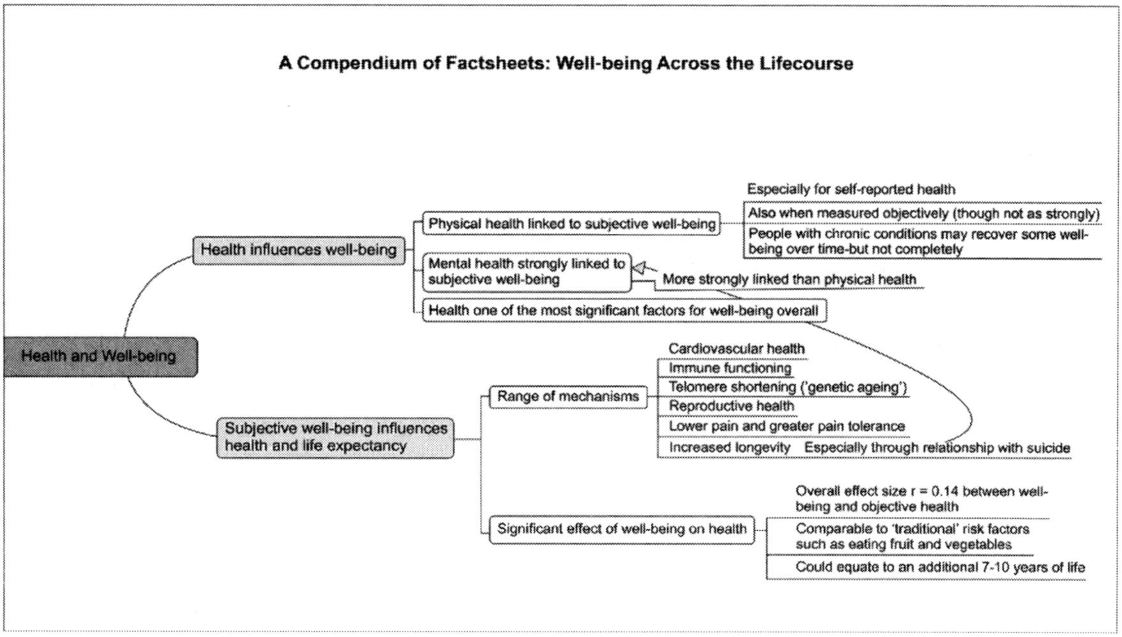

Fig. 1.1: A Compendium of Factsheets: Well-being across the Lifecourse.

Source: New Economics Foundation Stoll, L., Michaelson, J. & Seaford, C., 2012, Well-being evidence for policy: a review, new economics foundation, London and has been developed for inclusion in a working paper produced for the WHO Expert Group on Well-being, October 2012 retrieved from https://assets.publishing.service.gov.uk.

1.6 Scope of Geography of Health

The Geography of Health is an interdisciplinary field that examines the spatial dimensions of health, well-being, and healthcare provision. It draws from both natural and social sciences to provide a comprehensive understanding of the complex interactions between humans, their health, and their environment.

The link between the Geography of Health and natural sciences, such as biology, botany, zoology and ecology is evident in studying the distribution of diseases and health outcomes in relation to environmental factors. For example, geographers may analyze the impact of air pollution on respiratory health or the spread of vector-borne diseases like malaria in specific geographic regions. Natural science disciplines provide knowledge and methods to understand the physical aspects of health, the spread of diseases, and the implications of environmental factors. On the other hand, the Geography of Health also incorporates social sciences, such as sociology, anthropology, and economics. These disciplines help explore the social, cultural, and economic factors that influence health outcomes and healthcare access. Geographers may examine how social inequalities, cultural practices, or economic conditions impact the distribution of health resources and healthcare services across regions. Understanding these social dynamics is vital for addressing disparities, improving healthcare planning, and promoting equitable health outcomes.

The Geography of Health is closely associated with various branches of geography, as it explores the spatial aspects of health, diseases, and healthcare systems within the broader geographic context. Medical geography focuses specifically on the spatial distribution of diseases, healthcare resources, and health outcomes. It examines patterns of disease prevalence, investigates the factors contributing to disease transmission, and analyzes the accessibility and distribution of healthcare facilities. The Geography of Health can be seen as an extension of medical geography, as it encompasses a broader understanding of health and well-being beyond just diseases. The Geography of Health intersects with urban geography by exploring the health issues and healthcare delivery within urban areas. It investigates how urbanization influences health outcomes, such as the impact of urban environments on mental health or the presence of health inequalities in urban neighbourhoods. It also analyzes the spatial distribution of healthcare facilities in urban areas and their accessibility to different populations. Population geography examines the distribution, composition, and migration of populations. It is closely related to the Geography of Health because population characteristics play a significant role in determining health outcomes. Geographers analyze the relationship between population dynamics, demographic factors, and health indicators, such as the impact of aging populations on healthcare systems or the influence of population density on disease transmission. The Geography of Health intersects with environmental geography by exploring the relationship between the environment and health outcomes. Geographers investigate how various environmental factors, such as air and water quality, climate change, or access to green spaces, affect human health. They may analyze the spatial patterns of environmental hazards, the impact of natural disasters on public health, or the relationship between agriculture and food security. Geography of Health is closely linked to social and economic geography. The social structure and varied economic activities create various factors responsible for spread of certain communicable disease. The lifestyle of various castes, religions, genders etc. is also responsible for various lifestyle diseases. Various occupations and economic activities are responsible for non-communicable diseases too.

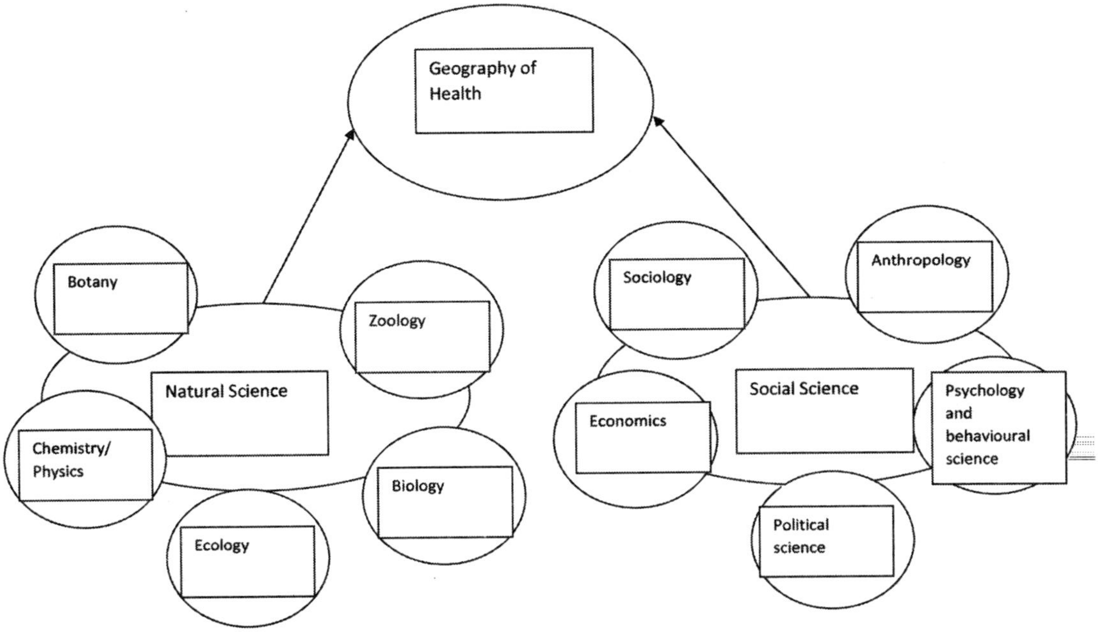

Fig. 1.2: Relationship of Geography of Health with Natural and Social Sciences.

Source: Compiled by Author.

The scope of health geography or medical geography is very vast as we could see its interrelationship with various other disciplines. Some of the areas where a health geographer can do impactful work are:

1. **Disease Mapping and Epidemiology:** Geographical analysis plays a crucial role in mapping disease patterns, identifying disease clusters, and studying disease transmission. For example, mapping the spread of infectious diseases like malaria, HIV/AIDS, or COVID-19 helps identify high-risk areas, understand population movement patterns, and guide public health interventions. Cartographic output of health indicators like health status, health policy, healthcare etc. requires experts. Geographers can align the both and create resources for other researches.
2. **Environmental Health:** Geographers examine the impact of environmental factors on health, such as air and water quality, access to sanitation, and exposure to pollutants. For instance, studying the relationship between proximity to industrial sites and respiratory diseases helps understand the spatial distribution of health risks. Environmental health is the most upcoming field of investigation since early 1990s. Therefore, geographers are better trained to handle related diseases, their distribution and assessments of health facilities. They can suggest the spatial solution or generate real world models at micro and macro level.
3. **Healthcare Accessibility and Utilization:** Geography of Health investigates how geographic factors influence access to healthcare services. This includes studying healthcare infrastructure, the distribution of healthcare facilities, and analyzing barriers to access faced

by different populations, such as rural communities or marginalized groups. Geographers can analyze healthcare facility locations, population distribution, and demographic data to identify areas with limited access to healthcare services. This information can help policymakers and health organizations target resources and develop strategies to improve accessibility.

4. **Health Disparities and Social Determinants of Health:** Geographers explore how social and economic factors shape health outcomes, highlighting the role of social determinants of health, including income, education, and race/ethnicity. For example, mapping areas with limited access to nutritious food (food deserts) can help understand the relationship between geography, socio-economic status, and chronic diseases like obesity. Geographers can help identify vulnerable populations, such as the elderly, low-income communities, or those living in remote areas, who may face unique challenges in accessing healthcare. By considering social and spatial factors, geographers can help develop targeted interventions and services to address their specific needs.
5. **Medical Tourism and Global Health:** The Geography of Health also investigates the globalization of healthcare, including the movement of patients seeking medical treatment across borders. This involves analyzing the factors influencing the flow of medical tourists, such as affordable healthcare options, quality of care, and cultural preferences. Geographers can identify and analyze potential destinations for medical tourism based on factors, such as healthcare infrastructure, accessibility, cultural compatibility, cost of living, environmental conditions, and political stability. This information can help medical tourists make informed decisions about where to seek treatment and support the development of medical tourism strategies.
6. **Urban Planning and Health:** Health geographers collaborate with urban planners to create healthier cities. They analyze the impact of urbanization on health, such as access to parks, healthcare facilities, transportation, and food environments. Geographers can work closely with healthcare providers, public health officials, policymakers, and community organizations. By collaborating, they can integrate spatial perspectives into healthcare planning and advocate for evidence-based policies that improve accessibility and utilization.Their spatial analysis helps inform urban design, land-use planning, and policies to create healthy, inclusive, and sustainable cities.

Health geographers are employed in various relevant fields now-a-days. The demand for experts in geography of health is increasing. Health geographers are involved in global health initiatives by analyzing health disparities and healthcare delivery systems across different regions. They study the social, economic, and environmental determinants of health globally. Their work informs international development projects, humanitarian assistance programmes, and policy interventions aimed at improving health outcomes worldwide. Health geographers contribute to healthcare planning and policy development at various levels, including national, regional, and local. By examining population demographics, healthcare facility locations, and accessibility, they assist in optimizing the distribution of healthcare resources. Their spatial analysis helps identify areas in need of additional healthcare services or improvements in healthcare delivery.

REFERENCES

Argyle, M. & Crossland, J. (1987). Happiness as a function of personality and social encounters. In F. Strack, M. Argyle, & N. Schwarz (Eds.), *Social encounters: Contributions to social interaction*, pp. 115-131, Hemisphere Publishing Corporation.

Benzeval, M., Judge, K., Whitehead, M., (eds.) (1995). *Tackling Health Inequalities: An Agenda for Action*, King's Fund, London.

Berkman, L.F., Kawachi, I. (2000). A historical framework for social epidemiology. In: Berkman, L., Kawachi, I., editors. *Social Epidemiology.* Oxford University Press, Oxford, pp. 3-12.

Briney, Amanda (2020). *Medical Geography, A History and Overview of Medical Geography*, Thoughtco retrieved from https: //www.thoughtco.com/medical-geography-overview-1434508

Clark, L.A. & Watson, D. (1991). Tripartite model of anxiety and depression: Psychometric evidence and taxonomic implications. *Journal of Abnormal Psychology*, 100(3), pp. 316-336.

Crisp, Roger (2017). *"Well-Being". The Stanford Encyclopedia of Philosophy,* Metaphysics Research Lab, Stanford University. Retrieved 5 December, 2020.

Curtis, S. (2016). *Geography and Health*, 2nd edition, Routledge.

Cutchin, M.P. (2007). The need for the "new health geography" in epidemiologic studies of environment and health. *Health Place*, September, 13(3): 725-42. doi: 10.1016/j.healthplace.2006.11.003. Epub 2007 Jan 5. PMID: 17208033; PMCID: PMC1880902.

Diener, E., Suh, E. (1997). Measuring Quality of Life: Economic, Social and Subjective Indicators. *Social Indicators Research*, 40: 189-216.

Diener, E. (2000). Subjective well-being: The science of happiness and a proposal for a national index. *American Psychologist*, 55(1), 34-43.

Dolfman, M.L. (1973). The concept of health: an historic and analytic examination in *Journal of School Health*, https: //doi.org/10.1111/j.1746-1561.1973.tb03740.x

Evangelos, C. Karademas (2007). Positive and negative aspects of well-being: Common and specific predictors, *Personality and Individual Differences*, Volume 43, Issue 2, July, pp. 277-287, https: //doi.org/10.1016/j.paid.2006.11.031.

Fleuret, S. and Atkinson, S. (2007). Well-being, health and geography: A critical review and research agenda, *New Zealand Geographer*, 63, 106-118, 10.1111/j.1745-7939.2007.00093.x

Graham, H., (ed.) (2000). *Understanding Health Inequalities*. Open University Press, Maidenhead. *Healthcare System in Ancient Science of Life*, Vol. No. V. No. 4, April 1986, pp. 216-227.

Hyma, B., Tamesh, A. and Iyengar, N.L.S. (1986). Geographical approach towards the study of *Healthcare System in Ancient Science of Life*, Vol. No. V. No. 4, April 1986, pp. 216-227.

Jones, K., Moon, G. (1993). Medical geography: taking space seriously, *Progress in Human Geography,* 17, 515-24.

Jones, K. and Moon, G. (1987). *Health, Disease and Society: A Critical Medical Geography*, Routledge Publication, accessed from https: //www.researchgate.net/publication/234015155_Health_Disease_and_Society_A_Critical_Medical_Geography

Kearns, R. & Moon, G. (2002). From medical to health geography: novelty, place and theory after a decade of change. *Progress in Human Geography*, 26(5), 605-625. https: //doi.org/10.1191/0309132502ph389oa

Koenig, Harold, G., Dana E. King, and Verna Benner Carson (2012). *Handbook of Religion and Health*, Second Edition.

Krause, Neal (2003). "Religious Meaning and Subjective Well-Being in Late-Life." *The Journals of Gerontology*: Series B. Also see Krause, Neal and Elena Bastida (2011). "Religion, Suffering, and Self-rated Health among Older Mexican Americans." *The Journals of Gerontology*: Series B.

Litva, A., Eyles, J. (1995). Coming out: exposing social theory in medical geography, *Health and Place,* 1, 5-14.

O'Keefe, Tim (6 October, 2019). "Cyrenaics". *Internet Encyclopedia of Philosophy.*

Park, Crystal, L. (2005). "Religion as a Meaning-Making Framework in Coping with Life Stress". *Journal of Social Issues.*

Schieman, Scott, Alex Bierman, and Christopher G. Ellison (2013). "Religion and Mental Health." In Carol S. Aneshensel, Jo C. Phelan, and Alex Bierman (eds.). *Handbook of the Sociology of Mental Health*, Second Edition.

Tuan, Y.F. (1974). *Topophilia*, Columbia University Press, New York.

Watson, D. & Tellegen, A. (1985). Towards a consensual structure of mood. *Psychological Bulletin*, 98(2), 219-235.

Chapter 2

Determinants of Human Health

Health and Well-being is the ultimate goal of one's life. Human health gets influenced by various factors. Natural factors like climate, soil, air and water impacts the health of people. Population growth, climate change, landuse change, economic and political set up also influence health of human beings. It is very difficult to identify single cause for diseases as there can be multiple factors that can affect one's health:

1. Geographical and Environmental Factors,
2. Socio-economic Factors,
3. Demographic Factors, and
4. Genetic Factors.

2.1 Terms Associated with Health

Before we discuss the factors in detail, let's focus on some important concepts that will further help to understand the relationship between various factors and the diseases:

1. **Health Risk:** According to WHO, health risk is something that increases your chance of developing a disease. Health risk refers to the likelihood of harm or injury that is associated with a particular activity or situation. For example, smoking, consuming unhealthy foods, excessive drinking, and lack of physical exercise can increase the risk of various health problems, like cancer, heart disease, diabetes etc.
2. **Health Exposure:** It is linked to contact. No matter how dangerous a substance or activity, without exposure, it cannot harm you. Over 400 years ago, a scientist said, "...nothing [is] without poisonous qualities. It is only the dose that makes a thing poison. On the other hand, health exposure is the degree to which an individual has come into contact with a harmful substance or situation. It can be either direct or indirect exposure, and could include things like pollution, radiation, infectious diseases, and toxins in the workplace (www.health.ny.gov).

To give examples:

- A person who smokes regularly is at a higher health risk of developing lung cancer or breathing issues.
- Prolonged exposure to air pollution may increase the health exposure and risk of developing respiratory illness such as asthma.
- A person who works in a chemical factory with inadequate safety measures is exposed to harmful toxins, thereby increasing the health exposure and risk of developing respiratory, skin or other related issues.

3. **The Dose:** It is the amount of a substance that enters or contacts a person. An important factor to consider in evaluating a dose is body weight. If a child is exposed to the same amount of chemical as an adult, the child (who weighs less) can be affected more than the adult. For example, children are given smaller amounts of aspirin than adults because an adult dose is too large for a child's body weight (www.health.ny.gov).
   Therefore, the greater the amount of a substance a person is exposed to, the more likely that health effects will occur. Large amounts of a relatively harmless substance can be toxic. For example, two aspirin tablets can help to relieve a headache, but taking an entire bottle of aspirin can cause stomach pain, nausea, vomiting, headache, convulsions or death (www.health.ny.gov).
4. **Routes of Exposure:** According to Department of Health, New York, there are three major means by which a toxic substance can come into contact with or enter the body. These are called routes of exposure.
   - **Inhalation (breathing):** It is linked to inhalation of gases, vapors, dusts or mists are a common route of exposure. Chemicals can enter lungs through the nose, air passages and can start irritation. They can get deposited in the airways and enter blood stream which gets absorbed through the lungs into the bloodstream. The blood can then carry these substances to the rest of the body.
   - **Direct Contact (touching):** Direct contact happens with the skin or eyes. It is also a route of exposure. Some substances are absorbed through the skin (touch) and enter the bloodstream. Wounded, cut or cracked skin will allow substances to enter the body more easily.
   - **Ingestion (swallowing):** Ingestion of food, drink, or other substances is another route of exposure. Chemicals that get in or on food, cigarettes, utensils or hands can be swallowed while eating. Children are at greater risk of ingesting substances found in dust or soil because they often put their fingers or other objects in their mouths. Lead in paint chips is a good example. Substances can be absorbed into the blood and then transported to the rest of the body (www.health.ny.gov).
5. **Length of Exposure:**
   - **Short term or Acute exposure** is a short contact with a chemical. It may last a few seconds or a few hours. For example, it might take a few minutes to clean windows with ammonia, use nail polish remover or spray a can of paint. The fumes someone might inhale during these activities are examples of acute exposures.
   - **Long term or Chronic exposure** is continuous or repeated contact with a toxic substance over a long period of time (months or years). If a chemical is used every

day on the job, the exposure would be chronic. Over time, some chemicals, such as PCBs and lead, can build up in the body. Chronic exposures can also occur at home. Some chemicals in household furniture, carpeting or cleaners can be sources of chronic exposure (www.health.ny.gov).

6. **Sensitivity:** It is important to note that all people are not equally sensitive to chemicals, and are not affected by them in the same way. There are many reasons for the differentials.
   - **Genetics:** People's bodies vary in their ability to absorb and break down or eliminate certain chemicals due to genetic differences.
   - **Allergies:** People may become allergic to a chemical after being exposed. Then they may react to very low levels of the chemical and have different or more serious health effects than non-allergic people exposed to the same amount. People who are allergic to bee venom, for example, have a more serious reaction to a bee sting than people who are not.
   - **Biological:** Factors such as age, illness, diet, alcohol use, pregnancy and medical or non-medical drug use can also affect a person's sensitivity to a chemical. Young children are often more sensitive to chemicals for a number of reasons. Their bodies are still developing and they cannot get rid of some chemicals as well as adults. Also, children absorb greater amounts of some chemicals (such as lead) into their blood than adults (www.health.ny.gov).

2.2 Geographical and Environmental Factors

Natural system and humans are interconnected. According to the ancient Indian Ayurvedic philosophy, human body is made up of 'panch tatava' or five elements: air, water, soil, fire and space. Geographical and environmental factors have a significant impact on human health. They may either contribute to well-being or pose threat to it.

2.2.1 *Climate*

The climate in a particular region can significantly affect human health. In tropical regions, for example, the warm and humid climate can encourage the growth of pathogens that cause diseases such as dengue fever and malaria. On the other hand, in colder regions, extreme cold can result in hypothermia and frostbite.

1. Extreme Heat: High temperatures can cause heat exhaustion and heatstroke, dehydration, and even death. Heatwaves have been linked to an increase in cardiovascular and respiratory diseases, as well as kidney problems. Extreme heat can have several negative effects on human health, ranging from minor issues such as dehydration and heat exhaustion to life-threatening conditions such as heatstroke. When the body is exposed to high temperatures for an extended period, it struggles to cool itself effectively, leading to several health problems. The human body responds to heat stress in two primary ways: redistributing blood flow towards the skin (vasodilation) to improve heat transfer from muscles to skin and subsequently to the environment, and secreting sweat onto the skin, which subsequently evaporates and removes body heat (Kenny, 2013). The brain regulates these physiological heat loss responses, with additional thermal input from temperature-sensitive nerve cells in the skin and throughout the body. This regulation can also be affected by non-thermal signals, such as from dehydration, metaboreceptors (a type of chemoreceptor that responds to metabolic products generated by exercising muscles), and cytokines (Fealey, 2013). Heat when exposed to high temperatures, the body tends to lose a lot of fluids through sweating, leading to dehydration. This can further cause symptoms like fatigue, headaches, dizziness, and heat exhaustion, which can be severe in some cases. Excessive heat also affects the respiratory system, making it difficult to breathe, particularly for people with respiratory diseases such as asthma, chronic obstructive pulmonary disease (COPD) and other lung and heart conditions. Extreme heat can also increase the risk of heart attacks, strokes, and other cardiovascular diseases, particularly in people with pre-existing conditions. Heatstroke is a life-threatening condition that can arise from prolonged exposure to extreme heat. It can cause severe symptoms like fever, confusion, seizures, and even unconsciousness. According to the World Health Organization, around 9,000 people died from heatstroke in India in 2017. Extreme heat can worsen the symptoms of people with chronic conditions, such as diabetes, multiple sclerosis, and other conditions. Often, these patients are relying on medications which might reduce sweating and impair the heart's ability to regulate body temperature.

It is, therefore, essential to take preventive measures like drinking enough water, staying indoors during peak sun hours, and lowering the body's core temperature to avoid the above-mentioned conditions.

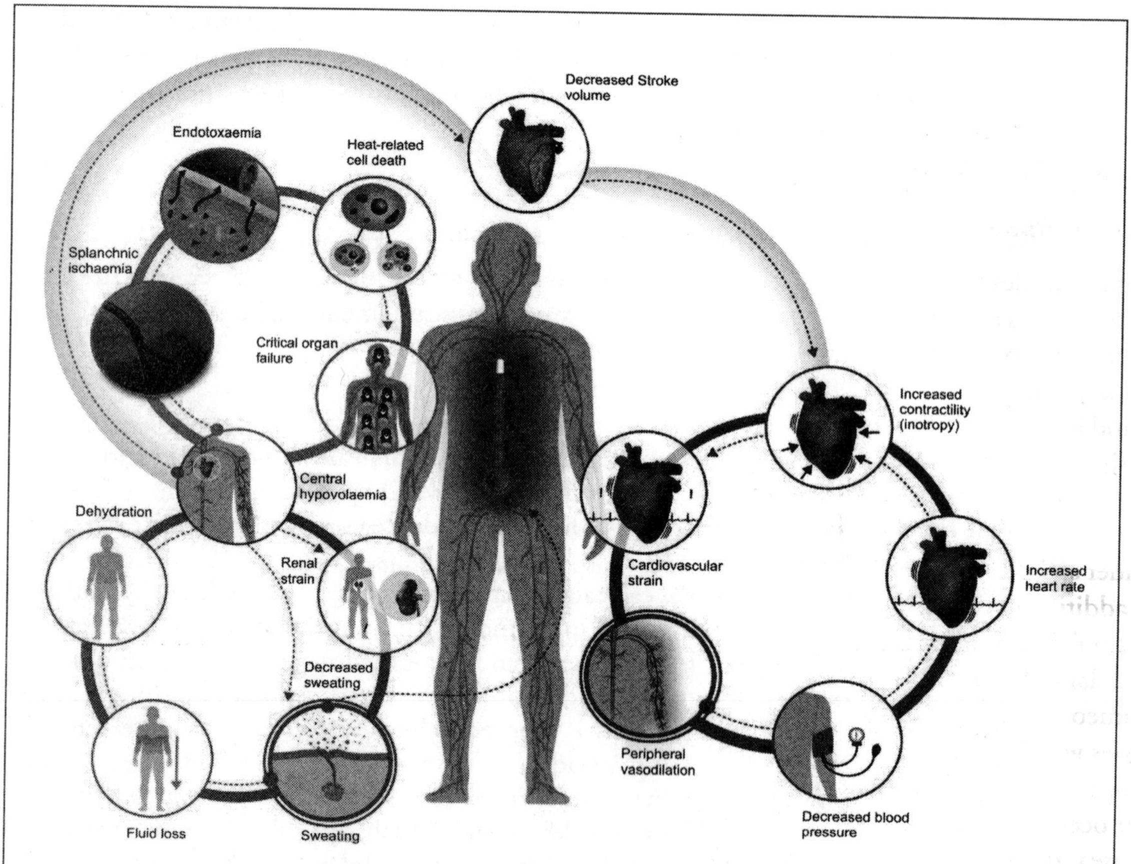

Fig. 2.1: Illustration of the physiological pathways of human heat strain.

Source: Ebi., K.L. *et al.*, (2021). Hot weather and heat extremes: health risks, Heat and Health 1, *The Lancet,* Vol. 398, August 21, 2021, www.thelancet.com

2. Extreme cold: Cold temperatures can cause hypothermia, frostbite, and respiratory issues. It can also worsen the symptoms of asthma and lead to heart attacks. Extreme cold can also have several negative effects on human health, ranging from minor issues like frostbite and hypothermia to life-threatening conditions like heart attacks and strokes. When the body is unable to maintain its core temperature, it can lead to hypothermia, which is a life-threatening condition. Symptoms of hypothermia include shivering, confusion, slurred speech, and difficulty in moving. Exposed skin and extremities can also get frostbite in extreme cold. It causes damage to the skin and tissues due to freezing. Extreme cold can also increase the risk of heart attacks, blood pressure fluctuations, and other cardiovascular diseases. Cold weather can also trigger joint pain and stiffness. Extreme low temperatures may even cause worsen the symptoms in people with arthritis and similar diseases. Cold, dry air particularly during winter could worsen the symptoms of asthma and other respiratory problems. Prolonged exposure to cold can also cause Raynaud's phenomenon, in which fingers, toes or other extremities become numb and tingly due to reduced blood flow.

Thus, just like extreme heat, extreme cold can also pose significant risks to human health throughout the cold weather regions and programmes like the Cold Weather Strategy implemented in the UK and several other countries can help to mitigate this impact. It is, therefore, essential to take preventive measures like staying warm and dry, wearing appropriate protective clothing, and avoid prolonged exposure for susceptible individuals to avoid the above-mentioned conditions.

2.2.2 *Altitude*

High altitudes can cause health problems due to reduced oxygen level. People living in high altitude areas are often at risk of altitude sickness, which can cause headache, dizziness, and in severe cases, pulmonary edema (Edema is swelling caused by too much fluid trapped in the body's tissues) or cerebral edema. Altitude or high altitude, referring to the height above sea level, often found in mountain areas, can have significant effects on human health. Elevation also appears to be significant; with Andes mountains standing out as largely free of Malaria in the tropical zone that otherwise seem to support malaria transmission (Hazen and Anthamatten, 2011). High altitude introduces environmental stressors that are distinct from sea level. Hypobaric hypoxia, colder and drier climates, and increased radiation challenge reproductive success (Moore, 2017). In addition to the direct effects of high altitude, the health of high-altitude residents (particularly in rural communities) is compounded by vulnerability to food and water insecurity associated with land degradation and the concurrence of conflict and climate change (Hock *et al.*, 2019; Romeo *et al.*, 2020). Population estimates for the number of humans residing at high altitude varies widely. With the decrease in atmospheric pressure and available oxygen at high altitudes, people may experience Acute Mountain Sickness (AMS) which is a collection of symptoms that can occur when we rapidly ascend to high altitudes. Common symptoms include headaches, nausea, dizziness, fatigue, and shortness of breath. At very high altitudes above 5500 metres, there is a high risk of fatal brain swelling or other severe forms of altitude sickness, which for instance affects climbers of Mount Everest every year. High Altitude Pulmonary Edema (HAPE) that can occur due to increased blood flow and pressure in the lungs. Fluid buildup in the lungs can cause the person to become very breathless and will require further medical attention for the patient. High Altitude Cerebral Edema (HACE) is more severe condition than AMS that could happen due to fluid buildup in the brain. It could cause mental disorientation, confusion, and severe headaches. At high altitudes, the body may lose water more quickly due to dryness and increased breathing rates, which can lead to dehydration. High altitude regions are often sunny, and reflection from snow on mountains can cause sunburns and snow blindness, which can cause corneal injury.

Therefore, when we travel to high altitude locations, it is essential to take adequate precautions. Ascending slowly, staying hydrated, and having proper clothing are some of the preventive measures that we can take. Additionally, the use of medications like acetazolamide can help prevent AMS and HACE when the body is not adjusting to the low oxygen levels. It is important to be mindful of the risks and take necessary measures to ensure a safe and healthy stay in mountain areas.

2.2.3 *Water Quality*

The quality of water available to people in a particular region can significantly affect human health. Poor water quality can lead to the spread of water-borne illnesses such as cholera and dysentery, which can be fatal if not addressed properly. Water quality has significant effects on human health, as people use water for drinking, cooking, bathing, and many other activities. Contaminated water can lead to water-borne illnesses, which can range from mild to severe and may have long-term effects on health. According to WHO, over 2 billion people live in water-stressed countries, which is expected to be exacerbated in some regions as a result of climate change and population growth. Globally, at least 2 billion people use a drinking water source contaminated with faeces. Microbial contamination of drinking-water as a result of contamination with faeces poses the greatest risk to drinking-water safety. While the most important chemical risks in drinking water arise from arsenic, fluoride or nitrate, emerging contaminants such as pharmaceuticals, pesticides, per- and poly-fluoroalkyl substances (PFASs) and microplastics generate public concern. Microbiologically contaminated drinking water can transmit diseases, such as diarrhoea, cholera, dysentery, typhoid and polio and is estimated to cause 4,85,000 diarrhoeal deaths each year (https://www.who.int/news-room/fact-sheets/detail/drinking-water).

Some prominent diseases or infections caused due to contaminated water are:

1. **Gastrointestinal Illnesses:** Polluted water can cause gastroenteritis, which can result in diarrhoea, vomiting, and stomach cramps, leading to dehydration and nutritional deficiencies, particularly common in developing countries where access to clean drinking water is limited.
2. **Intestinal Worms:** Parasitic worms such as tapeworms and roundworms found in contaminated water, can lead to symptoms like stomach aches, diarrhoea, and malnutrition that can affect children's growth and cognitive development.
3. **Heavy Metal Poisoning:** Heavy metals, such as lead, cadmium, mercury, and arsenic can cause severe illnesses when ingested through water or food grown with polluted water.
4. **Cancer:** Long-term exposure to industrial and agricultural waste containing chemicals such as benzene, lead, and pesticides, have been associated with cancer instances in several instances around the world.

5. **Neurological Disorders, including Parkinson's Disease, Alzheimer's Disease, and Developmental Delays:** Contaminated water may also contain harmful chemicals that could affect neurological systems of the human body, endangering fetal and child neuro-development.

For instance, it is reflected by the Flint Water Crisis (2014-2019) where lead contamination in the public water supply caused significant health problems in children exposed to lead, including developmental delays, learning challenges, and behavioural concerns. In Bengal, India, groundwater influenced by arsenic exposure is leading to chronic arsenicosis and cancer in the long term.

Therefore, the quality of water we consume is vital for our health and well-being. It is necessary to have proper water management, filtration systems, laws and regulations that are enforced to preserve, protect and purify sources of water, like using safe and sustainable treatments, lowering chemical pollutants, conducting regular health tests on water quality. Access to safe and clean water should be made possible for everyone as part of their fundamental right to healthy living. Safe drinking water with required minerals can enhance human health in a magical way.

UNEP study [Water Quality: International Decade for Action 'Water for Life' 2005-2015 (un.org)] shows that increased levels of nitrate at river mouths are found in parts of Russia and Europe. Everyday, 2 million tons of sewage and other effluents drain into the world's waters. Every year, more people die from unsafe water than from all forms of violence, including war. The most significant sources of water pollution are lack of inadequate treatment of human wastes and inadequately managed and treated industrial and agricultural wastes. The quality of water necessary for each human use varies, as do the criteria used to assess water quality. For example, the highest standards of purity are required for drinking water, whereas it is acceptable for water used in some industrial processes to be of less quality (un.org). The acronym WASH (Water, Sanitation and Hygiene) is used as a reminder for the critical connections between water and health. Therefore, it is important to consider water and hygiene as an essential components for disease management.

2.2.4 *Landuse and Landcover Change*

Human activity has changed the face of the global landscape. These changes in landuse and cover have, in turn, altered the dynamics of infectious disease transmission in numerous ways. They have created new habitat and breeding sites for disease vectors which, in many cases, favour disease transmission. They have altered exposure pathways by changing the way organisms (including humans) interact with each other. They have led to changes in the genetics, and thereby, the virulence, and infectiousness of pathogens. They have also changed the lifecycle of pathogens and vectors and the species composition of whole communities of disease-relevant organisms. Not surprisingly, these changes have occurred coincident with a rise in new or reemerging infectious diseases (Myers, 2011). Landuse changes can create suitable habitats for disease-carrying vectors, such as mosquitoes and ticks. For instance, deforestation can lead to increased contact between humans and vectors carrying diseases like malaria, dengue fever, and Lyme disease. The expansion of agricultural lands and urbanization can also alter ecosystems and increase the risk of zoonotic diseases, such as the transmission of diseases from animals to humans like COVID-19. Deforestation and agricultural activities can contribute to water pollution through soil erosion, pesticide run-off, and excessive nutrient discharge. Contaminated water sources can lead to water-borne diseases, such as diarrhoea, cholera, and typhoid.

In a study published in *Scientific American*, it was found that in Central Valley, California, USA, intensive agricultural practices and landuse changes in California's Central Valley have caused air pollution issues. The region experiences high levels of ozone and particulate matter due to livestock emissions, vehicle exhaust, and dust stirred up by land tillage. This has led to increased rates of respiratory diseases, including asthma and chronic obstructive pulmonary disease (COPD), among individuals living in the area. In a similar study it was found that in Sub-Saharan Africa land cover changes, such as rapid urbanization and deforestation, have contributed to the spread of vector-borne diseases in many parts of Sub-Saharan Africa. For example, in urban areas like Nairobi, Kenya, increased landuse change has created suitable breeding grounds for mosquitoes, leading to the spread of diseases like malaria and dengue fever (Refer Table 2.1). The loss of natural spaces due to landuse changes has been linked to negative impacts on mental health. Urban environments with limited access to green spaces have been associated with increased rates of depression, anxiety, and stress. Studies have shown that exposure to nature and green spaces can have a positive impact on mental well-being.

Table 2.1: Mechanisms of altered infectious disease exposure resulting from environmental change

Mechanism by which environmental change alters disease transmission	**Examples**	**Diseases known to be impacted by this mechanism**
Changes in density or identity of disease-related organisms	Deforestation or irrigation projects improve breeding habitat and survival of certain anopheline mosquitoes that transmit malaria in Africa, Latin America, and Asia.	Malaria, schistosomiasis, dengue, Japanese encephalitis, filariasis, trypansomiasis, leishmaniasis, cholera, plague, Rift Valley fever, dracunculosis, onchocerciasis, hantavirus, hemorrhagic viruses, Chagas disease, Oropouche/Mayaro virus harmful algal blooms.
	Deforestation in Cameroon favours one snail species over another, thereby increasing human exposure to pathogenic schistosomes.	
	Sea surface warming and nutrient loading lead to proliferation of *Vibrio cholerae* and disease outbreaks.	
Changes in Exposure Pathways	Incursions into wildlife habitat can lead to new exposure to zoonotic disease as seen in Ebola, simian retroviruses, and, possibly, HIV.	Malaria, trypanosomiasis, cryptosporidiosis, giardiasis, Ebola, simian retroviruses, HIV, dengue, filariasis, Chagas disease, plague, leptospirosis, typhus, diarrhoeal disease, food poisoning.
	Dense urban settlements with poor sanitation, waste disposal, or water treatment can lead to increased exposure to many diseases including diarrhoeal disease, dengue, and leptospirosis.	

(*Contd.*)

Mechanism by which environmental change alters disease transmission	Examples	Diseases known to be impacted by this mechanism
Changing the environment in which organisms live creates genetic alterations which can increase disease transmission	Livestock management relying on extensive use of antibiotics in concentrated animal feeding operations (CAFOs) leads to the emergence of pathogens resistant to numerous antibiotics.	Antibiotic resistant bacteria, influenza, SARS.
	Confinement of different animal species in wet markets or pig-duck farms can lead to genetic rearrangements resulting in increased virulence or altered infectivity.	
Changes in life-cycle of vectors or pathogens	Deforestation causes increased ambient temperature in homes and breeding sites which shortens gonotrophic cycles, reduces development time, and increases survivalship of anopheline mosquitoes in Kenya.	Malaria.
Changes in species composition of communities of organisms	Biodiversity loss in Northeastern forests of the United States increases exposure to Lyme Disease.	Lyme Disease, West Nile virus, malaria, hantavirus, Guanarito, Junin, Machupo, bartonellosis, Nipah virus, St. Louis encephalitis.
	Altered species composition of wetlands in Belize in response to nutrient loading creates favourable habitat for a more effective malaria vector.	

Source: Myers, S.S., 2011.

2.2.5 *Air Quality*

Human health can be negatively impacted by exposure to pollutants in the environment. For example, air pollution caused by industrial activities, vehicle traffic, or wildfires can contribute to respiratory problems, such as asthma, bronchitis, and lung cancer. Air pollution can have several negative effects on human health, as it often contains harmful chemicals, particles, and other pollutants that can cause short and long-term health problems. Urbanization and industrial landuse changes often result in increased pollution levels, especially in cities. High levels of air pollution, such as particulate matter (PM2.5), have been linked to respiratory problems, cardiovascular diseases, and even premature death. According to the World Health Organization (WHO), outdoor air pollution caused an estimated 4.2 million premature deaths in 2016. Some prominent health issues associated with air pollution are:

1. **Respiratory Diseases:** Air pollution can lead to respiratory diseases such as asthma, chronic obstructive pulmonary disease (COPD), and lung cancer. Harmful pollutants such as particulate matter, ozone, sulphur dioxide, and nitrogen oxide can cause inflammation in the lungs and result in severe respiratory problems.

2. **Cardiovascular Diseases:** Air pollution can also contribute to heart disease, stroke, and other cardiovascular problems. Fine particles from car exhaust can penetrate deep into the lungs and blood vessels, causing inflammation, and increasing the risk of heart attacks and strokes.

The Great Smog of London in 1952 was a severe air pollution event that occurred in London, England. Lasting from December 5th to December 9th, the smog resulted in one of the deadliest environmental disasters in history.

Causes: The primary causes of the Great Smog were industrial emissions and domestic coal burning. During that time, coal was widely used for heating and power generation, and weather conditions contributed to the stagnant air and low-lying fog that acted as a blanket, trapping pollutants close to the ground.

Duration and Severity: The Great Smog lasted for five days, during which London experienced unusually cold weather. The smog was thick and dark, reducing visibility to only a few metres. The pollutant concentrations were estimated to be significantly higher than normal, reaching dangerous levels.

Health Impacts: The dense smog caused a range of health problems. The most affected individuals were the elderly, young children, and individuals with pre-existing respiratory conditions. The pollution led to an increase in respiratory infections, such as bronchitis and pneumonia. There was also a notable surge in hospital admissions and deaths, particularly due to respiratory and cardiovascular issues.

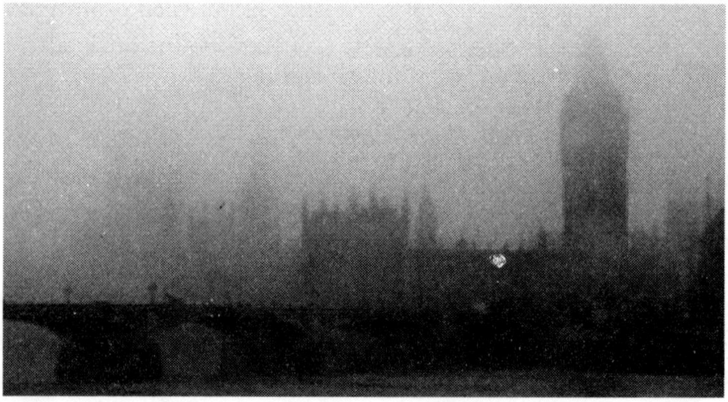

Source: www.history.com

Death Toll: The exact number of deaths caused directly by the Great Smog remains uncertain. Initial reports estimated around 4,000 deaths during the event, but subsequent studies indicated a higher toll. Research conducted later by scientists suggested that the smog may have led to approximately 12,000 premature deaths in the long term due to related health complications.

Response and Legislation: The devastating impact of the Great Smog prompted the British government to take action. The Clean Air Act was passed in 1956, which aimed to regulate industrial emissions, enforce smoke control areas, and encourage the use of cleaner fuels. The legislation provided a framework for reducing air pollution in the UK over subsequent decades.

3. **Neurological Disorders:** Long-term exposure to air pollution particularly by fine particulate matter, has been linked to an increased risk of cognitive decline, Alzheimer's disease, Parkinson's disease, and behavioural disorders which calls for further research and monitoring.
4. **Pregnancy and Child Health:** Exposure to air pollutants during pregnancy could lead to complications such as low birth weight, preterm births, respiratory problems, coronary heart disease, and even death. According to Medanta.org, The Dangers of Exposure to Air Pollution during Pregnancy can lead to the following risks:
   - *Low Birth Weight:* Air Pollution can cause babies to have low birth weight. While the exact reason is unknown, this is likely due to a restriction of nutrient delivery through the placenta.
   - *Preterm Birth:* Air pollution can cause premature birth, and can thus lead to neurological disorders and permanent physical disabilities in newborn babies.
   - *Autism:* A Harvard study revealed that a child with autism was twice as likely to be delivered by woman who was exposed to high particulate matter pollution during their third trimester.
   - *Asthma:* Asthma during pregnancy can lead to a condition called preeclampsia, causing elevated blood pressure and decreased function of the liver and kidneys. If untreated, asthma can cause your baby to suffer from lack of oxygen. This can result in poor growth, premature birth, and low birth weight.
   - *Risk of Miscarriage:* Studies have found links between prolonged exposure to outdoor air pollution and miscarriages. Outdoor air pollution is also likely to cause lower fertility rates in men and women.
5. **Cancer:** Air pollution contains several carcinogenic chemicals such as benzene, formaldehyde, and polycyclic aromatic hydrocarbons (PAHs), which can cause different forms of cancer, such as lung cancer, bladder cancer, and mesothelioma.

New Delhi, India, experienced hazardous air pollution from last 5-6 years, in the month of November due to stubble burning in peripheries, that triggers public health emergencies due to high PM2.5 or PM10 (particulate matters) and nitrogen oxide levels, which leads to increasing respiratory diseases, cancer, pregnancy complications and lower life expectancy. To manage the impact of this pollution schools are kept closed for few days so that the harmful gases do not affect children. It is important to take necessary measures to reduce air pollution such as promoting clean energy, reducing vehicular emissions, initiating green endeavours, public awareness, and regulatory enforcement, as prevention is the most effective and cost-efficient strategy to manage the health implications of air pollution.

2.2.6 *Natural Disasters*

Geographical factors like earthquakes, floods, hurricanes, and tsunamis can cause considerable damage to homes, buildings, and infrastructure. They can also lead to injuries and illnesses due to direct exposure, lack of access to medical care, and contamination of water supplies. Natural disasters can have severe impacts on human health, by compromising water, food, and healthcare infrastructure, leading to starvation or exposure to environmental hazards. Here are some examples of health issues that could arise during or after natural disasters:

1. **Physical Injuries:** Natural disasters such as floods or hurricanes can cause physical injuries in survivors, from an impact, or from being trapped and displaced in the wreckage of destroyed infrastructures. In 2010, a devastating earthquake struck Haiti, resulted in an estimated 2,30,000 deaths and over 3,00,000 injuries. The Great East Japan Earthquake in 2011 caused over 15,000 deaths and more than 6,000 injuries. Similarly, the Indian Ocean Tsunami in 2004 caused by an under sea earthquake led to an estimated 2,30,000 deaths across 14 countries, with injuries sustained by thousands of survivours.
2. **Respiratory Diseases:** Dust, smoke, ash, and other particulate debris that could arise during disasters could significantly impact indoor and outdoor air quality, leading to respiratory issues like coughing, irritation, pneumonia, asthma, and other similar conditions.
3. **Waterborne Illnesses:** Floods, hurricanes, and other natural disasters can cause damage to water supply systems, causing unsafe drinking water. Exposure to contaminated water could lead to diseases like cholera, typhoid, and dysentery.
4. **Mental Health Issues:** Natural disasters can cause anxiety, depression, PTSD (Post Traumatic Stress Disorder), and other mental health issues among survivors. Displacement, loss of property, and uncertainty, could traumatize people and lead to worsened mental health or disorders.
5. **Vector-Borne Diseases:** Spread through vectors like mosquitoes, natural disasters could increase illnesses that could spread in flood-prone areas, like dengue, malaria, and other similar diseases. In 2019, heavy floods in South Sudan resulted in a significant rise in malaria cases. The country reported over 1.6 million malaria cases and 1,562 deaths attributed to the disease. Similarly, floods in India, particularly in states like Assam and Bihar, often lead to a surge in malaria cases. In 2019, Assam recorded over 1,60,000 malaria cases. The Aedes mosquito, which thrives in stagnant water, is also responsible for the transmission of the Zika virus. In 2015-16, Brazil faced a significant outbreak of Zika virus. The flooding caused by heavy rains contributed to the proliferation of mosquitoes, resulting in thousands of cases, including neurological complications and birth defects in newborns.
6. **Malnutrition:** Disasters can affect food supplies by damaging crops or disrupting food delivery systems, leading to food insecurity and malnutrition or starvation. During famines, malnutrition results when the population does not have access to enough food or have access to only low-nutrient food sources, resulting in the body being denied essential nutrients. Malnutrition associated with famine includes symptoms, such as weight loss, fatigue, and other noticeable health decline symptoms. This leads to the body's degradation and deteriorating health, particularly affecting children, pregnant, and breastfeeding women who are more prone to malnutrition's effects. Somalia has experienced recurrent droughts, which have been exacerbated by conflicts and political instability. Droughts have led to failed crops, livestock deaths, and severe food shortages, causing malnutrition and widespread famine. Cyclone Idai struck Mozambique in 2019, causing widespread devastation and displacing thousands of people. The cyclone destroyed crops, livestock, and infrastructure, leading to food shortages and malnutrition in the affected areas.

The Bhuj earthquake, also known as the Gujarat earthquake, struck the state of Gujarat in India on January 26, 2001. It was a massive quake with a magnitude of 7.7 that caused extensive damage to infrastructure and resulted in significant human casualties.

1. Injuries and Death: The earthquake caused widespread destruction of buildings and infrastructure, leading to many people being trapped or crushed under debris. The immediate impact resulted in numerous injuries, both minor and severe, including fractures, lacerations, and crush injuries. Sadly, thousands of people lost their lives in the disaster.

2. Mental Stress: Earthquakes can have a profound psychological impact on survivors. The Bhuj earthquake caused significant trauma and mental distress among the affected population. People experienced fear, anxiety, grief, and post-traumatic stress disorder (PTSD) due to the loss of loved ones, displacement, and the destruction of their homes and communities.

3. Malnutrition: The destruction of infrastructure and disruption of the food supply chain due to the earthquake led to food shortages and limited access to nutritious food. The lack of access to adequate food resources increased the risk of malnutrition, especially among vulnerable groups such as children, pregnant women, and the elderly.

4. Other Health Issues: Besides injuries and malnutrition, the earthquake gave rise to various health issues. The collapse of sanitation systems and contamination of water sources increased the risk of water-borne diseases such as diarrhoea, cholera, and typhoid. In overcrowded temporary shelters, there was an increased likelihood of respiratory infections and the spread of communicable diseases.

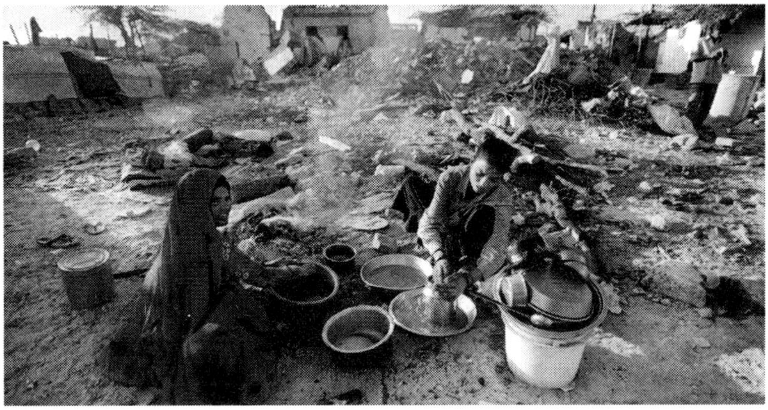

Source: Outlookindia.com

5. Long-term Consequences: The impact of the Bhuj earthquake extended beyond the immediate aftermath. The displacement of people, destruction of livelihoods, and loss of infrastructure resulted in long-term socio-economic consequences. The affected communities faced challenges in rebuilding their lives, accessing healthcare, education, and employment opportunities, which further contributed to mental stress, poverty, and social displacement.

Natural disasters can have significant impacts on human health—physical, mental, and emotional. It is, therefore, essential for authorities to initiate protective measures before, during, and after a natural catastrophe. These measures include developing and enforcing building codes, proper urban planning, early warning systems, and developing community-level preparedness to ensure that food and safe drinking water are available to all affected individuals while medical treatments and psychosocial support services are standard for people who need them.

2.3 Socio-economic Factors

Socio-economic factors such as income, education, occupation, and social status can have a significant impact on human health. Below are some of these factors that can influence health:

2.3.1 *Income Level*

People with lower income levels tend to have poorer health outcomes compared to those with higher income levels. This is because low income can limit access to healthy food, healthcare, safe housing, and other resources that promote good health. Income can have a significant impact on a person's health, as it can determine access to healthcare services, nutritious food, safe housing, and other factors that contribute to overall well-being. Income influences health and longevity through various clinical, behavioural, social, and environmental mechanisms. Isolating the unique contribution of income to health can be difficult because this relationship intersects with many other social risk factors. Poor health also contributes to reduced income, creating a negative feedback loop sometimes referred to as the health-poverty trap (www.healthaffairs.org).

- **Higher Incomes:** People with higher incomes often have better access to healthcare services, including preventative care, screenings, and treatment options. This can help them catch and treat health issues before they become more serious. Lower income individuals may not be able to afford healthy food options, which can lead to malnutrition, obesity, and other health issues. With more disposable income, individuals can buy more fresh produce and high-quality food. People with low incomes may live in unsafe or overcrowded housing, which can lead to health issues like respiratory problems, allergies, and infections. Higher-income individuals can afford safe and healthy housing options. Financial stress can lead to chronic stress, which can raise the risk of mental health issues, high blood pressure, heart disease, and stroke. Higher-income individuals may have more financial stability and less stress. Though on contrary, many scholars consider the term "diseases of affluence", i.e "diseases of rich people" or rich countries which are associated with higher income like many non-communicable diseases. Diseases like type 2 diabetes. Hypertension and obesity were earlier considered to be in this category. Currently, such diseases are also prevalent in developing countries and middle and low income group people.
- **Poverty**: Poverty and health are closely linked. Considering absolute poverty, it has been defined as "a condition characterized by severe deprivation of basic human needs, including food, safe drinking water, sanitation facilities, health, shelter, education, and information. It depends not only on income but also on access to services." On the other hand, overall poverty is a "lack of income and productive resources to ensure sustainable livelihoods; hunger and malnutrition; ill health; limited or lack of access to education and other basic services; increased morbidity and mortality from illness; homelessness

and inadequate housing; unsafe environments and social discrimination and exclusion. It is also characterized by a lack of participation in decision-making and civil, social, and cultural life. It occurs in all countries: as mass poverty in many developing countries, pockets of poverty amid wealth in developed countries, loss of livelihoods as a result of economic recession, sudden poverty as a result of disaster or conflict, the poverty of low-wage workers, and the utter lack of people who fall outside family support systems, social institutions and safety nets" (Alqassim and Setouhy, 2022). Poverty can have a significant impact on human health in various ways. Poverty can impact people's health at all stages of life in several ways and impacts overall life expectancy. In England, for example, between 2009 and 2013, the life expectancy for those in the most deprived areas compared to the least deprived areas was 7.9 years greater for men and 5.9 years greater for women (www.news-medical.net). According to World Bank, poverty is a major cause of ill health and a barrier to accessing healthcare when needed. This relationship is financial: the poor cannot afford to purchase those things that are needed for good health, including sufficient quantities of quality food and healthcare. But, the relationship is also related to other factors related to poverty, such as lack of information on appropriate health-promoting practices or lack of voice needed to make social services work for them.

- **Malnutrition:** Poverty can lead to malnutrition as people living in poverty may not have access to nutritious food options. According to the World Health Organization, 45 per cent of deaths among children under the age of five are caused by malnutrition, and the majority of those children live in low-income households. On average, babies born in the most deprived areas in the UK weigh 200g less than those born in more affluent areas, which may subsequently impact cognitive development. Babies living in poverty are also more likely to die within the first year of birth and were more likely to be bottle-fed. Seventy-three per cent of women in the most deprived areas were shown to initiate breastfeeding compared to 89 per cent of women in the least deprived areas (www.news-medical.net).
- **Infectious Diseases:** People living in poverty may be more susceptible to infectious diseases due to poor living conditions and inadequate access to healthcare and sanitation. For example, Tuberculosis (TB) is more prevalent in areas of poverty due to poor living conditions and overcrowding. Neglected tropical diseases affect over one billion people, almost all in the poorest and most marginalised communities. You may not have heard of diseases such as leprosy, lymphatic filariasis, onchocerciasis, schistosomiasis, soil-transmitted helminths and trachoma, but they can cause severe pain and life-long disabilities—and mean enormous productivity losses. However, efforts to tackle them have usually taken a back seat to the bigger killers (www.healthpovertyaction.org).
- **Mental Health:** Poverty can also negatively impact mental health, causing stress, anxiety, and depression, which can manifest into physical symptoms. Those living in poverty are at an increased risk of suicide and other mental health disorders. Inequality and deprivation in society leads to mental harassment. It leads to resentment and feeling of alienation. Such people tend to suffer many mental problems like extreme anger, anxiety, depression etc. Such people, who are unable to manage mental stress and do not have money to

access any expert help, gets into drugs, alcohol and crime. Poverty can be both cause and consequence of mental health.

- **Environmental Pollution:** People living in poverty may be exposed to environmental pollution, which can lead to various health issues. For example, air pollution is more prevalent in areas of poverty, which can lead to respiratory problems. Environmental health is deeply significant to poverty, important concern for the poor (Cairncross and Kolsky, 2003). Poor people often live in areas with the worst environmental conditions; they have lower resistance to infection; they pay more for environmental health services; and when they fall ill, they lose income and even their jobs.... Problems such as unsafe water, sanitation, and poor hygiene; air pollution; and inadequate vector control are major contributors to the worldwide disease burden. Poor communities are disproportionately affected by these issues, which seem likely to worsen with climate variability and change. Ill health resulting from these problems affects school attendance, incomes, and communities' efforts to improve their long-term quality of life. Progress on this important agenda and in the quality of life of the poor is essential for sustainable development (www.cbd.int).
- **Lack of Access to Healthcare**: People in poverty may not have access to healthcare and preventative services. They may avoid visiting doctors due to the cost of medical bills, which can lead to medical issues from untreated conditions. Marginalised groups and vulnerable individuals are often worst affected, deprived of the information, money or access to health services that would help them prevent and treat disease (www.healthpovertyaction.org). According to WHO (2017), at least half of the population of the world lack access to safe healthcare facilities. Out of pocket expenditure is very high, i.e., around 800 million people spend more than 10 per cent of their budget on health expenses. "Investments in health, and more generally investments in people, are critical to build human capital and enable sustainable and inclusive economic growth (WHO, 2017).

Extreme poverty interacts with health in many ways and undermines a whole range of human capabilities, possibilities and opportunities (Muller, 2005). It is important to focus on basic necessities of poor and marginal sections of society. Education, sanitation and food and water security should be considered as a priority by policymakers. Environmental health needs to be targeted to improve the conditions of poor in the society.

2.3.2 *Education*

Higher levels of education are often associated with better health outcomes. Education can improve health literacy, promote healthy behaviours, and increase access to job opportunities that offer health benefits. There is a strong correlation between education level and human health. Having higher levels of education can lead to better health outcomes in many ways.

1. **Better job Opportunities:** The knowledge based world requires highly educated people. Education helps to develop skills and competence to survive in the world. People who are well qualified have a better scope to earn. Qualification is directly linked to better job and better job is directly linked to more earnings. People who earn more live in better conditions and have high standard of living. They can afford best healthcare facilities.

They can purchase healthy and fresh food and medicines. Conversely people who are uneducated do not get good jobs and earn less. Poor earnings lead to unsafe housing, water and sanitation facilities. The poor conditions impact their health and they are unable to afford the expenditure required for healthcare.

2. **Disease Prevention:** Education can play a vital role in disease prevention. Educated individuals tend to have higher rates of vaccinations, regular check-ups with doctors, and general health knowledge. This can lead to early detection and prevention of illnesses. Education helps people to read and understand better. They attend various workshops, seminars or read newspaper and blogs to enhance their knowledge about the diseases. They also recognise the significance of vaccination and other government programmes to prevent certain diseases. Low health literacy can hinder disease prevention efforts. Incorporating health education into the curriculum can teach students about various diseases, their causes, symptoms, and preventive measures. This equips them with the necessary knowledge to protect themselves and others, promoting healthy behaviours from an early age.
3. **Better Mental Health:** There is a strong link between education and mental health. Education provides people with crucial problem-solving skills that can help reduce stress, anxiety, and depression. Furthermore, higher levels of education help to reduce the risk of developing certain mental health disorders such as Alzheimer's. In a study conducted by *British Journal of Psychiatry, 2015,* the relationship between educational attainment and common mental disorders (CMDs) was investigated in a large sample of individuals from the UK. It reported that lower educational attainment was associated with higher rates of CMDs, with those who had not completed high school being at a significantly higher risk. JAMA Psychiatry, 2014 carried out a research to explore the association between educational achievement and lifetime risk of mental disorders in a population-based sample from the US National Epidemiologic Survey on Alcohol and Related Conditions. They found that lower educational achievement was significantly associated with increased risk of several mental disorders, including mood and anxiety disorders.
4. **Access to Healthcare:** People with higher levels of education are more likely to be aware of available healthcare options and benefits. With better knowledge and resources, educated patients tend to be more engaged with their medical care, resulting in better health outcomes. They are aware about government schemes and the way to get benefit. They have health insurance and life insurance to secure their future. As mentioned earlier, the educated people have a higher probability to earn more and therefore, they have access to better healthcare facilities and hospitalization facility at the time of emergency.
5. **Safer and Healthier Behaviours:** Educated individuals are more likely to make healthier choices and adopt safer behaviours, such as limiting alcohol and drug use, maintaining proper safety practices, and paying attention to their overall wellness. Less educated people are living in unhealthy areas of the cities. The food and water they consume is not safe at times. They live in congested places and lack proper sanitation facilities. Rural and low-income areas, which are more populated by people with less education, often suffer from shortages of primary care physicians and other healthcare providers and facilities. Higher crime rates, exposing residents to greater risk of trauma and deaths from violence and the

stress of living in unsafe neighbourhoods. People with less education, particularly males, are more likely to be incarcerated, which carries its own public health risks (societyhealth.vcu.edu). Well educated people are considered to be more responsible and carry healthy behaviour. They know to segregate wet, dry and hazardrous waste. They are more careful while disposing of the e-waste. They also educate their children and family about the same. Such behaviours help to mitigate the unhealthy conditions in the area they live in. Now-a-days educated people are heading their neighbourhoods and are managing the resources in a better manner. They are working on creating zero waste zones and green spaces. They also participate in tree plantation drives around their houses and offices as they understand the significance of green space. They do not litter or spit on roads. Their daily behaviour becomes very relevant to improve the conditions of their area.

6. **High Life Expectancy/Longevity:** Education is often cited as a significant factor in increasing life expectancy. In some countries, a link has been found between healthcare and education, with higher education levels leading to longer lifespans. In tandem with the decrease of mortality, the populations have experienced significant increases in educational attainment (Lutz *et al.,* 2014a). Between 1970 and 2009, for instance, the average number of years of education rose by 3.6 years for people aged 25 and older in 175 countries (Gakidou *et al.,* 2010). A great deal of research acknowledges the strong impact of socio-economic resources on various health outcomes, suggesting socio-economic conditions as a "fundamental cause" of inequalities in health and mortality (Link and Phelan, 1995). Many studies have shown that highly educated people stand to benefit first and most from the prevailing drivers of decreasing mortality, particularly with regard to the risk factors of cardiovascular diseases (Hummer and Lariscy, 2011; Mirowsky and Ross, 2003). Lleras-Muney (2005) estimated—with data for the USA in 1960—that one more year of education increased average life expectancy at age 35 by as much as 1.7 years. Further, Woolf *et al.* (2007) estimated that eliminating education-specific inequalities in mortality would save even more lives than medical advances (Luy *et al.,* 2019).

By improving awareness, providing individuals with problem-solving skills and greater access to healthcare resources, education can ultimately lead to better health outcomes.

2.4 Occupation/Work Spaces

A workplace or place of employment is a location where people perform tasks, jobs and projects for their employer. Types of workplaces vary across industries and can be inside a building or outdoors. Workplaces can be mobile, and some people may work in different locations on various days. The type of job that a person does can impact his health in a significant way. For example, people in manual labour jobs may be at higher risk of injury or exposure to harmful substances than those in office jobs. Additionally, jobs that do not offer health insurance or paid sick leave can limit access to healthcare and time for self-care.

(a) Certain occupations can expose individuals to occupational hazards, such as exposure to harmful chemicals or particulates like nuclear plants or refineries, loud noises, and physically demanding work like masons. Over time, exposure to these hazards can lead to chronic health problems such as respiratory diseases, hearing loss, and joint pain.

(b) Certain occupations can lead to stress, burnout, and other mental health issues. Jobs that are high-pressure, involve long hours or irregular schedules, or require frequent interactions with difficult people can take a toll on an individual's emotional well-being. Over time, this can result in conditions, such as depression, anxiety, and even addiction.

(c) Finally, occupation can also impact one's lifestyle choices, including diet, exercise, and sleep habits. Certain professions, such as shift work, may make it difficult to maintain a healthy lifestyle, leading to an increased risk of obesity, heart disease, and other chronic health problems.

A recent ILO report estimated that 2 million occupational fatalities occur across the world every year (ILO, 2003b), the highest proportions of these deaths being caused by work-related cancers, circulatory and cerebrovascular diseases, and some communicable diseases. The overall annual rate of occupational accidents, fatal and non-fatal, is estimated at 270 million. Some 160 million workers suffer from work-related diseases and about two-thirds of those are away from work for four working days or longer as a result. After work-related cancers, circulatory diseases and certain communicable diseases, accidental occupational injuries are the fourth main cause of work related fatalities.

Some vulnerable groups seem to be particularly at health risk :

2.4.1 *Women*

The special position of women workers needs attention. The gender division of labour has an impact on women's safety and health in the workplace, which goes well beyond reproductive hazards. As one union points out: Health and Safety is male dominated. 86 per cent of Health and Safety Inspectors are male. Resources are traditionally invested far more on "male" industries, rather than areas of industry where women work. Safety standards are based on the model of a male worker. Tasks and equipment are designed for male body size and shape. This can lead to discrimination in a number of areas (GMB, 1998). According to a report by The National Institute for Occupational Safety and Health (NIOSH), homicide is the leading cause of injury death for women in the workplace. Homicide accounts for 40 per cent of all workplace death among female workers. Workplace homicides are primarily robbery-related, and often occur in grocery/convenience stores, eating and drinking establishments, and gasoline service stations. Female workers are also at risk for non-fatal violence. Women were the victims in nearly two-thirds of the injuries resulting from workplace assaults. Most of these assaults (70%) were directed at women employed in service occupations, such as healthcare, while an additional 20 per cent of these incidents occurred in retail locations, such as restaurants and grocery stores (www.cdc.gov/niosh/docs). Women reproductive health is generally ignored by various organizations. Very few women represent the higher levels in any organization this leads to lack of understanding and empathetic view of policy makers. The policies made by governments or private organizations either lack or are ignored especially during pregnancy or post-partum period. The organizations also do not consider importance of paid maternity leaves, dedicated rooms for breastfeeding, creche facilities on the campus, and right up to a true women's cell to help deal with women's health issues.

2.4.2 *Home-Based Workers*

There are many home-based workers, in both developed and developing countries. Some countries regard them as ordinary employees, subject to normal safety and health legislation. In other countries, they are not included in legislation. But countries that ratify the Home Work Convention, 1996 (No. 177), must ensure protection in the field of occupational safety and health equal to that enjoyed by other workers. Prolonged sitting or poor ergonomics can lead to back pain, neck strain, eye strain, and repetitive strain injuries, like carpal tunnel syndrome. They can also experience isolation, lack of social interaction, and blurred boundaries between work and personal life can contribute to stress, anxiety, depression, and feelings of loneliness. Working from home often involves less physical activity and more prolonged sitting, which can increase the risk of obesity, cardiovascular diseases, and metabolic disorders. The convenience of working from home can lead to unhealthy eating habits, such as snacking on unhealthy food or irregular meal times. Irregular work hours, excessive screen time, and stress can disrupt sleep patterns, leading to insomnia or poor quality sleep. Constant exposure to screens, improper lighting, and inadequate breaks can cause eye strain, dry eyes, and other vision-related issues. There can be difficulty in setting boundaries between work and personal life which can result in increased stress, burnout, and difficulties in maintaining healthy relationships.

2.4.3 *Part-time Workers*

They are another group who may suffer from not being covered by safety and health provisions. They do not get benefits like the regular workers.

Part-time work may offer less stable income and limited job benefits, leading to financial stress and difficulties in accessing healthcare services. This can have negative impacts on health outcomes and increase the risk of chronic conditions. Part-time workers may struggle with balancing work and personal responsibilities, which can contribute to increased stress levels and adverse health effects. Research has shown a link between part-time work and higher levels of psychological distress, including symptoms of anxiety and depression. Lack of job security and inconsistent work schedules may contribute to these challenges. Part-time and contingent workers may be at higher risk of workplace accidents and occupational hazards due to less comprehensive training and safety protocols. Many health promotion initiatives, such as wellness programmes, are typically targeted towards full-time employees. Part-time workers may have limited access to these resources, potentially impacting their health behaviour and outcomes. This is why the Part-Time Work Convention, 1994 (No. 175), stipulates that "measures shall be taken to ensure that part-time workers receive the same protection as that accorded to comparable full-time workers in respect of: ... (b) occupational safety and health." Part-time workers often face challenges in accessing employer-sponsored health insurance benefits, as many policies require a minimum number of hours worked. This can result in inadequate healthcare coverage and limited access to necessary medical services.

2.4.4 *Migrant Workers*

In 2000, economically active migrants were estimated to number some 81 million. For many of them, working conditions are abusive and exploitative: forced labour, low wages, poor working environment, a virtual absence of social protection, the denial of freedom of association and union rights, discrimination, xenophobia and social exclusion all rob workers of the potential benefits of working in another country (ILO, 2004). The safety and health risks associated with such conditions are compounded by the kinds of work that most migrants do, namely hazardous and risky jobs, particularly in agriculture and construction.

In Europe, occupational accident rates are about twice as high for migrant workers as for native workers, and there is no reason to believe that the situation is not different in other parts of the world. Language barriers, exposure to new technology, family disruption, poor access to healthcare, stress and violence are some of the specific problems faced by migrant workers that make them particularly vulnerable to safety and health risks at the workplace.

According to IMO, migrants' health vulnerabilities can occur throughout the migration cycle. The conditions in which they travel, restricted access to health services upon arriving to destination country, exploitation, poor living and working conditions, discrimination, the geographical distance from their families and support system, are some of the aspects of the migration process that can impact the health of labour migrants and lead to the deterioration of their health status. Many migrant workers are employed in high risk and hazardous sectors such as mining, and construction. These kinds of jobs usually involve long hours and hard physical labour, which can result in increased occupational accidents. A study conducted among Nepalese migrant workers in Malaysia, Qatar and Saudi Arabia reported poor health and safety regulations, intense productivity pressure and risky practices, such as working without safety equipment. These have led to severe injuries including lost fingers and permanent disabilities (Adhikary *et al.*, 2019). Migrant those are in an irregular migration status endure dangerous working conditions and fear drawing attention to them and losing their jobs, or being deported. Furthermore, migrant workers are often not allowed to form and join trade unions, which may be an additional obstacle to raising concerns about their health and safety in the workplace. In addition, sexual exploitation has been widely reported in particular in the context of female labour migrants working in informal sector, such as domestic work (www.iom.int/health-labour-migrants). Male migrant workers stay at a higher risk of occupational injuries, mainly because of their employment in high-risk industries, such as mining and construction. For example, a study in Saudi Arabia comparing occupational injuries among insured Saudi Arabian labourers with those among insured migrant labourers, using data from a health insurance database, concluded that 93.5 per cent of the injured were migrant workers and only 6.5 per cent were from the host population (Abbas *et al.*, 2018). While in European Union, the most commonly reported work-related health problems among refugee and migrant workers relate to musculoskeletal, respiratory and mental health. Migrant workers also feel stressed due to mental harassment as well as unusual working conditions (Simon *et al.*, 2015). In a study conducted in Sweden, migrants who were temporarily employed were at increased risk of psychological distress compared with those who had permanent jobs or were self-employed (Sidorchuk *et al.*, 2016). Geography and type of employment often influence, and can increase, the risk of malaria for refugee and migrant populations (Canavati, S. *et al.*, 2016; WHO, 2017; Tatem *et al.*, 2017). In the Greater Mekong subregion of South-east Asia, migrants employed as rubber tappers, forest workers, miners, military personnel and farmers often work near border regions and forest fringe areas that are highly receptive to malaria, such as the Thailand-Myanmar border. Similarly, throughout the regions, refugees and migrants consistently have a higher prevalence of hepatitis than their host country counterparts. In the WHO African Region and WHO Region of the Americas, cholera and diarrhoeal diseases affect refugee and migrant groups, with a particularly high prevalence reported in children under 5 years of age: for example, children in refugee camps in Kenya who are younger than 5 years were reported as having a risk of cholera that was 51 per cent higher than for children aged 5 years and older (Kisera *et al.*, 2020).

Climate change and the increased number of conflicts mean increasing numbers of people are on the move. The impact of anthropogenic climate change is already felt across 80 per cent of the world's land area, which holds 85 per cent of the world's population. It is predicted that over 200 million additional people will be forced to move by 2050 (WHO, 2020).

2.4.5 *Workers in the Informal Economy*

Informal workers are much more likely than formal workers to be exposed to poor working environments, low safety and health standards, and environmental hazards, and to suffer poor health or injury as a result. Most informal workers have little or no knowledge of the risks they face and how to avoid them. The very nature of the informal economy makes it almost impossible for governments to collect the vital statistics needed to take appropriate remedial action, and, since much informal work takes place in homes, inspectorates cannot investigate working conditions or get information and advice to the people who need it. High exposure to risks combined with low coverage of social protection place most informal economy workers in a very vulnerable situation.... Vulnerability to diseases and poor health therefore result from a combination of undesirable living and working conditions. It is well established that gender inequality is more prevalent in the informal economy, where women are concentrated in the lower end and earn significantly less than men. It is also in the informal economy that child labour and bonded labour are most prevalent and most difficult to address (www.ilo.org).

The extension of fundamental rights and social protection to workers in the informal economy has been a major concern for the ILO in recent years. Following the preparation of a report on the subject (ILO, 2002a), a general discussion was held at the 90th Session of the ILC in 2002, which resulted in the adoption of a resolution (ILO, 2002b) and a basis for a future plan of action.

In India, nearly two-thirds of the contribution to the net domestic product is by the unorganized sector (labour.nic.in). According to the National Sample Survey Organization (NSSO, 1999-2000), 370 million workers constituted 92 per cent of the total unorganized workforce in the country (labour.nic.in). The large majority of the working population in the informal sector is outside the purview of any formal health insurance cover such as Central Government Health Scheme, Employees' State Insurance Scheme etc. This raises concern with regard to the catastrophic out-of-pocket (OOP) spending especially by households in the informal sector. In the absence of an integrated public healthcare or universal social health insurance system, catastrophic OOP spending are likely to plunge a sizeable section of even the well-off to abysmal poverty levels (Krishna *et al.*, 2004; Sakthivel and Karan, 2009).

2.4.6 *Child Labour*

Many children are still involved in hazardous work, although the numbers are falling: the worldwide total was estimated at 126 million in 2004, a considerable drop from an estimated

171 million in 2000. According to UNICEF, roughly 160 million children were subjected to child labour at the beginning of 2020, with 9 million additional children at risk due to the impact of COVID-19. This accounts for nearly 1 in 10 children worldwide. These children are many times employed illegally or they do not have knowledge about their rights and health benefits or are not given the same. They go through physical and mental stress in their very tender age. Children employed on work happen to miss schools and therefore, lack basic education. Lack of education blocks their future growth too. At times there is a fear of trafficked, especially if they are migrating alone or taking irregular routes with their families. Such children are exposed to violence and sexual assault too. According to Global Estimates of Child Labour 2017, there are 73 million children involved in hazardous work that directly endangers their health and safety. Hazardous work can cause death, serious illness or injury, permanent disability or psychological damage, as a direct consequence of poor safety and health standards, exploitation or abuse (international-partnerships.ec.europa.eu).

Children can work in dangerous conditions in all sectors, including agriculture, mining, construction, manufacturing, the service industry, retail and domestic service. However, agriculture is where the highest incidence of child labourers are found (71%) and it is a sector particularly prone to dangerous conditions, especially for children (Fig. 2.2). For example, hazardous work in cotton production is among the worst forms of child labour, as children are exposed to harmful pesticides (as indicated by ILO Convention 182 on the Worst Forms of Child Labour, which was universally ratified in 2020).

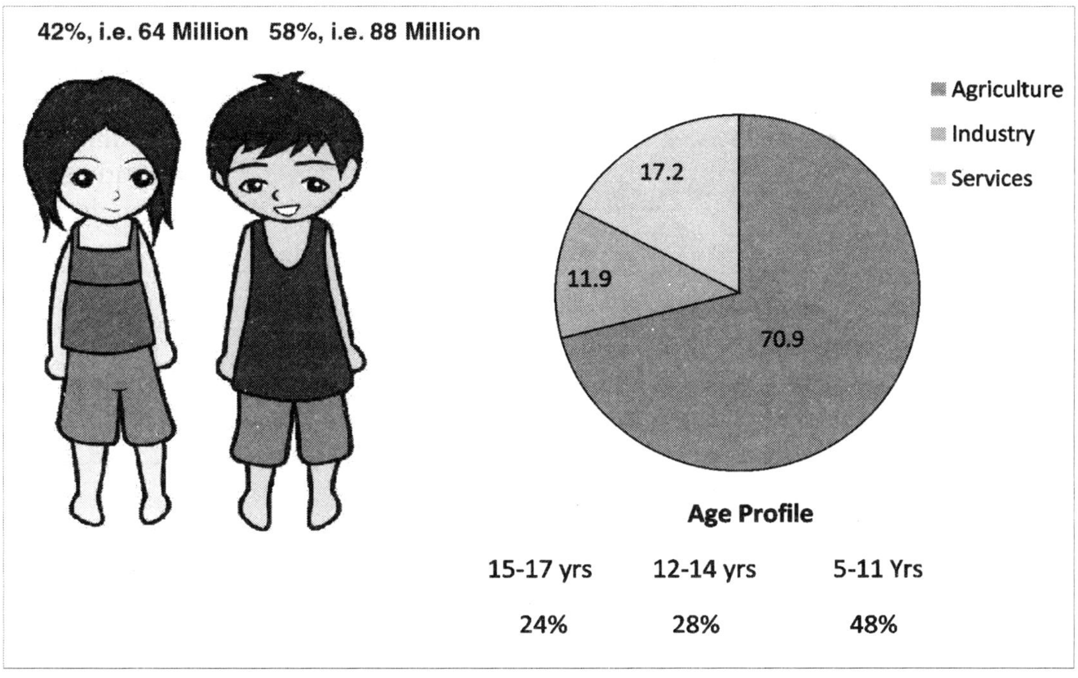

Fig. 2.2: Children employed in sectors.

Source: Author Adopted from ILO data.

2.4.7 *The Ageing Population*

According to WHO, world population aged 60+ will be around 2 billion in 2050 from 900 million in 2015. The old people of the world workforce raises many concerns, including some relating to occupational safety and health. The ILO has always been committed to the protection of ageing workers, and has been active specifically in elaborating international labour standards in invalidity, old age and survivors' insurance. But most of the time they are being neglected and do not get pay and benefits like other employees. India, the second most populous nation in the world, is also facing remarkable increase in ageing population, reportedly 8.6 per cent (104 million) of the total population in 2011 (Mini and Thankappa, 2016). This figure is expected to escalate to about 20 per cent and, in terms of absolute numbers, the country will be a home for 319 million older individuals by 2050 (UN, 2019). Soon this older population will surpass the young population below 14 years (Bose and Banerjee, 2019). Unfortunately, the majority of the Indian older population are unable to access healthcare services after the retirement age (60 years and above) due to paucity and poor coverage of universal health and pension programmes. Therefore, to manage the livelihood and healthcare needs, older people are compelled to work after the retirement age (Rajan, 2010). Census of India (2011) figures illustrate that a large proportion (33 million) of older people are working after the retirement age, especially in informal sector. However, informal sector provides financial support to only marginal level of workforce after the retirement (Reddy, 2016). Even in formal sector, nearly 10 per cent of the population engaged in selected organized workplaces receive the benefit of social or voluntary health insurance schemes (Balarajan *et al.*, 2011). The absence of proper financial and healthcare schemes can hamper the health conditions of older people indulged in economic activities. It makes older workforce as one of the most vulnerable groups in India.

Table 2.2: Type of Occupations and associated health hazards

Type of occupations/jobs	Associated prominent health hazards
Construction workers	Physical injuries from falls, electrocution, or being struck by objects, backache, spine issues, skin problems, eye problems, respiratory issues.
Miner	Exposure to harmful gases, dust, and asbestos leading to lung diseases.
Farmer	Chronic exposure to pesticides leading to respiratory and neurological issues.
Nurse	Risk of physical injuries from lifting patients and exposure to infectious diseases.
Fire fighter	Exposure to smoke and chemicals leading to respiratory issues and burns.
Welder	Inhalation of metal fumes and UV radiation leading to respiratory and eye problems.
Lab technician or scientists	Exposure to hazardous chemicals and biological agents leading to chemical poisoning or infection.
Truck driver	Risks associated with long hours of sitting, sedentary lifestyle, and road accidents, AIDS.
Soldiers	Injuries, wounds or killed, physical and psychological trauma, Post-Traumatic Stress Disorder (PTSD), Exposure to environmental hazards like extreme climates, chemical substances, and infectious diseases.
Doctors	Infectious diseases, sleep deprivation and fatigue.
Engineers	Accidental injuries, Exposure to hazardous materials leading to cancer, musculoskeletal disorders and strain injuries.
IT Professionals	Eye strain, carpal tunnel syndrome, and posture-related problems, anxiety and depression.

2.5 Socio-Cultural Factors

Individuals who hold a higher social status, such as those with higher education and income levels, may have better access to healthcare and resources that promote good health. They may also have less stress and better mental health outcomes than those with a lower social status. A healthy lifestyle refers to a series of behavioural patterns through which individuals maintain and promote good health based on certain motivations, norms, abilities, and knowledge about what constitutes healthy, stress relieving, or pleasurable behaviours (Cockerham, 2005). Culture consist of values, attitudes, habits and customs, acquired by learning which starts with the earliest experiences of childhood, much of which is not deliberately taught by anyone and which so thoroughly internalized that it is unconscious but 'goes deep' (Cassel, 1957). Socio-cultural factors can have a significant impact on an individual's health, as it influences the quality and access to various resources and opportunities that can affect a person's overall well-being. The following are some ways in which social status can influence an individual's health:

2.5.1 *Dietary Habits and Preferences*

Cultural dietary preferences can impact health outcomes. The relationship between ethnicity and nutrition may be of evolutionary significance. Food beliefs may have beneficial or detrimental effects on health status. The study of acculturating populations may elucidate the pathogenesis of nutrition-related chronic diseases (Reddy and Anitha, 2015). For instance, in regions where traditional diets consist of whole foods, vegetables, and lean proteins, such as the Mediterranean diet, individuals may have lower rates of obesity, heart disease, and certain cancers. Conversely, regions with diets high in processed foods and sugary beverages may experience higher rates of obesity, diabetes, and related health issues. The traditional Japanese diet, also known as Washoku, consists of fish, seafood, rice, vegetables, soy products (tofu, miso), and green tea. This diet is associated with a low prevalence of obesity, cardiovascular diseases, and certain types of cancer, likely due to its low saturated fat and high nutrient content. Similarly, in Islamic dietary laws, known as *Halal*, prescribe specific guidelines for food consumption. Muslims are encouraged to avoid pork and alcohol and to consume meat that adheres to specific slaughtering practices. It is believed in their culture that observing *Halal* principles can promote food safety, cleanliness, and mindfulness in food consumption. In India, Ayurvedic principles of diet emphasize balance and individualization in food choices. This traditional Indian diet focuses on seasonal, vegetarian dishes with herbal spices such as turmeric, ginger, and cumin. It aims to maintain physical and mental well-being by considering an individual's body type or *doshas*. Ayurvedic principles have been associated with improved digestion, reduced inflammation, and overall health.

2.5.2 *Beliefs and Cultural Practices*

Cultural beliefs and practices can influence health behaviours and decision-making. For example, in some regions, beliefs about traditional medicine can affect individuals' adherence to modern medical treatments. Many cultures have traditional healing practices that differ from conventional Western medicine. Researchers have investigated the impact of these practices on physical health outcomes. A study published in *Evidence-Based Complementary and Alternative Medicine* examined the effectiveness of traditional Tibetan medicine in treating chronic diseases.

Pregnant women in many Asian cultures are advised that if they eat blackberries their baby will have black spots, or that if they eat a twin banana they will give birth to twins. Such ethnocentric beliefs have their foundation in folklore and traditional practices. The Vietnamese traditionally believe that disease is caused by an imbalance of the humoral forces of *yin* and *yang*. When ill, Vietnamese commonly use herbal medicines and a set of indigenous folk practices referred to as "southern medicine" in an effort to restore the *yin/yang* balance. These practices, from the Western viewpoint, were once thought to pose barriers to health (encyclopedia.com). The findings suggested potential benefits for conditions such as cardiovascular disease and diabetes. In some communities, cultural norms related to body image may contribute to eating disorders or disordered eating behaviours. Numerous studies have explored the link between religious or spiritual beliefs and mental health outcomes. For example, a study published in the *Journal of Clinical Psychology* showed that individuals with higher levels of religious beliefs and practices had lower levels of depression and anxiety. Similarly, other studies have found that spiritual practices can contribute to better coping mechanisms, resilience, and improved overall well-being. In a study published in *PubMed* journal in 2008, it was found that the Arab Muslim population is one of the dramatically increasing minorities in the United States. In addition to other factors, religion and cultural background influence individuals' beliefs, behaviours, and attitudes towards health and illness. The author describes health beliefs and practices of the Arab Muslim population in the United States. That population is at an increased risk for several diseases and faces many barriers to accessing the American healthcare system. Some barriers, such as modesty, gender preference in healthcare providers, and illness causation misconceptions, arise out of their cultural beliefs and practices. Other barriers are related to the complexity of the healthcare system and the lack of culturally competent services within it (Yosef, 2008). Cultural practices can also impact exposure to environmental risks. For example, in regions where indoor air pollution from traditional cooking methods is prevalent, such as parts of Asia and Africa, respiratory diseases can be more common. Similarly, high risk of thigh and abdomen cacer is detected in Kashmir because people use *Kangri* (a pot containing burning coal) to keep themselves warm. The habit of smoking is well associated with oral cancer etc.

2.5.3 *Gender Roles*

Cultural expectations around gender roles can impact health outcomes. In many parts of the world, women face barriers to accessing healthcare due to cultural norms and restrictions. This can lead to delayed diagnosis, inadequate preventive care, and higher maternal mortality rates. According to WHO, Harmful gender norms—especially those related to rigid notions of masculinity—can also affect boys and men's health and well-being negatively. For example, specific notions of masculinity may encourage boys and men to smoke, take sexual and other health risks, misuse alcohol and not seek help or healthcare. Such gender norms also contribute to boys and men perpetrating violence—as well as being subjected to violence themselves. They can also have grave implications for their mental health (www.who.int). According to National AIDS Control Organization (NACO), the trans community is at an increased risk of mental health issues due to transphobia, discrimination and violence.

2.5.4 *Social Support System*

Cultural norms around family and community can influence social support systems, which are vital for mental health and well-being. In some cultures where strong family ties are emphasized, individuals may have access to a strong support network, reducing stress and improving overall health. On the other hand, in cultures where seeking help for mental health issues is stigmatized, individuals may suffer in silence. Research has also demonstrated the link between social relationships and many different aspects of health and wellness (APA, 2023). Poor social support has been linked to depression and loneliness and has been shown to alter brain function and increase the risk of alcohol use, cardiovascular disease, depression or suicide. On the other hand, if social support system is good it can help people to manage mental stress at the time of crisis.

People with high social status often have access to strong social networks that provide emotional and practical support, which helps to improve their overall health. An individual with a low social status may lack support structures, increasing their risk of experiencing feelings of social isolation and depression.

2.5.5 *Discrimination and Social Inequalities*

Discrimination or mistreatment based on religious, racial, or sexual orientation leads to poor mental health and increases the risk of premature mortality. LGBTQ+ individuals are at higher risk of depression, anxiety, and substance use disorders in insecure environments where they face stigma even in accessing healthcare services. Discrimination can also influence individuals' health indirectly, even when they are unaware that it has happened. Discrimination due to race, gender, gender identity, and sexual orientation determine access to healthcare and the social determinants of health, including contact with the criminal justice system. While loss of jobs, financial stress, and loss of a loved one to death or incarceration are all stressors any individual may face, they are experienced earlier and at higher rate for populations experiencing discrimination. Reduced access to health and social resources also affects the families of individuals being discriminated against (Davis, 2020). Trauma-related symptomology such as hypervigilance is also associated with discrimination related to race, transgender status, and sexual orientation. Hypervigilance, or a heightened awareness and anticipation of protecting oneself against additional trauma, is a key feature of post-traumatic stress disorders and is one of the proposed pathways through which trauma leads to poor cardiovascular and metabolic health, substance abuse, and sleep disturbances (Davis, 2020). Discriminatory attitude of a society can lead to lack of access to health services for many. It can also lead to discrimantory violence which can lead to injury and death.

Social cultural factors play a critical role in shaping an individual's physical and mental health condition. Educational opportunities, income and job security, reliable social networks, and freedom from discrimination are various indicators of a high social status that enable better health and well-being.

2.6 Demographic Factors

Demography is the scientific study of the profile and habits of populations, e.g. their age, gender, fertility, mortality and migration patterns. Demography of a place depends upon mortality, fertility and migration. Basic understanding of demography is essential for public health practitioners because the health of communities and individuals depends on the dynamic relationship between the numbers of people, the space which they occupy and the skills they have acquired (Badrinath and Gillam, 2012).

2.6.1 *Age*

Age is a significant factor in human health, as older adults are more vulnerable to several illnesses and disabilities. According to the World Health Organization, the leading causes of death globally in 2019 are, by and large, age-related diseases. It was found that worldwide, people aged 60 years and above accounted for 46 per cent of COVID-19 deaths (March 2021). The incidence of cancer increases significantly with age. Globally, cancer is the second leading cause of death in people aged 70-74 years (WHO). According to the CDC, the mortality rate from heart disease increased with age. Older adults are at a higher risk of experiencing falls, which can cause severe injuries.

2.6.1.1 *Children*

- **Infant Mortality:** Children under the age of one are particularly vulnerable, with infant mortality rates varying widely globally. According to the WHO, in 2019, 38.9 per cent of all under-five deaths occurred in the neonatal period (the first 28 days of life), and 75 per cent of these deaths occurred during the first week of life.
- **Malnutrition:** Globally, malnutrition is a significant health challenge for children, leading to impaired physical and cognitive development. According to UNICEF, in 2020, over 149 million children under the age of five were stunted (too short for their age) due to malnutrition.
- **Infectious Diseases:** Children's immune systems are still developing, so they are more vulnerable to infectious diseases like diarrhoea, pneumonia, and measles. According to the WHO, in 2019, diarrhoea and pneumonia remain the leading causes of death in children under 5 years old globally.
- **Mental Health:** Children can be vulnerable to mental health challenges like anxiety and depression. According to a 2021 study by the WHO, at least one in seven children aged 2-9 years have experienced mental health difficulties.
- **New Threats to Children:** According to WHO, children are vulnerable to adverse health effects from indoor and outdoor air pollution which causes an estimated 7 million deaths per year (2016). Over 250 million children are at risk of not meeting their development potential (2017). There are 124 million children and adolescents affected by obesity (2016).

2.6.1.2 *Older Adults*

At the biological level, ageing results from the impact of the accumulation of a wide variety of molecular and cellular damage over time. This leads to a gradual decrease in physical and mental capacity, a growing risk of disease and ultimately death. These changes are neither linear nor consistent, and they are only loosely associated with a person's age in years. The diversity seen in older age is not random (www.who.int).

- **Chronic Diseases:** Older adults are more prone to chronic conditions such as heart disease, cancer, and diabetes. According to the CDC, about 80 per cent of older adults have at least one chronic condition, and 68 per cent have two or more.

- **Falls and Injuries:** Falls are a significant health challenge for older adults, leading to injuries and loss of independence. According to the CDC, 1 in 4 Americans aged 65+ falls each year, and falls are the leading cause of fatal and non-fatal injuries among older Americans.
- **Dementia:** Dementia and Alzheimer's disease are significant health challenges among older adults, causing memory loss and cognitive decline. According to the World Alzheimer Report, 2019, about 50 million people globally are living with dementia, and this number is expected to triple by 2050.

Both children and older adults are more prone to certain health challenges, which can have significant consequences for their quality of life and well-being. It is essential to address these issues through targeted public health initiatives, including preventative measures such as vaccines and lifestyle interventions, to improve the health outcomes for these age groups.

2.6.2 *Gender*

Gender differences are evident when it comes to human health. Here are some examples that show how gender impacts health:

2.6.2.1 *Female Health*

Globally, women have a higher life expectancy than men. According to WHO, women live about six to eight years longer than men on average. Women are at higher risk of developing autoimmune diseases, such as lupus and rheumatoid arthritis. Females of different age groups face various health issues. Here are some examples, along with data, that illustrate the major health issues linked to females across different age groups.

- **Adolescent Women:** *Reproductive health:* Adolescent females often face reproductive health challenges such as unplanned pregnancies and sexually transmitted infections (STIs). According to the WHO, an estimated 12 million adolescent females are infected with an STI annually.
- **Mental Health:** Adolescent females are more prone to mental health issues, including depressions and anxiety, with suicide becoming one of the leading causes of death among adolescents globally. According to the CDC, in 2020, suicide was the second leading cause of death among females aged 15-24 in the US.
- **Eating Disorders:** Adolescent females are more prone to eating disorders such as anorexia and bulimia. According to the National Eating Disorders Association, an estimated 10 million females in the US will develop an eating disorder at some point in their lives.
- **Reproductive Age Women:** *Reproductive health*: Reproductive-age females often face challenges related to reproductive health such as infertility, miscarriages, and complications during pregnancy and childbirth. According to the WHO, approximately 830 women die from preventable causes related to pregnancy and childbirth everyday globally. Polycystic Ovary Syndrome/disease (PCOS) is a problem with hormones that happens during the reproductive years. PCOS affects around 8-13 per cent of reproductive aged women and up to 70 per cent of affected women remain undiagnosed. PCOS is associated with many physical and mental issues with women.

- **Breast Cancer:** Breast cancer is the leading cause of cancer-related deaths in females globally. According to the WHO, an estimated 6,27,000 women died from breast cancer in 2018, with 2.3 million new cases diagnosed.
- **Middle-aged Women:**
  Cardiovascular Disease: Cardiovascular disease (CVD) is an increasing health concern for middle-aged females, with risk factors such as high blood pressure, obesity, and lack of physical activity. According to the American Heart Association, heart disease kills approximately one woman every minute in the US.
  Menopause: Menopause transition, which usually occurs between the ages of 45-55 years, can cause various symptoms such as hot flashes, mood swings, and insomnia. According to the North American Menopause Society, approximately 6,000 women in the US reach menopause daily.
- **Older Women:**
  Osteoporosis: Older females are more prone to osteoporosis, a bone disease that increases the risk of fractures. According to the International Osteoporosis Foundation, 1 in 3 women worldwide over the age of 50 will experience osteoporotic fractures.
  Dementia: Dementia and Alzheimer's disease are growing health concerns for older females, with females making up the majority of the 50 million people worldwide living with dementia. According to the Alzheimer's Association, about two-thirds of Americans with Alzheimer's disease are female.
  Women of different age groups face diverse health challenges that require targeted prevention, diagnosis, and treatment approaches. Raising awareness, promoting healthy lifestyles, and strengthening health systems are essential to improving females' health outcomes across different age groups.

2.6.2.2 *Male Health*

Men are more prone to mental health disorders such as depression and anxiety. Men are generally more likely to engage in risky behaviours—such as smoking, excessive alcohol consumption, and drug use—than women, leading to significant health complications.

Males of different age groups face various health issues. Here are some examples along with data that illustrate the major health issues linked to males across different age groups.

(a) Adolescents

- **Substance Abuse:** Adolescent males are more prone to substance abuse, including alcohol and drug use, leading to a higher risk of injuries and accidents. According to the CDC, in 2020, 14.1 per cent of males aged 12-17 reported using an illicit drug in the past month.
- **Mental Health:** Adolescent males are also more likely to experience mental health challenges such as depression and anxiety, with suicide being the third leading cause of death among males aged 15-24 years in the US. According to the CDC, in 2020, suicide was the second leading cause of death among males aged 15-24 in the US.
- **Violence:** Adolescent males are more likely to engage in violent behaviour and become victims of violent crimes. According to the Bureau of Justice Statistics, males aged 18-24 are most likely to be victims of violent crime in the US.

(b) Reproductive Age Men

- **Reproductive Health:** Reproductive-age males face health challenges such as infertility, sexually transmitted infections, and prostate cancer. According to the American Cancer Society, prostate cancer is the most common non-skin cancer among males in the US, with an estimated 2,48,530 new cases diagnosed in 2021.
- **Cardiovascular Disease:** Cardiovascular disease (CVD) is a leading cause of death among middle-aged males, with risk factors such as high blood pressure, smoking, and diabetes. According to the American Heart Association, CVD is responsible for one in three deaths among males in the US.

(c) Middle-aged Men

- **Mental Health:** Middle-aged males are often reluctant to seek help for mental health issues, increasing their risk of suicide. According to the National Institute of Mental Health, in 2020, suicide was the seventh leading cause of death among males aged 45-54 in the US.
- **Cancer:** Middle-aged males are prone to various cancers such as lung, colon, and prostate cancer. According to the American Cancer Society, an estimated 3,17,760 new cases of lung cancer will be diagnosed among men in 2021 in the US.

(d) Older Men

- **Osteoporosis:** Older males are more prone to osteoporosis, leading to a higher risk of fractures. According to the International Osteoporosis Foundation, 1 in 5 men worldwide over the age of 50 will experience osteoporotic fractures.
- **Dementia:** Dementia and Alzheimer's disease are growing health concerns for older males, with males making up about one-third of the 50 million people worldwide living with dementia. According to the Alzheimer's Association, about one in ten Americans aged 65 and older has Alzheimer's disease.

Overall, males of different age groups face diverse health challenges that require targeted prevention, diagnosis, and treatment approaches. It is essential to raise awareness, promote healthy lifestyles, and strengthen health systems to improve males' health outcomes across different age groups.

Thus, age and gender are significant drivers of human health, with various factors such as lifestyle, biology, environmental exposure, and access to healthcare services impacting an individual's health. It is essential to consider demographic factors when designing health policies and interventions to better address the specific needs of different age and gender groups.

2.6.3 *Density of Population*

Population density refers to number of people per square area. The density of population can significantly impact health issues, as it affects the spread of infectious diseases, access to healthcare services, and availability of environmental resources. Both density of population and proximity to man-made activities, as well as the natural environment, concentrate risk for humans (Fitzpatrick and LaGory, 2011). Population density is, therefore, a measure of "the degree of pressure on natural resources" as well as an indicator reflecting the level of human activity within a specific bounded landscape (Agovino *et al.,* 2018). Exposure to contaminants from soil, water or air coupled with social or economic vulnerability and population density may increase potential harm to health at a subclinical or clinical level (Carnegie, 2022).

2.6.3.1 *Infectious Diseases*

Higher population density can lead to an increased risk of infectious diseases as it increases person-to-person contact, making it easier for infections to spread. For instance, in 2020, the COVID-19 pandemic hit several large urban areas with a high population density the hardest, such as New York City. Influenza outbreaks are more frequent and severe in high-density cities, with higher case fatality rate (CFR) in urban areas versus rural areas. There are many examples of how the density of population can impact the spread of infectious diseases, for example, the COVID-19 pandemic is an ongoing example of how a highly infectious disease can spread rapidly throughout densely populated areas. The nature of the virus' transmission through respiratory droplets, along with high population density, has increased the risk of transmission in several urban communities. For instance, densely populated New York City was an early epicenter of the COVID-19 pandemic in the United States. According to NYDH "More populous counties in New York State consistently showed higher levels of COVID-19 diagnoses and hospitalizations." Tuberculosis (TB) is another example of a highly infectious disease that can spread quickly in densely populated areas, especially in cities. People living in crowded conditions, such as prisons, slums, and migrant worker communities, are at higher risk of TB infection. For example, in Mumbai, India, where the population density is high, TB is a significant concern. According to a 2016 study, Mumbai accounts for 25 per cent of all TB cases in the country, the majority of which are found in slum areas where overcrowding and poor living conditions increase the risk of transmission.

In both of these infectious diseases examples, high population density creates ideal conditions for the spread of infections. Efforts to control the spread of these diseases must consider the density of the population and other factors that increase the risk of transmission. Campaigns to increase public awareness of the dangers of infectious diseases and promoting personal hygiene such as mask-wearing, regularly washing hands, and social distancing can make a significant difference in controlling the spread of infectious diseases.

2.6.3.2 *Non-communicable Diseases*

Non-communicable diseases do not spread like communicable ones. But in areas with high density there is pressure on natural and man-made resources, employment opportunities, educational competencies etc. All these factors influence decisions of individuals. High competition means more hardwork and sometimes more hours of working. It also means poor dietary habits and lack of exercise. This is the reason of developing more non-communicable or lifestyle diseases in most dense areas. On the other hand, a high population density is synonymous with mixed landuse, high street connectivity, and short distances to destinations and transit (Sarkar *et al.*, 2017; Yin *et al.*, 2020). People living in neighbourhoods with higher population densities usually travel by active modes and have higher levels of physical activity, resulting in a lower likelihood of obesity and a higher level of health (Stevenson *et al.*, 2016). This argument is supported by many studies conducted in developed countries (Lopez, 2007; Pouliou and Elliott, 2010). Therefore, policymakers and planners in developed countries recommend densification to shape healthy cities and improve people's health (Stevenson *et al.*, 2016). However, a high population density is also related to impoverished areas, congestion, and air pollution (Frank and Engelke, 2005), which are the main causes of obesity and other diseases. There are several gaps in the literature on the relationship between population density and health. First, major studies are based on low-density contexts (e.g. North America), lacking evidence from high-density contexts, particularly from China as a whole (Sun and Yin, 2018). Second, most studies assume that the association between population density and health is linearity instead of non-linearity, which may not fit the real world situation (Galster, 2018). Third, many studies are cross-sectional and thus fail to identify causal relationships (Feng *et al.*, 2010).

2.6.3.3 *Access to Healthcare Services*

High population density areas can be associated with inadequate healthcare services. As more people living in a single geographic area are in need of medical services, access to healthcare services may be limited due to an insufficient number of medical professionals or facilities, leading to overcrowded emergency departments, hospitals, and limited resources allocated to primary care. For example, a 2018 study showed that people residing in rural and less densely populated areas of the United States had worse healthcare access and outcomes compared to their counterparts in high-density urban areas. Climate refugees displaced in densely populated urban settings, such as people who have been forced to migrate because of environmental challenges, also face barriers to accessing healthcare and other basic necessities.

Access to quality healthcare services is a significant challenge for many people in high-density regions of Africa. One example of poor healthcare services in high-density regions of Africa is the limited number of hospitals and medical facilities. The few available medical facilities are often overcrowded, understaffed, and ill-equipped to handle the large patient populations. Additionally, healthcare services are often located far away from residential areas, making access to health services for routine check-ups or emergency care challenging. Another issue is the high cost of medical care, which is often unaffordable for the majority of the population. This situation forces many people to rely on traditional healers and other informal healthcare providers, increasing the risk of misdiagnosis, delayed treatment, and complications. The high population density also contributes to the spread of infectious diseases, a persistent health problem in many African countries. The lack of basic hygiene and sanitation in public spaces, such as market places, streets, and water sources, increases the risk of transmission of infectious diseases such as malaria, cholera, and typhoid. Furthermore, healthcare workers are scarce, making it challenging to provide sufficient healthcare to the population. Many qualified and skilled healthcare professionals leave the continent for better opportunities and working conditions, leaving behind a limited number of healthcare workers.

2.6.3.4 *Environmental Challenges*

High population density can lead to environmental issues such as air pollution, water pollution, and poor living conditions, all affecting chronic diseases such as asthma, cancer, and heart and lung diseases. For instance, in 2019, a study by WHO revealed that 91 per cent of the global population lived in areas where air pollution levels were higher than deemed safe by the organization's guidelines. This problem is particularly acute in densely populated urban areas, where pollution is concentrated. While many enthusiasts for centralisation and urbanisation argue this allows for resources to be used more efficiently, in developing countries this mass movement of people heading towards the cities in search of employment and opportunity often outstrips the pace of development, leading to slums, poor (if any) environmental regulation, and higher levels of centralised pollution. Even in developed nations, more people are moving to the cities than ever before. The pressure placed on growing cities and their resources such as water, energy and food due to continuing growth includes pollution from additional cars, heaters and other modern luxuries, which can cause a range of localised environmental problems (Rover and Butler, 2023).

The problems in densely populated areas are waste disposal, sanitation facilities, air pollution, water pollution etc. Several studies show that these environmental challenges pose serious health issues. For example, The Impact of Population Density on a City's Environmental Sustainability by Cervero and Kockelman (1997) explores the relationship between population density and environmental sustainability using data from various cities. It examines how increased density affects transportation, landuse, and resource consumption. Sun and Liu study on "The Relationship between Population Density and Air Pollution in U.S. Cities" analyze the connection between population density and air pollution levels across different cities in the United States. It highlights how higher population density can lead to increased emissions, air pollution, and associated health hazards. In light of this, public health strategies must take into account population density and its impact on health, including proper planning of healthcare resources, efforts to increase access to health services, and improved environmental strategies to combat negative health outcomes.

2.7 Genetic Factors

Although there are many possible causes of human disease, family history is often one of the strongest risk factors for common disease complexes such as cancer, cardiovascular disease (CVD), diabetes, autoimmune disorders, and psychiatric illnesses. A person inherits a complete set of genes from each parent, as well as a vast array of cultural and socio-economic experiences from his/her family. Family history is thought to be a good predictor of an individual's disease risk because family members most closely represent the unique genomic and environmental interactions that an individual experiences (Kardia *et al.*, 2003). Genetic factors play a crucial role in many health issues and diseases.

2.7.1 *Genetic Disorders*

Harmful change to a gene or mutation in genes from one generation to another can cause genetic disorders. Genetic disorders can be:

- **Chromosomal:** This type affects the structures that hold your genes/DNA within each cell (chromosomes). With these conditions, people are missing or have duplicated chromosome material. Down syndrome (associated with developmental delays, mild to moderate intellectual disability, and characteristic physical features), Prader-Willi syndrome (loss of function of specific genes on chromosome 15. In newborns, symptoms include weak muscles, poor feeding, and slow development), Williams syndrome (affects many parts of the body. Facial features frequently include a broad forehead, underdeveloped chin, short nose, and full cheeks), Angelman syndrome (affects the nervous system, symptoms include a small head and a specific facial appearance, severe intellectual disability, developmental disability, limited to no functional speech, balance and movement problems, seizures, and sleep problems) etc.

- **Complex (Multifactorial):** These disorders stem from a combination of gene mutations and other factors. Many genes and variants contribute to it. Even your environment contributes to it. Often these individual contributions are so small that they are hard for scientists to really disentangle. They include chemical exposure, diet, certain medications and tobacco or alcohol use. Some diseases caused by this are: Rheumatoid arthritis (RA), AS, multiple sclerosis, psoriasis and psoriatic arthritis, scleroderma, SLE, and type 1 diabetes mellitus (T1D).
- **Single-gene (Monogenic):** This group of conditions occurs from a single gene mutation. There are an estimated 10,000 different types of single-gene diseases (also called monogenic diseases), which are diseases caused by mutations in a single gene. The World Health Organization estimates that 10 out of every 1000 people are affected. This means that between 70 million and 80 million people in the world are living with one of these diseases (WHO, 2021; Worldometre, 2021). Achondroplasia (short limbed dwarfism), Beta Thalassemia (blood disorder), Cyst fibrosis (thick mucus that affect respiratory and reproductive system), Huntington disease (Neurological disorder) etc. are monogenic diseases.

2.7.2 *Genetic Disorders and Regions*

Some genetic disorders are prevalent primarily in some particular regions of the world. The regional presence of such disorders are discussed below:

- **Cystic Fibrosis:** This is a genetic disorder that affects the respiratory, digestive, and reproductive systems. It is caused by mutations in the CFTR gene, which regulates the flow of salt and fluids in and out of cells. This is most common in people of European ancestry, although it also occurs in other populations.
- **Huntington's Disease:** This is a neurological disorder that causes progressive degeneration of brain cells. It is caused by mutations in the HTT gene, which produces a protein called Huntington. It is most common in Europe and North America and less common in Asia.
- **Sickle Cell Anaemia:** This is an inherited blood disorder that affects the production of hemoglobin, the protein that carries oxygen in the blood. It is caused by mutations in the HBB gene, which codes for the beta-globin subunit of hemoglobin. This is most common in sub-Saharan Africa, but it also occurs in significant numbers in the Middle East, India, and parts of the Mediterranean.
- **Breast Cancer:** While most cases of breast cancer are not caused by inherited genetic mutations, some individuals may have a higher risk due to mutations in the BRCA1 or BRCA2 genes. These genes are involved in DNA repair and help prevent the development of cancer. Mutations in the BRCA1 and BRCA2 genes are most commonly found in people of Ashkenazi Jewish ancestry, but they also occur in other populations.

- **Alzheimer's Disease:** While the exact causes of Alzheimer's disease are not fully understood, genetic factors are thought to play a role. Mutations in genes such as APOE and PSEN1 have been associated with an increased risk of developing the disease. This disease is more common in Europe and North America and least common in Sub Saharan Africa.
- **Thalassemia:** Thalassemia is a blood disorder involving lower than normal amount of oxygen carrying protein. This is most common in people of Mediterranean, Middle Eastern, Asian, and African ancestry.
- **Hemochromatosis:** This is most common in people of European descent.

Table 2.3: Presence of Genetic disorders in the world

Genetic disorder based diseases	Prominent regions of their presence
Cystic Fibrosis	European descent, with the highest prevalence observed in individuals from Northern European regions.
Sickle Cell Disease	Individuals of African, Middle Eastern, Mediterranean, and Indian descent. It is more prevalent in regions with a history of malaria.
Tay-Sachs Disease	Individuals of Ashkenazi Jewish descent, with a higher prevalence in Jewish communities from Eastern Europe and the United States.
Hemochromatosis	Individuals of Northern Europe, specifically Celtic, descent. It is more prevalent in regions such as Ireland and Scotland.
Thalassemia	Individuals of Mediterranean, Middle Eastern, and South Asian descent. Regions like Italy, Greece, Cyprus, and India have a higher occurrence of this disorder.
Achondroplasia	This form of dwarfism is not limited to any specific region and can occur in all populations worldwide.
Huntington's Disease	People of European descent, with a higher occurrence in populations of Western European origin.
Sickle Cell anaemia	Most common in sub-Saharan Africa, but it also occurs in significant numbers in the Middle East, India, and parts of the Mediterranean.

Source: Created by author based on various sources of information.

More than 600 genetic disorders are treatable (Bick *et al.*, 2021). Around 1 in 50 people is affected by a known single-gene disorder, while around 1 in 263 is affected by a chromosomal disorder. Around 65 per cent of people have some kind of health problem as a result of congenital genetic mutations (Kumar *et al.*, 2001). There is a wealth of data available on the genetic factors responsible for diseases worldwide. Large-scale studies such as the Human Genome Project and the Exome Aggregation Consortium (ExAC) have generated extensive databases of genetic variants and their associations with various diseases.

2.8 Other Causes in Contemporary World (Climate Change and Food Insecurity)

2.8.1 *Climate Change and Health Issues*

In the 1970s and 1980s, the term "global warming" was commonly used to describe the trend of rising temperatures on Earth. This term focused on the increase in average temperatures as a result of burning fossil fuels and other human activities. By the 1990s, there was a growing understanding that the impacts of global warming were not limited to just rising temperatures, but also included changes in precipitation patterns, sea level rise, and more frequent extreme weather events. As a result, the term "climate change" came into use to reflect these broader impacts. In recent years, there has been a greater emphasis on the role of human activities in driving climate change. The term "anthropogenic climate change" is increasingly used to emphasize that climate change is primarily caused by human activities such as burning fossil fuels, deforestation, and agriculture.

According to NOAA (National Oceanic and Atmospheric Administration), aerosols released by volcanic eruptions, ocean currents, Earth's orbital changes, solar variations etc. are some of the natural climate change factors. Other factors that impact climate change are linked to human factors namely urbanization, industrialization, vehicular emissions, landuse change etc. Human factors are responsible for giving impetus to the natural processes, thus posing greater challenges not only to the environment but also to human health.

1. **Rising Temperatures:** According to data from NASA, the global temperature has risen by 1.18°C (2.12°F) since the late 19th century, with the majority of this increase occurring in the last few decades. 2020 tied with 2016 as the warmest year on record, and the past 10 years are the warmest decade since record-keeping began.
2. **Decreasing Arctic Sea Ice:** The Arctic sea ice extent has decreased significantly in recent years, with the minimum extent in 2020 tying for the second-lowest on record, according to the National Snow and Ice Data Centre. This loss of sea ice has significant impacts on Arctic ecosystems, as well as affecting global climate patterns.
3. **Increased Frequency of Extreme Weather Events:** There has been an increase in the frequency of extreme weather events such as heatwaves, droughts, and intense rainfall events in recent years. For example, in 2020, the US experienced 22 billion-dollar weather and climate disasters, tied with 2011 for the most such events in a single year, according to NOAA.
4. **Rising Sea Levels:** Global sea levels have risen by about 8-9 inches (21-24 cm) since 1880, according to data from NOAA. This rise is primarily due to the expansion of seawater as it warms and melting of glaciers and ice sheets. Sea level rise has significant implications for coastal regions, including increased flooding and erosion.
5. **Changes in Animal and Plant Behaviour:** Changes in climate are causing changes in the timing of seasonal events for many plant and animal species. For example, studies have shown that migratory birds are arriving earlier in the spring, and some flowers are blooming earlier. These changes have implications for ecosystems and food webs.

According to WHO, between 2030 and 2050, climate change is expected to cause approximately 2,50,000 additional deaths per year, from malnutrition, malaria, diarrhoea and heat stress. The direct damage costs to health (i.e. excluding costs in health-determining sectors such as agriculture and water and sanitation), is estimated to be between USD 2-4 billion/year by 2030 (www.who.int). Climate change causes various health issues like:

1. **Heat-related Illness and Death:** As global temperatures rise, heatwaves and extreme heat events are becoming more frequent and severe. This can lead to heat exhaustion, heatstroke, and other heat-related illnesses, which can be fatal in extreme cases. Extreme weather events, such as heat waves, hurricanes, and floods can cause a range of health problems, from dehydration and heat exhaustion to injury and illness from flooding and

evacuation. In particular, heatwaves can put vulnerable populations at risk, including the elderly, children, and those with respiratory or cardiovascular conditions. As temperatures rise, the risk of heatstroke and other heat-related illnesses increases, particularly for those who do not have access to air-conditioning.

Heat islands occur when urban areas experience higher temperatures than surrounding rural areas due to factors such as the absorption and retention of heat by buildings and pavement, lack of vegetation, and waste heat from vehicles and buildings. According to a report by the US Global Change Research Programme, urban areas will experience more extreme heat events, leading to more heat-related illnesses and deaths. In addition to higher temperatures, climate change can also bring changes in precipitation patterns, leading to drought conditions in some areas. This can increase the demand for water in urban areas, leading to more use of air conditioners, which in turn intensify heat islands. According to the National Oceanic and Atmospheric Administration (NOAA), urban areas are warming at a rate of twice that of rural areas. In some cities, heat islands can be up to 22°F hotter than surrounding areas.

The EPA has found that exposure to extreme heat can lead to serious health problems, including heat exhaustion and stroke. Climate change is expected to increase the frequency and intensity of extreme heat events, making the impacts of heat islands even more significant.

2. **Increased Air Pollution and Health Issues:** Climate change can lead to increased air pollution, as higher temperatures and changing weather patterns can worsen air quality. This can exacerbate respiratory conditions like asthma and chronic obstructive pulmonary disease (COPD). Rising temperatures lead to more smog and air pollution. Higher temperatures make it easier for pollutants to combine and form smog. Ozone and particulate matter are among the pollutants that can cause respiratory problems such as asthma. According to the National Climate Assessment, the number of days with unhealthy levels of smog in the US is projected to increase by 70 per cent by 2050. Climate change increases the risk of wildfires, which release large amounts of air pollutants including carbon monoxide, fine particulate matter, and volatile organic compounds. In 2020, the wildfires in California alone produced as much air pollution as a year's worth of car emissions.

   According to the EPA, air quality in the US has improved over the past several decades, but climate change is expected to offset these gains. Extreme heat events, for example, can increase the production of ground-level ozone, which can cause respiratory problems and worsen existing lung conditions. In 2019, the US experienced a 10 per cent increase in air pollution, which was largely due to wildfires in California and the Western US. The smoke from these fires led to a record number of unhealthy air quality days in some parts of the country. A study by the US Government Accountability Office found that climate change is expected to increase run-off of nutrients from farmland, leading to poorer water quality. This could affect the health of fish and other aquatic life, as well as drinking water supplies.
3. **Allergies and Infectious Diseases:** Changing climate conditions can also lead to increase in insect-borne diseases like dengue fever, malaria, and Lyme disease. Warmer temperatures

can also lead to longer pollen seasons, worsening allergies and asthma. Rising temperatures due to climate change can extend the pollen season, leading to longer allergy seasons for people who suffer from allergies. A study published in *The New England Journal of Medicine* found that in some US cities, the pollen season has increased by up to 27 days over the past two decades. A study published in the journal *Clinical and Experimental Allergy* found that climate change is already making pollen allergies worse in some geographic areas, and that this trend is likely to continue. By the year 2040, it is estimated that the prevalence of pollen allergies will have increased by nearly 70 per cent in some regions of the US.

Climate change can affect the distribution and abundance of vector-borne diseases such as Lyme disease, malaria, and dengue fever. Mosquitoes, ticks, and other disease-carrying insects thrive in warmer temperatures, and as these temperatures become more common, so too will the risk of disease transmission. For example, a report by the Centers for Disease Control and Prevention (CDC) found that the incidence of Lyme disease has tripled in the US over the past two decades, partly due to climate change. Climate change can exacerbate air pollution, which is a known risk factor for respiratory infections such as influenza and pneumonia. Increased exposure to air pollution due to climate change can lead to higher incidence and severity of these infections. According to the World Health Organization, the geographic range of dengue fever has expanded significantly in recent years due to climate change. The disease, which is transmitted by mosquitoes, is now found in more than 100 countries, and is responsible for an estimated 50 to 100 million infections each year.

Research conducted by the Harvard T.H. Chan School of Public Health found that even a small increase in particulate matter air pollution can lead to a significant increase in respiratory infections in children. This study highlights the importance of reducing air pollution levels to protect public health, especially in the face of ongoing climate change.

4. **Mental Health Impacts:** Climate change can have significant impacts on mental health. Extreme weather events, such as hurricanes, floods, and wildfires, can cause trauma, stress, and anxiety in affected individuals. Climate change can also lead to a loss of livelihoods and displacement, resulting in financial insecurity and social isolation. People who experience extreme weather events such as hurricanes, floods, and wildfires can experience significant trauma and stress. This can lead to anxiety, depression, and other mental health issues. For example, after Hurricane Katrina in 2005, there was a significant increase in rates of post-traumatic stress disorder (PTSD) and other mental health issues among affected populations. A report by the American Psychological Association found that extreme weather events such as hurricanes, wildfires, and floods can lead to significant mental health impacts, including depression, anxiety, and PTSD. The report calls for increased awareness of the mental health impacts of climate change and greater efforts to address mental health needs after extreme weather events.

Climate change can lead to social displacement, such as when rising sea levels force people to move to new areas. This can result in the loss of community and disconnection from social networks, which can lead to feelings of isolation and loneliness. This can have a negative impact on mental health. A study published in the journal *Global Environmental*

Change found that social displacement due to climate change can lead to a range of mental health impacts, including depression, anxiety, and PTSD. The study calls for greater attention to the mental health needs of climate refugees and others who are displaced due to climate change. A review of research on the mental health impacts of climate change found that environmental degradation and loss of species can lead to "ecological grief", which can negatively impact mental health. The review calls for greater attention to the emotional and psychological impacts of climate change as part of efforts to address the issue. As climate change leads to environmental degradation and loss of species, it can cause distress to people who care about the environment and nature. This can lead to feelings of despair, hopelessness, and grief, which can negatively impact mental health.

5. **Water-borne Diseases:** Climate change can impact the quality and availability of water, leading to an increased risk of water-borne diseases like cholera, typhoid fever, and Hepatitis A. Extreme weather events such as floods and hurricanes can lead to increased run-off of pollutants into waterways. This can cause an increase in water-borne diseases such as cholera, dysentery, and cryptosporidiosis. Following a severe flood in Pakistan in 2010, there were over 3,00,000 cases of diarrhoea reported, and over 21,000 cases of acute watery diarrhoea in Zimbabwe following Cyclone Idai in 2019. As water temperature rise due to climate change, it can affect the distribution and transmission of water-borne diseases. For example, warmer water can help pathogens such as Vibrio bacteria thrive, leading to an increase in cases of infections such as cholera. Changes in rainfall patterns due to climate change can affect the quantity and quality of water available for human use. Droughts can lead to water scarcity and increased risk of water-borne diseases due to inadequate sanitation and hygiene, while heavy rainfall events can cause sewage overflows and flooding, which in turn increases the risk of water-borne diseases.

According to the World Health Organization (WHO), climate change is expected to increase the incidence of water-borne diseases worldwide. The WHO estimates that climate change will cause an additional 2,50,000 deaths per year from malnutrition, malaria, diarrhoea, and heat stress between 2030 and 2050.

A study by the US CDC found that in the US, water-borne disease outbreaks are most commonly associated with extreme precipitation events, drought, and other severe weather events. These events can lead to the spread of diseases such as Hepatitis A, cryptosporidiosis, and giardiasis. Warmer temperatures have been linked to increase in Vibrio infections, which can cause serious illness and death. A study published in the journal *PLOS Neglected Tropical Diseases* found that the risk of Vibrio infection in the US has already increased by 74 per cent due to climate change.

2.8.2 *Food Insecurity, Nutrition and Health*

Food is the basic necessity of every human being. Nutrition is an integral part of food. Food insecurity is defined as a household-level economic and social condition of limited or uncertain access to adequate food (USDA, 2022). Food insecurity adversely affects human health, which means food security and nutrition are crucial to improving people's health outcomes. Both food insecurity and health outcomes are the policy and agenda of the 2030 Sustainable Development Goals (SDGs) (Beyene, 2023).

After remaining relatively unchanged since 2015, the prevalence of undernourishment (SDG Indicator 2.1.1) jumped from 8.0 in 2019 to around 9.3 per cent in 2020 and continued to rise in 2021. It is estimated that between 702 and 828 million people in the world (corresponding to 8.9 and 10.5 per cent of the world population, respectively) faced hunger in 2021. One in five people in Africa (20.2 per cent of the population) was facing hunger in 2021, compared to 9.1 per cent in Asia, 8.6 per cent in Latin America and the Caribbean, 5.8 per cent in Oceania, and less than 2.5 per cent in Northern America and Europe (FAO, 2022).

Food security is affected by availability, accessibility, affordability, stability of food. Poverty is a significant driver of food insecurity. Low-income households often cannot afford enough food for themselves and their families, particularly if they have other financial pressures like high rent or medical bills. People who are unemployed or underemployed often struggle to put food on the table. The lack of consistent income can make it difficult to buy enough groceries every month. Inflation is another important variable that obstruct food security. In some areas, the cost of food is simply unaffordable for many people. This can be compounded by other factors like a lack of access to transportation to get to affordable grocery stores or farmers markets. Disasters like hurricanes, droughts, and floods can destroy crops and disrupt food supply chains, leading to significant food shortages and higher prices. Ongoing conflicts in regions around the world can make access to food incredibly difficult. It can also force people to flee their homes and become refugees, further exacerbating food insecurity.

According to the Food and Agricultural Organization of the United Nations (FAO), as of 2019, an estimated 690 million people around the world were experiencing food insecurity. Additionally, a 2021 report from Feeding America found that the COVID-19 pandemic had led to a sharp increase in food insecurity in the United States, with more than 42 million people (including 13 million children) living in food-insecure households.

Food insecurity can lead to a range of health issues due to inadequate access to sufficient, nutritious food. Here are some examples of how food insecurity can impact health:

1. **Malnutrition and Deficiencies:** When individuals are food insecure, they cannot consume enough high-quality, nutrient-rich foods to meet their bodies' needs. This can lead to micronutrient deficiencies, such as low levels of iron or vitamin A, which can cause anaemia, weakened immune systems, and other health issues. Food insecure often do not have access to a variety of nutritious foods that provide the nutrients to their bodies need for proper growth and development.

   (a) *Iron Deficiency:* People who are food insecure are often unable to consume enough iron-rich foods, such as meat and leafy greens. As a result, they may develop iron-deficiency anaemia, which can cause fatigue, weakness, and impaired cognitive function.

   (b) *Vitamin A Deficiency:* Food-insecure individuals may not have access to vitamin A-rich foods, such as dark leafy greens and orange vegetables. This can lead to visual impairment, increased susceptibility to infections, and delayed growth.

   (c) *Stunted growth:* Children who experience chronic food insecurity may suffer from stunted growth due to a lack of sufficient nutrients. According to the FAO, an estimated 144 million children under the age of five around the world are stunted due to malnutrition.

(d) *Wasting:* Similarly, children who experience acute food insecurity (i.e. not having enough food for a short period of time) may experience wasting, which is characterized by severe weight loss and muscle wasting. According to the FAO, an estimated 47 million children under the age of five around the world were wasted in 2019 due to malnutrition.

(e) *Cognitive and Behavioural Issues:* Malnutrition resulting from food insecurity can also negatively impact cognitive function and behaviour. Children who experience chronic malnutrition may struggle with memory, attention, and learning, while adults may experience mental health issues such as depression and anxiety.

2. **Obesity and Other Lifestyle Diseases:** Food insecurity can also lead to overconsumption of cheap, high-calorie, low-nutrient foods, such as junk food, due to financial constraints. This can result in weight gain and an increased risk of type 2 diabetes.

   (a) *Obesity:* Food insecurity is associated with a higher risk of obesity. According to a study by the CDC, food insecurity increases the odds of being obese by 1.6 times. This is because when people do not have access to healthy foods, they often rely on cheaper, less nutritious options that can lead to weight gain. According to Feeding America, a non-profit organization that addresses food insecurity in the United States, food-insecure individuals are 50 per cent more likely to develop diabetes and twice as likely to experience depression than those who are food-secure. Additionally, malnutrition resulting from food insecurity can lead to impaired cognitive development and a reduced ability to learn and succeed in school.

   (b) *Diabetes:* Food insecurity is also linked to a higher risk of developing type 2 diabetes. A study by the American Diabetes Association found that food insecurity was associated with a 30-40 per cent increased risk of developing diabetes.

   (c) *Cardiovascular Disease:* Food insecurity is also linked to an increased risk of cardiovascular disease. A study published in the *Journal of General Internal Medicine* found that food insecurity was associated with a 2-fold increase in the risk of heart attack or stroke.

3. **Mental Health:** Food insecurity can also have negative impacts on mental health, including depression and anxiety. According to a study published in the *Journal of Hunger and Environmental Nutrition*, food insecurity is associated with a higher risk of depression and poor mental health. In a study of 47 countries, researchers found that food insecurity was associated with a higher risk of depression. People experiencing food insecurity were 1.5 times more likely to experience depression compared to those who were food secure. A global survey conducted by the World Health Organization found that food insecurity was associated with a higher risk of anxiety. People experiencing food insecurity were more likely to report feelings of anxiety compared to those who were food secure. Food insecurity was associated with a higher risk of suicidal ideation. People experiencing food insecurity were more likely to think about suicide compared to those who were food secure.

REFERENCES

Abbas, M., Kashif, M., Balkhyour, M., Ahmad, I., Asam, Z-U-Z, Saeed, R. (2018). Trends in occupational injuries and diseases among Saudi and non-Saudi insured workers. *East Mediterr Health J.*, 24(10): 1010-17. doi: 10.26719/2018.24.10.1010.

Adhikary, P., Keen, S., van Teijlingen, E. (2019). Workplace accidents among Nepali male workers in the Middle East and Malaysia: a qualitative study. *J Immigr Minor Health*, 21(5): 1115-22. doi: 10.1007/s10903-018-0801-y

Agovino, M., Aprile, M.C., Garofalo, A., Mariani, A. (2018). Cancer mortality rates and spillover effects among different areas: A case study in Campania (southern Italy) *Soc. Sci. Med.*, 204: 67-83. doi: 10.1016/j.socscimed.2018.03.027.

Ahmad, Alqassim and Maged, El-Setouhy, Impact of Poverty on Health, in *Healthcare Access—New Threats, New Approaches,* Edited by Ayse Emel Onal, IntechOpen, DOI: 10.5772/intechopen.108704

Badrinath, P., & Gillam, S. (2012). Demography. In S. Gillam, J. Yates, & P. Badrinath (Eds.), *Essential Public Health: Theory and Practice* (pp. 29-42). Cambridge: Cambridge University Press. doi: 10.1017/CBO9781139059442.007

Beyene, S.D. (2023). The impact of food insecurity on health outcomes: empirical evidence from sub-Saharan African countries. *BMC Public Health*, 23, 338. https: //doi.org/10.1186/s12889-023-15244-3

The State of Food Security and Nutrition in the World 2022 (fao.org)

Bick, David, Bick, Sarah L., Dimmock, David P., Fowler, Tom A., Caulfield, Mark J., Scott, Richard H. (March 2021). "An online compendium of treatable genetic disorders". *American Journal of Medical Genetics. Part C, Seminars in Medical Genetics,* 187 (1): 48-54. doi: 10.1002/ajmg.c.31874. ISSN 1552-4876. PMC 7986124. PMID 33350578.

Canavati, S.E., Quintero, C.E., Lawford, H.L.S., Yok, S., Lek, D., Richards, J.S. *et al.* (2016). High mobility, low access thwarts interventions among seasonal workers in the Greater Mekong Sub-region: lessons from the malaria containment project. *Malar J.*, 15(1): 434. doi: 10.1186/s12936-016-1491-3. 553

Carnegie, E.R., Inglis, G., Taylor, A., Bak-Klimek, A., Okoye, O. (2022 Feb. 24). Is Population Density Associated with Non-Communicable Disease in Western Developed Countries? A Systematic Review. *Int J Environ Res Public Health*, 19(5): 2638. doi: 10.3390/ijerph19052638. PMID: 35270337; PMCID: PMC8910328.

Chowdhury, P., Mohanty, I., Singh, A., Niyonsenga, T. (2023, Feb. 22). Informal sector employment and the health outcomes of older workers in India. *PLoS One*, 18(2): e0266576. doi: 10.1371/journal.pone.0266576. PMID: 36812213; PMCID: PMC9946227

Cockerham, W.C. (2005). Health lifestyle theory and the convergence of agency and structure. *J. Health Soc. Behav.*, 46: 51-67. doi: 10.1177/002214650504600105

Davis, B.A. (2020). *Discrimination: A Social Determinant of Health Inequities in Health Affairs,*10.1377/forefront.20200220.518458

Fealey, R.D. (2013). Interoception and autonomic nervous system reflexes thermoregulation, in: Aminoff, M.J. Boller, F. Swaab D.F., *Handbook of clinical, neurology*. Elsevier, Amsterdam, pp. 79-88.

Feng, J., Glass, T.A., Curriero, F.C. *et al.* (2010). The built environment and obesity: A systematic review of the epidemiologic evidence. *Health and Place*, 16(2): 175-190.

Fitzpatrick, K.M., LaGory, M. (2011). *Unhealthy Cities Poverty, Race, and Place in America*. Routledge; New York, USA.

Frank, L.D., Engelke, P. (2005). Multiple impacts of the built environment on public health: Walkable places and the exposure to air pollution. *International Regional Science Review,* 28(2): 193-216.

Gakidou, E., Cowling, K., Lozano, R., & Murray, C.J.L. (2010). Increased educational attainment and its effect on child mortality in 175 countries between 1970 and 2009: a systematic analysis. *The Lancet*, 376(9745), 959-974.

Galster, G.C. (2018). Non-linear and threshold effects related to neighbourhood: Implications for planning and policy. *Journal of Planning Literature*, 33(4): 492-508.

Hayward, M.D., Hummer, R.A., & Sasson, I. (2015). Trends and group differences in the association between educational attainment and U.S. adult mortality: implications for understanding education's causal influence. *Social Science & Medicine*, 127, 8-18.

Hock, R. *et al.*, "High mountain areas" in IPCC Special Report on the Ocean and Cryosphere in a Changing Climate, H.-O. Pörtner *et al.*, Eds. (Intergovernmental Panel on Climate Change, 2019), pp. 131-202.

Hummer, R.A., & Lariscy, J.T. (2011). Educational attainment and adult mortality. In R.G. Rogers & E.M. Crimmins (Eds.), *International handbook of adult mortality* (pp. 241-261). Dordrecht, Heidelberg, London, New York: Springer.

John Cassel (1957). Social and cultural implications of food and food habits, *American Journal of Public Health*, 47; 732-740.

Kardia, S.L., Modell, S.M., Peyser, P.A. (2003). Family-centred approaches to understanding and preventing coronary heart disease. *American Journal of Preventive Medicine*, 24(2): 143-151.

Kisera, N., Luxemburger, C., Tornieporth, N., Otieno, G., Inda, J. (2020). A descriptive cross-sectional study of cholera at Kakuma and Kalobeyei refugee camps, Kenya in 2018. *Pan Afr Med J.*, 37: 197. doi: 10.11604/pamj.2020.37.197.24798

Kumar, Pankaj; Radhakrishnan, Jolly; Chowdhary, Maksud A.; Giampietro, Philip F. (2001-08-01). "Prevalence and Patterns of Presentation of Genetic Disorders in a Pediatric Emergency Department", *Mayo Clinic Proceedings*, 76 (8): 777-783. doi: 10.4065/76.8.777. ISSN 0025-6196. PMID 11499815.

L.G. Moore (2017). Measuring high-altitude adaptation. *J. Appl. Physiol.* 123, 1371-1385 (2017).

Labour.nic.in [Internet]. Building and Other Construction Workers (Regulation of Employment and Working Conditions) Act, 1996. [last accessed on 2010, June 30]. Available from: http: //labour.nic.in/dglw/building_works.html.

Labour.nic.in [Internet]. Informal sector in India: Approaches for social security. [last accessed on 2010, May 15]. Available from: http://labour.nic.in/ss/INFORMALSECTORININDIA-Approaches for Social Security.pdf

Land Use Change and Human Health - PMC (nih.gov)

Link, B.G., & Phelan, J. (1995). Social conditions as fundamental causes of disease. *Journal of Health and Social Behaviour*, 35 (extra issue), 80-94.

Lleras-Muney, A. (2005). The relationship between education and adult mortality in the United States. *Review of Economic Studies*, 72(1), 189-221.

Lopez, R.P. (2007) Neighbourhood risk factors for obesity. *Obesity*, 15(8): 2111-2119.

Luy, M., Zannella, M., Wegner-Siegmundt, C. *et al.* (2019). The impact of increasing education levels on rising life expectancy: a decomposition analysis for Italy, Denmark, and the USA. *Genus*, 75, 11. https: //doi.org/10.1186/s41118-019-0055-0

Müller, O, Krawinkel, M. (2005). Malnutrition and health in developing countries [review]. *CMAJ*, 173(3): 279-86.

Population mobility and malaria. Geneva: World Health Organization; International Organization for Migration; 2017 (http: //apps.who.int/iris/handle/10665/255816, accessed 3 April, 2022.

Pouliou, T., Elliott, S.J. (2010). Individual and socio-environmental determinants of overweight and obesity in Urban Canada. *Health and Place* 16(2): 389-398.

Poverty, Health & Environment Placing Environmental Health on Countries' Development Agendas, 2008, published by Joint Agency paper by Asian Development Bank, Austrian Development Agency, German Federal Ministry for Economic Cooperation and Development, WHO *et al.*, retrieved from https: //www.cbd.int/financial/doc/Pov-Health-Env-CRA.pdf

Rajan, S.I. (2010). *Demographic ageing and employment in India*, Bangkok: International Labour Organization, Regional Office for Asia and the Pacific (ILO Asia-Pacific Working paper series).

Reddy, S., Anitha, M. (2015). Culture and its Influence on Nutrition and Oral Health. *Biomed Pharmacol J*, 8(October Spl Edition).

Reddy, A.B. (2016). Labour force participation of elderly in India: patterns and determinants. *International Journal of Social Economics*, 43(5): 502-16. doi: 10.1108/ijse-11-2014-0221

Romeo, R., F. Grita, F. Parisi, L. Russo, Vulnerability of Mountain Peoples to Food Insecurity: Updated Data and Analysis of Drivers (Food and Agriculture Organization, Rome, 2020), 3.

Rover, S. and Butler, C. (2023). Population and Environment—a Global Challenge, Australian Academy of Science retrieved from https: //www.science.org.au/curious/earth-environment/population-environment

Rowell, L. (1983). Cardiovascular aspects of human thermoregulation. In *Circ Res*, 52: 367-379.

Sakthivel, S. and Anup Karan (2009). "Deepening Health Insecurity in India: Evidence from National Sample Surveys since 1980s", *Economic & Political Weekly*, Vol. XIV, No. 40.

Samuel, S. Myers (2011). *Landuse Change and Human Health in Integrating Ecology and Poverty Reduction, 2012*, ISBN : 978-1-4419-0632-8

Sarkar, C., Webster, C. (2017). Healthy cities of tomorrow: The case for large scale built environment-health studies. *Journal of Urban Health,* 94(1): 4-19.

Simon, J., Kiss, N., Łaszewska, A., Mayer, S. (2015). Public health aspects of migrant health: a review of the evidence on health status for labour migrants in the European Region. Copenhagen: WHO Regional Office for Europe (Health Evidence Network Synthesis Report No. 43; https: //apps.who.int/iris/handle/10665/326345, accessed 29 March, 2022).

Stevenson, M., Thompson, J., de Sá TH, *et al.* (2016). Land use, transport, and population health: Estimating the health benefits of compact cities. *The Lancet,* 388: 2925-2935.

Sun, B., Yin, C. (2018). Relationship between multi-scale urban built environments and body mass index: A study of China. *Applied Geography,* 94: 230-240.

Tatem, A.J., Jia, P., Ordanovich, D., Falkner, M., Huang, Z., Howes, R. *et al.* (2017). The geography of imported malaria to non-endemic countries: a meta-analysis of nationally reported statistics. *Lancet Infect Dis.,* 17(1): 98-107. doi: 10.1016/S1473- 3099(16)30326-7

U.S. Department of Agriculture, Economic Research Service. (n.d.). *Definitions of food security.* Retrieved March 10, 2022, from https: //www.ers.usda.gov/topics/food-nutrition-assistance/food-security-in-the-u-s/definitions-of-food-security/

Woolf, S.H., Johnson, R.E., Phillips, R.L., & Philipsen, M. (2007). Giving everyone the health of the educated: an examination of whether social change would save more lives than medical advances. *American Journal of Public Health,* 97(4), 679-683.

World Health Organization. Aging and Health 2018 [updated 5 February 2018; cited 2018, 25 July]. http: //www.who.int/news-room/fact-sheets/detail/ageing-and-health.

World Health Organization. Genes and Human Diseases. Accessed July 1, 2021. https: //www.who.int/genomics/public/geneticdiseases/en/index2.html

World report on the health of refugees and migrants. Geneva: World Health Organization; 2022. Licence: CC BY-NC-SA 3.0 IGO, ISBN: 978-92-4-005446-2; ISBN 978-92-4-005447-9

Worldometer. Current world population. Accessed July 1, 2021. https: //www.worldometers.info/world-population/

Yin, C., Cao, J., Sun, B. (2020). Examining non-linear associations between population density and waist-hip ratio: An application of gradient boosting decision trees. *Cities,* 107: 102899.

Yosef, A.R. (2008 July). Health beliefs, practice, and priorities for healthcare of Arab Muslims in the United States. *J Transcult Nurs.*, 19(3): 284-91. doi: 10.1177/1043659608317450. PMID: 18445762.

Chapter

3

Development, Environment and Human Health

Development is a process of change. The first conceptualization is that 'development' is a process of structural societal change. Thomas (2000, 2004) refers to this meaning of development as 'a process of historical change'. The key characteristics of this perspective are that it is focused on processes of structural societal change, it is historical and it has a long-term outlook. This means that a major societal shift in one dimension, for example from a rural or agriculture-based society to an urban or industrial-based society (what is sometimes called the shift from 'traditional' to 'modern' characteristics), would also have radical implications in another dimension, such as societal structural changes in the respective positions of classes and groups within the relations of production for example (by which we mean the relationship between the owners of capital and labour). This means that development involves changes to socio-economic structures—including ownership, the organization of production, technology, the institutional structure and laws (Deane, 1965). The dimensions of development are extremely diverse, including economic, social, political, legal and institutional structures, technology in various forms (including the physical or natural sciences, engineering and communications), the environment, religion, the arts and culture. Some readers may even feel that this broad view is too restricted in its scope. Indeed, one might be forgiven for feeling that "there is just too much to know now (as, indeed, there always was)" (Corbridge, 1995: x).

Modernization Theory (1950s-1960s) defines development as the process of economic growth and technological advancement that would lead to the modernization of society. Dependency (1960s-1970s) theory saw development as a process in which developing countries were dependent on developed countries for resources, leading to unequal power relations and exploitation. Human Development (1980s-1990s) approach emphasized the role of social and political factors in development, such as education, healthcare, and gender equality, to achieve human well-being and capabilities. Sustainable Development (1990s-present) approach aims for development that balances economic growth, social well-being, and environmental conservation to meet the needs of the present without compromising future generations. Post-Development

(1990s-present) approach challenges the dominant development discourse and argues for alternative ways of achieving well-being that are not founded on Western concepts of progress and modernity.

It is important to note that these definitions coexist and overlap, and different actors and institutions may prioritize one approach over the others. There have been several types of economic revolutions and development throughout world history. Most important ones are Agricultural revolution, industrial revolution, Information technology revolution, globalization and urbanization.

3.1 Impacts of Agricultural Revolution

This was a major economic shift that occurred around 10,000 BCE when humans started to cultivate crops and domesticate animals. This led to the rise of settled societies and the development of specialized labour. The agricultural revolution was a major turning point in human history, and it had a significant impact on economic growth. It led to Specialization and Surplus. The shift from nomadic hunting and gathering to settled agriculture allowed people to produce more food than they needed to survive. With this surplus, people could trade or sell their produce for other goods or services, which led to the development of specialized labour and the growth of market economies. It was a driving force to urbanization. The rise of settled societies allowed for the growth of towns and cities, which became centres of trade and commerce. People who lived in cities could engage in more specialized labour, such as crafts, trade, and services, which further fuelled economic growth. It highlighted the importance of technology. Agricultural societies developed new technologies to improve crop yields and increase efficiency, such as the plough, irrigation systems, and domesticated animals, which also paved the way for further technological advancements. Massive population growth also took place after agricultural revolution. The ability to produce more food led to population growth, which in turn encouraged people to develop better ways of producing and distributing goods. This led to increased innovation and competition, further driving economic growth.

Thus, the agricultural revolution allowed for the development of complex societies, specialized labour, and the growth of market economies, all of which paved the way for further economic growth and development in human history. The Agricultural Revolution in Britain proved to be a major turning point, allowing population to far exceed earlier peaks and sustain the country's rise to industrial pre-eminence. It is estimated that total agricultural output grew 2.7-fold between 1700 and 1870 and output per worker at a similar rate. The Agricultural Revolution gave Britain the most productive agriculture in Europe, with 19th-century yields as much as 80 per cent higher than the Continental average. The increase in the food supply contributed to the rapid growth of population in England and Wales, from 5.5 million in 1700 to over 9 million by 1801, although domestic production gave way increasingly to food imports in the 19th century as population more than tripled to over 32 million. The rise in productivity accelerated the decline of the agricultural share of the labour force, adding to the urban workforce on which industrialization depended. The Agricultural Revolution has, therefore, been cited as a cause of the Industrial Revolution (https://courses.lumenlearning.com/).

Agricultural development has positively affected human health in numerous ways.

3.1.1 *Improved Nutrition*

Agricultural development has led to the availability of a variety of nutritious foods such as fruits, vegetables, and whole grains that are essential for a balanced diet. Increased crop yields and modern farming practices have made these foods accessible and affordable to people all over the world, helping to improve nutrition and reduce malnutrition. Between 1960 and 1990, the share of undernourished people in the world fell significantly (Eiselen, 2009). Improved availability and decreased staple food prices dramatically improved energy and protein consumption of the poor (Hazell, 2010). Biofortification (breeding micronutrients into staple crops, such as the vitamin A-enhanced, orange-fleshed sweet potato) offers a new solution for improving nutrition outcomes, particularly for the rural poor, who depend on their own production for a large proportion of their daily caloric intake (Ecker *et al.*, 2011).

3.1.2 *Increased Food Security*

Agricultural development has helped in providing a more stable food supply by increasing productivity and reducing market volatility. This helps to prevent food shortages and minimize the risk of famine, which can have significant public health implications. For example in India, rice and wheat production increased manifold. The production of rice has increased from 34.48 million tonnes in Triennium Endings (TE) 1962-63 to 112.47 million tonnes in TE 2018-19. The rice yield per hectare has also improved from 1013 kilogram (kg) in 1960 to 2578 kilogram in 2017-18. Same time, the wheat production also increased substantially from 11.28 million tonnes in TE 1962-63 to 99.18 million tonnes in TE 2018-19 (GoI, 2019). The developing world witnessed an extraordinary period of food crop productivity growth over the past 50 years, despite increasing land scarcity and rising land values. Although populations had more than doubled, the production of cereal crops tripled during this period, with only a 30 per cent increase in land area cultivated (Pingali, 2012).

3.1.3 *Increased Access to Healthcare*

Agricultural development has helped to improve access to healthcare by creating jobs and generating income in rural areas. This has a significant impact on the health and well-being of communities, especially those in developing countries where access to healthcare is limited.

Negative environmental and health impacts of agricultural revolution were deep rooted and significant The Green Revolution, which took place from the 1940s to the 1960s, led to significant increases in food production in various parts of the world. While it helped to alleviate hunger and malnutrition in many developing countries, it also had detrimental effects on the environment.

Some negative environmental impacts of the Green Revolution include:

3.1.4 *Soil Degradation*

The increased use of chemical fertilizers and pesticides led to soil degradation over the years, particularly in areas used for monoculture. This soil degradation can reduce soil fertility, increase erosion, and soil acidity. For example, in Punjab, India, where green revolution was most significant, soil nutrient depletion at an alarming rate has been a major concern. Soil is a critical component of our ecosystem, and it plays a vital role in supporting human health. Soil degradation, which is the decline in quality and productivity of the soil, can have several negative impacts on human health. Soil degradation can lead to a decline in the nutritional quality of crops. When soil quality is poor, crops may not receive enough nutrients, which can lead to stunted growth and reduced yield. The reduction in crop yields can result in food insecurity and malnutrition, which can have long-term impacts on human health. Soil degradation can lead to soil erosion, which can cause sedimentation in water bodies. The soil particles can make the water turbid, and nutrients and chemicals from soil degradation can pollute the water. The polluted water can cause water-borne diseases like cholera, typhoid, and dysentery. Degradation of soil can result in dust emissions, which can cause respiratory problems. Soil particles that are small enough to be inhaled deep into the lungs can cause respiratory illnesses like asthma, bronchitis, and lung cancer. The buildup of toxins in the soil when it is contaminated, the toxic chemicals can be absorbed by crops, animals, and humans. For instance, heavy metals such as lead and cadmium can accumulate in soil and are potentially toxic to humans. Soil degradation can create favourable habitats for disease-carrying organisms like mosquitoes. In turn, these vectors can transmit diseases such as malaria, dengue fever, and yellow fever to humans.

3.1.5 *Water Scarcity*

The Green Revolution relied heavily on water irrigation systems, which led to the depletion of water resources in some areas. For instance, some areas in Mexico, where irrigation systems were introduced, water level started depleting in the underground aquifer. Water is essential for human survival, and when there is a shortage of water, dehydration can occur. Dehydration can lead to a host of health problems, including fatigue, headaches, dizziness, and confusion. In severe cases, dehydration can lead to kidney failure or even death. Water scarcity can also result in an increase in water-borne diseases, as people resort to using contaminated water sources such as rivers, ponds, or wells. Drinking contaminated water can result in water-borne diseases such as cholera, typhoid, and dysentery, which can cause diarrhoea, dehydration, and in severe cases, death. Water scarcity can result in inadequate sanitation and hygiene practices, which can lead to health problems. In developing countries, many people lack access to clean water for basic hygiene, leading to the spread of diseases such as trachoma, which is an eye infection that can eventually lead to blindness.Water scarcity in long run, can lead to reduced food production, which can impact food security. When there is not enough water for irrigation, crop yields can decline, leading to food shortages. Malnutrition, hunger, and related health problems can occur when people cannot access sufficient amounts of nutritious food. Water scarcity can contribute to conflicts over water resources, leading to societal instability and violence. Such conflicts can result in the displacement of communities and increased vulnerability to health problems such as malnutrition and water-borne diseases. Thus water scarcity has severe negative impacts on human health. It is essential to implement water conservation and management practices to address these issues so that communities can prevent water scarcity, reduce the spread of water-borne diseases, and improve overall health and well-being. The use of wastewater in agriculture raises major public health concerns, mainly due to the often high concentration of pathogenic micro-organisms. Water-borne parasites are a major health concern in this regard, especially in endemic areas, mainly due to the high environmental resistance of eggs/cysts combined with a low infectious dose (Kpoda, 2022).

3.1.6 *Biodiversity Loss and Related Diseases*

The monoculture approach adopted by the Green Revolution focused on only a few high-yielding crop varieties at the expense of traditional crop varieties and local biodiversity. This has led to a loss of genetic diversity, reducing the resilience of crops to pests and diseases. For instance, the introduction of high-yielding varieties in rice led to a decline of traditional varieties in Thailand.

The loss of biodiversity can impact human health in various ways. For example, Zoonotic diseases, also known as zoonoses, are diseases that can be transmitted from animals to humans. Loss of biodiversity can increase the emergence and spread of zoonoses. When natural habitats are destroyed, animals are forced to move closer to human settlements, which increase the likelihood of disease transmission. For example, Ebola and COVID-19 are believed to have originated from interactions between wildlife and humans. Biodiversity is essential for the production of food, and the loss of biodiversity can reduce food security. When there is a loss of diversity in plant and animal species in an ecosystem, it can result in the loss of important food sources. This can lead to malnutrition, famine, and other health problems. Moreover, many medicines and pharmaceuticals are derived from plants and animals. The loss of biodiversity reduces the availability of these resources, which can hinder the development of new drugs and treatments for human diseases. For example, the Madagascar periwinkle is a plant that produces compounds used to treat leukemia, and the loss of this plant could impact the development of new treatments for the disease.

3.1.7 *Excessive use of Chemicals and Toxification*

Pesticides are chemicals used to kill pests such as insects, rodents, and weeds on crops. These chemicals are toxic and can cause cancer, immune system problems, and neurological disorders. For example, in India, farmers who have been exposed to pesticides have a higher risk of developing leukemia and other cancers. Chemical fertilizers are used to increase the yield of crops. They contain chemicals like nitrogen, phosphorus, and potassium that can harm humans and the environment. Overusing fertilizers can lead to eutrophication, which is the excessive growth of algae in water bodies that causes oxygen depletion and fish kills. In China, overuse of fertilizers has led to high levels of nitrogen and phosphorus in rivers, causing health problems for people who rely on these rivers for drinking water. At many places in the world antibiotics are used in animal agriculture to promote growth and prevent disease. However, overuse of antibiotics has resulted in antibiotic-resistant bacteria, which can cause infections in humans that are difficult to treat. This problem is a worldwide concern, and countries like Denmark have already banned the use of antibiotics in animal agriculture.

Genetically modified organisms (GMOs) are crops that are genetically engineered to be resistant to pests and herbicides. These crops have been controversial due to their potential health and environmental impacts. For example, in France, a study showed that rats fed with GMO corn had higher rates of tumors and kidney and liver problems than rats fed with non-GMO corn. Thus, the use of chemicals in agriculture poses a significant risk to human health worldwide. As consumers, it is essential to be aware of the potential negative impacts of these chemicals and to advocate for sustainable and organic farming practices.

The state of Punjab in India has been a subject of interest regarding the impact of agricultural development on cancer cases. Punjab has witnessed a significant transformation in its agricultural practices over the past few decades, with the introduction of the Green Revolution in the 1960s and the subsequent use of chemical inputs, intensive irrigation, and mechanization. The widespread use of pesticides, fertilizers, and irrigation practices has raised concerns about their long-term effects on human health and the environment.

The excessive use of pesticides to protect crops from pests has been a common practice in Punjab. Farmers and agricultural workers are frequently exposed to these chemicals, which may have toxic effects and potential links to cancer development. The state relies heavily on groundwater for irrigation, which has led to over-exploitation and contamination. The presence of heavy metals, nitrates, and other pollutants in the water supply could potentially lead to health issues, including an increased risk of cancer. The Green Revolution in Punjab promoted the cultivation of high-yield varieties of rice and wheat, leading to a monoculture system. This lack of crop diversification can deplete soil fertility and increase pesticide usage, potentially impacting the overall environmental and public health. There has been a lack of awareness among farmers and the general population about the potential health risks associated with intensive agricultural practices. This has limited the adoption of alternative, sustainable farming methods and the use of protective measures among farmers.

Punjab has the highest number of cancer patients in India. The "Cancer Train" in Punjab refers to a train that runs from the state of Punjab in India to Bikaner in Rajasthan, primarily used by cancer patients seeking treatment. It gained attention due to the large number of individuals using this mode of transportation to access cancer treatment facilities. The Cancer Train was needed for several reasons like Lack of Local Treatment Facilities. Punjab, particularly the Malwa region, faced a scarcity of specialized cancer treatment centres. Patients had limited access to quality healthcare within the state, leading them to travel in search of appropriate medical facilities. Seeking cancer treatment can be financially burdensome. Patients from Punjab found it more cost-effective to travel to Bikaner, where charitable hospitals provides subsidized or free cancer treatment, including chemotherapy and radiotherapy. Bikaner had a cluster of well-established hospitals specializing in cancer treatment, attracting patients from neighbouring regions, including Punjab. These hospitals had experienced oncologists and better medical infrastructure than the available options in Punjab.

3.1.8 *Excessive Irrigation*

For the purpose of meeting the demand for energy and food, the construction of irrigation and dam system is undertaken. However, creation of water resources can have negative impacts on human health especially through the transmission of diseases from vectors such as Schistosomiasis and Malaria (Wale *et al.*, 2019). Untreated or partially treated wastewater, which is a negative externality of urban water use, is widely used for irrigation in water scarce regions in several countries including India. While the nutrients contained in the wastewater is considered as beneficial to agriculture, the contaminants present in it pose environmental and health risks (Srinivasan and Reddy, 2009). According to scholars like Bob Savoie and Jamie Bartram, improper irrigation practices, such as using contaminated water sources or inefficient water management, can lead to the spread of water-borne diseases like diarrhoeal diseases, cholera, and schistosomiasis. Studies by Christopher Barrett and Marc F. Bellemare (2010) have shown that irrigation can enhance agricultural productivity, increase food availability, and improve nutrition in communities reliant on irrigation-based agriculture. This is particularly significant in arid and semi-arid regions where irrigation can lead to the cultivation of a wider variety of crops. Scholars including David Molden and John P. McCornick (2007) have highlighted the environmental consequences of irrigation, such as an increased demand for water resources, depletion of aquifers, and altered ecosystems. These consequences can indirectly impact human health by affecting water availability and quality. Research by Susanne Scheierling and others (2012) indicates that improper irrigation techniques, such as excessive waterlogging, can lead to conditions like skin diseases, respiratory problems, and musculoskeletal disorders. These health issues can arise when irrigation water or practices directly affect individuals working in irrigated areas.

In this region, inadequate sanitation, poor water quality, and improper wastewater management in irrigation can contribute to the spread of water-borne diseases such as diarrhoeal diseases, cholera, and schistosomiasis. Similarly in areas of intensive rice cultivation, such as parts of Southeast Asia, the stagnant water associated with paddy fields can serve as breeding grounds for disease-carrying mosquitoes, leading to an increased risk of mosquito-borne diseases like dengue fever and malaria.

Table 3.1: Common diseases due to agricultural activities

Diseases due to agricultural activities	Prominent causes
Pesticide Poisoning	Exposure to excessive or inappropriate use of pesticides in agriculture can lead to poisoning in humans and animals.
Respiratory Diseases	Inhalation of dust particles, molds, and airborne pathogens during agricultural activities can cause respiratory diseases, including chronic obstructive pulmonary disease (COPD) and asthma.
Zoonotic Diseases	Zoonotic diseases, such as avian influenza (bird flu) and swine flu, can spread from animals to humans through farming practices and close contact, including improper handling of livestock.
Water-borne Diseases	Agricultural run-off laden with fertilizers, pesticides, and animal waste can contaminate water sources, leading to water-borne diseases like cholera and giardiasis.
Tick-borne Diseases	Farmers, agricultural workers, and outdoor enthusiasts are at risk of contacting tick-borne diseases like Lyme disease, caused by tick bites in rural areas.
Silicosis	Exposure to crystalline silica dust, often found in certain crops like rice, can cause lung disease called silicosis among agricultural workers involved in handling or processing these crops.
Skin Disorders	Frequent exposure to sunlight, various chemicals, and irritants during farm work can contribute to skin disorders such as contact dermatitis, skin cancer, and pigmentation issues.
Noise-Induced Hearing Loss	Agricultural machinery, such as tractors, combine harvesters, and chainsaws, produce high levels of noise that can result in hearing loss among farmers and farm workers.
Musculoskeletal Disorders	Repetitive and physically demanding tasks in agriculture, like heavy lifting, carrying loads, and prolonged manual labour, can lead to musculoskeletal disorders like back pain and joint problems.
Food-borne Illnesses	Improper handling, processing, or storage of agricultural products can contribute to the spread of food-borne diseases, such as Salmonella and E. coli infections.

Source: Compiled by author from various sources.

3.1.9 *Regional Prevalence of Certain Diseases Linked to Farming Activities*

Certain diseases associated with agriculture are more prominent in specific regions of the world due to various factors. These diseases may or may not be directly linked to agriculture but are found in areas which are either rural or are involved in farming activities.

1. **Malaria:** While not directly related to agriculture, the disease is often prevalent in regions where agriculture thrives. Mosquito breeding sites can form in the stagnant water created by irrigation systems and rice fields.
2. **Chagas Disease:** Common in rural areas of Latin America, Chagas disease is transmitted by triatomine bugs, which often reside in cracks and crevices of poorly constructed homes commonly found in agricultural regions.
3. **Dengue Fever:** Tropical and subtropical regions with high agricultural activity often experience outbreaks of dengue fever due to increased mosquito breeding grounds in irrigation systems and standing water near farmland.
4. **Leptospirosis:** This bacterial infection is more prevalent in regions with extensive agricultural activities, especially those involving direct contact with animal urine-contaminated water sources. It is common in Southeast Asia, Central and South America, and some African nations.
5. **African Trypanosomiasis (Sleeping Sickness):** Found in rural areas of Sub-Saharan Africa, this disease is spread by tsetse flies that inhabit areas with livestock and grazing fields.
6. **Rift Valley Fever:** Primarily affecting livestock, this viral disease spreads to humans through contact with infected animals or consumption of contaminated animal products. It is found in Africa, especially regions with livestock farming and irrigation practices.
7. **Histoplasmosis:** This fungal infection is associated with agricultural practices involving contaminated soil or bird droppings, and it is prevalent in certain regions of North and Central America, Africa, and Asia.
8. **Valley Fever:** Primarily found in arid regions of the Americas, including the south-western United States and parts of Mexico, this fungal infection often affects agricultural workers who inhale dust-borne spores while working in fields.

3.2 Impacts of Industrial Revolution

This was a period of significant economic growth and change that took place from the late 18th to mid-19th century. It was characterized by the widespread adoption of new technologies, such as the steam engine, and the shift from handmade goods to mass production. Industrialization is a period in history that led to significant economic growth and change. Industrialization increased efficiency and brought about a shift from manual labour to machine-based production, which greatly increased efficiency and productivity. For instance, the invention of the steam engine allowed for mass production of goods and services, leading to overall economic growth. The widespread adoption of machines in manufacturing led to the mass production of goods that were once considered expensive or exclusive, such as textiles and steel. These products became more affordable and accessible to regular people, which drove demand and further economic growth. Industrialization led to the development of new industries, such as transportation (railways, steamships), communication (telegraphs, telephones), and energy (coal, oil), which created new jobs and industries that were never possible before. Just as agriculture revolution led to urbanization, industrialization also led to people's movement to the cities. The rise of factories and greater job opportunities in urban areas brought large numbers of people from rural areas, creating densely populated cities and towns. This concentration of people stimulated the growth of businesses and commerce, leading to more economic growth.

Industrialization has brought prosperity around the world by promoting economic growth, creating jobs, and improving living standards. The industrial revolution in the United States helped the country to become a major economic power in the world. The mass production of consumer goods, such as cars and appliances, created new industries and jobs that lifted many people out of poverty. The country also benefited from its technology and innovation, which helped it to build a modern infrastructure and develop advanced industries such as aerospace, pharmaceuticals, and electronics. Similarly, following World War II, Japan rapidly industrialized and rose to become one of the world's largest economies. Japan's industrialization was driven by its manufacturing sector, which focused on producing quality consumer goods such as electronics, cars, and robotics. By investing in research and development, Japan has continued to innovate and become a leader in new industries such as green technology. Overall, industrialization transformed the way people lived and worked, creating new opportunities and industries that propelled economic growth forward.

The industrial revolution, which began in England in the late 18th century and spread worldwide, had both negative and positive impacts on human health. Although the industrial revolution has been associated with negative health impacts such as pollution and occupational hazards, there were significant positive impacts on human health as well. Some of the positive impacts of the industrial revolution on human health include:

3.2.1 *Improved Sanitation*

During the industrial revolution, cities became densely populated, leading to the spread of infectious disease. In the 1830s, Dr. William Henry Duncan, a government health official in Liverpool, England, surveyed living conditions and found that a third of the city's population lived in cellars of houses, which had earthen floors and no ventilation or sanitation. As many as 16 people were living in a single room and sharing a single privy. The lack of clean water and gutters overflowing with sewage from basement cesspits made workers and their families vulnerable to infectious diseases such as cholera (www.history.com). In the latter half of the nineteenth century, Britain monopolized the international market for sanitaryware, pipes and fittings. Britain led a sanitary revolution, supported by legislation, offering a holistic approach to health. Consequently, between 1850 and 1900, life expectancy increased by ten years from 43 to about 53 years (Bailey, 2022). However, advancements in technology led to improved sanitation practices, such as the implementation of sewage systems, which helped reduce disease transmission. During the industrial revolution, many cities implemented sewage systems to improve sanitation. The first comprehensive sewage system was created in London in the 1860s, which helped reduce the spread of diseases like cholera and typhoid fever. Similarly, the installation of sewage systems in other industrial cities such as Paris, Manchester, and New York City helped reduce the spread of water-borne diseases. Industrial cities began implementing regulations to ensure that food handlers and restaurants met minimum hygiene standards. By the end of the 19th century, cities such as Chicago and New York City had established boards of health which were responsible for enforcing public health regulations. This led to improvements in sanitation and a reduction in infectious diseases. Chlorination of water supplies and disinfection of surfaces were important innovations in the improvement of sanitation in industrial cities. These techniques helped reduce the spread of infectious diseases such as tuberculosis. Disinfection processes were implemented in many cities during and after the Industrial Revolution to improve public health. Industrialization led to overcrowded living conditions in cities, which led to the spread of infectious diseases. However, the construction of better-quality housing with sanitation facilities such as indoor toilets and running water helped improve living conditions and reduce the spread of diseases. Industrialization led to an increase in waste production, leading to problems with disposal. Industrial cities addressed this problem by implementing waste management systems, which helped reduce pollution and the spread of diseases caused by waste products. The industrial revolution led to significant advancements in medicine and medical technology. Industrialization allowed for the mass production of drugs and medical devices, and also led to increased research and development in medicine.

3.2.2 *Advances in Medicine*

The industrial revolution contributed to significant advances in medicine and medical technology. For example, anesthesia, vaccines, and antibiotics were developed during this period, which greatly improved medical treatment and reduced mortality rates. The industrial revolution made it possible to mass-produce drugs, leading to increased availability and affordability. For example, the mass production of the smallpox vaccine led to its widespread use and the eventual eradication of the disease. By 1896, over 10 million people had been vaccinated against smallpox in England alone. One of the most significant medical breakthroughs of the 20th century was the discovery of antibiotics, which were developed during the industrial era. Penicillin was discovered in 1928 by Alexander Fleming, and it became widely available during World War II. Antibiotics revolutionized medicine, and they continue to save countless lives everyday.

Advances in industrial technology also led to the development of medical devices such as X-rays, ultrasound machines, and magnetic resonance imaging (MRI) machines. These devices improved patient care by allowing doctors to diagnose and treat illnesses with more accuracy and precision. The industrial revolution also led to significant growth in medical research. In 1902, the Rockefeller Institute for Medical Research was founded with the goal of advancing medical research and finding cures for infectious diseases. The institute made several breakthroughs, including the discovery of the polio virus in 1908. The advancements in medicine during the industrial revolution contributed to a significant reduction in mortality rates. For example, in England and Wales, the death rate for children under five decreased from 154 deaths per 1,000 births in 1850 to 131 deaths per 1,000 births in 1900. New medical inventions exhibited at the first London International Exposition of 1851 included bloodletting instruments and artificial legs, hands, teeth and noses, as well as laryngoscopes and various cutting instruments. Artificial legs and hands were developed for soldiers who had lost their legs or hands in war (www.ndl.go.jp).

Table 3.2: List of some selected major inventions in medical field after industrial revolution

Inventions	Year
Stethoscope: Invented by René Laennec, the stethoscope revolutionized diagnostic medicine by allowing physicians to hear internal sounds of the body, aiding in the diagnosis of various conditions.	1816
Anesthesia: The use of general anesthesia in surgery was pioneered by William Morton, leading to pain-free surgical procedures and improved patient outcomes.	1846
X-rays: Wilhelm Conrad Roentgen discovered X-rays, allowing for non-invasive imaging of the human body and revolutionizing the field of diagnostic radiology.	1895
Insulin: Frederick Banting and Charles Best discovered insulin, leading to effective treatment for diabetes and significantly improving the quality of life for millions of individuals.	1921
Penicillin: Alexander Fleming's discovery of penicillin revolutionized the field of antibiotics, providing an effective treatment for bacterial infections and saving countless lives.	1928
Polio Vaccine: Developed by Jonas Salk, the polio vaccine dramatically reduced the incidence of polio worldwide, leading to the near eradication of the disease.	1955
Heart-Lung Machine: Developed by John Gibbon Jr., the heart-lung machine made open-heart surgery possible by temporarily replacing the function of the heart and lungs during the procedure.	1953
Artificial Pacemaker: Invented by Wilson Greatbatch, the artificial pacemaker regulates the heart's electrical activity, providing life-saving treatment for irregular heart rhythms.	1950s
Magnetic Resonance Imaging (MRI): The invention of the MRI by Raymond Damadian and Paul Lauterbur enabled non-invasive imaging of soft tissues, aiding in diagnoses across various medical specialities.	1970s
Human Genome Project: This collaborative effort to map and sequence the human genome has paved the way for advancements in personalized medicine, genetic testing, and targeted therapies for various genetic disorders.	(1990-2003)
3D-Printed Organs and Tissues: Researchers have made progress in 3D printing functional organs and tissues, such as hearts and kidneys, using bioinks made from patient-specific cells. Although still in the experimental stage, this technology holds great promise for transplantation and regenerative medicine.	2019 onwards

Source: Compiled by author from various sources.

3.2.3 *Improved Food Industry and System*

Advancements in agriculture and transportation technology led to increased food production and availability. The industrial revolution also led to the creation of new food preservation methods, which helped improve nutrition and reduce malnutrition. The development of machines and advanced techniques in the food industry resulted in increased efficiency and productivity. Machines like the combine harvester, which allowed for quicker and more efficient harvesting of crops, significantly reduced the amount of time and labour required to cultivate and produce food. The invention of canning, refrigeration and other preservation methods allowed for food to be stored for longer periods of time, making it easier to transport and sell. This innovation also changed the way people ate, allowing people to access a variety of foods year-round. The use of assembly line techniques in the food industry enabled mass production of goods. This allowed companies to produce large quantities of food at lower costs, making food more affordable and accessible to the masses like the production of packaged foods, like cereals and snacks. The Industrial Revolution introduced new transportation systems, making global trade easier and faster. This allowed for the distribution of exotic and speciality foods worldwide, making them available to people who wouldn't have otherwise had access to them. Developed world and countries have adopted the industrial process within their food supply chain process effectively and that allowed them to enhance their whole food systems with increased food productivity and effective distribution of the foods. The developed world has a significant increase in their food storage and has been able to effectively manage the growing demands of food even in the modest seasons (McMichael, 2012). The drivers of urbanization, production and processing technology, transport technology, and political forces that have played a large part in shaping current food systems will continue to be relevant (Hueston and McLeod., 2012).

3.2.4 *Improved Working Condition*

Although industrial work was initially dangerous and often hazardous, legislation and regulations were put in place to improve worker safety. This led to better working conditions, such as the reduction of physical strain, which helped reduce work-related injuries and illnesses. Industrialization led to the implementation of various laws which help improve working conditions. For example, the Factory Act of 1833 enforced standard working hours for children, and the Ten Hours Act of 1847 also established a nominal 10-hour workday for women and young people. Now it is one labour = 8 hours. Industrialization led to the development of new technologies that reduced the monotony of manual labour, such as machines, assembly lines and other systems that made the work environment more enjoyable. The Industrial Revolution saw significant improvements in sanitation practices. Moreover, the installation of running water and sewage systems, cleaner living environments, and a focus on hygiene in the workplace reduces the spread of diseases and illnesses. Industrialization led to the development of medical advancements which help improve the health of workers. With the increase in production and trade, workers had greater access to affordable healthcare and improvements in medical facilities. The formation of trade unions helped establish workers' rights, ensuring they had representation in negotiations with employers for improved working conditions, safety measures, and better pay.

Table 3.3: Acts and initiatives to improve health conditions of workers in different countries

Year	Region or country	Act/Initiative
1833	United Kingdom	Factory Act of 1833 (United Kingdom): This Act was one of the first legislative efforts to address labour conditions in factories. It limited the working hours of children aged 9-13 to 9 hours per day and required factory owners to provide education for child workers. This can help them to manage physical and mental stress.
1919	International	International Labour Organization: The ILO was established as part of the Treaty of Versailles after World War I. It is a specialized agency of the United Nations and focuses on promoting social justice, decent work, and internationally recognized labour standards.
1948	Universal	United Nations Universal Declaration of Human Rights: Article 23 of the Universal Declaration of Human Rights recognizes the right to work under favourable conditions, including fair wages, reasonable working hours, and the right to join trade unions.

(*Contd.*)

Year	Region or country	Act/Initiative
1970	United States	Occupational Safety and Health Act: This Act established the Occupational Safety and Health Administration (OSHA) to set and enforce standards for workplace safety and ensure the health and well-being of American workers.
1972	Japan	Occupational Safety and Health Law: This law addresses occupational safety and health issues such as risk assessment, prevention of workplace accidents, health examinations, and employee training. It sets forth obligations for employers and workers to ensure a safe working environment.
1974	United Kingdom	Health and Safety at Work Act: This legislation places a duty on employers to ensure the health, safety, and welfare of their employees and others affected by their work activities. It outlines the responsibilities of employers, employees, and enforcing authorities in ensuring a safe working environment.
1985	Canada	Canada Labour Code, Part II : The Part II of the Canada Labour Code sets out occupational health and safety standards for federally regulated industries and undertakings. It outlines employer responsibilities for workplace health and safety and employee rights to refuse dangerous work.

Source: Compiled by author from various sources.

In India, the main legislation governing occupational health and safety is the Factories Act, 1948. The Factories Act is applicable to factories engaging a specified number of workers and covers various aspects of occupational health and safety. It mandates certain provisions related to the welfare, health, and safety of workers in factories. There are health and safety provisions. The Act requires factories to provide and maintain adequate measures for the health and safety of workers. It covers areas such as cleanliness, lighting, ventilation, temperature, drinking water, disposal of waste and effluents, and prevention of fire. The Act includes provisions for the welfare of workers, including requirements for first aid facilities, canteens, shelters, restrooms, and sanitary facilities. The Act provides regulations for factories engaging in hazardous processes or using hazardous substances. It requires employers to take necessary precautions for the safe handling, storage, and transportation of such substances. The Act also empowers factory inspectors to require periodic health examinations of workers employed in specified occupations or processes. It aims to ensure that workers engaged in hazardous work are periodically examined to detect and prevent occupational diseases. The Act further mandates the reporting of accidents, dangerous occurrences, and occupational diseases in factories. It lays down the procedures for reporting and investigating such incidents and requires the submission of annual reports on accidents to the factory inspector.

3.2.5 *Increased Access to Education*

Before the industrial age, provision of formal schooling virtually everywhere was scarce—dependent on tuition and fees, voluntarist, and usually limited to males. Education belonged to the church in feudal Europe, and with seven out of every ten workers engaged in agriculture, the slender surplus enabled only small percentages of people to earn their bread through the written word (Bloch, 1963; Cipolla, 1993). The industrial revolution sparked prolonged, rising rates of productivity, first in the British economy and then in continental Europe, the northern United States, and Upper Canada (Madrick, 2002). As educational access widened, the education of women increased, the study of the classical curriculum declined, and by the twentieth century, the importance of schooling for both national economic development and individual mobility took on the status of an "education gospel" (Grubb & Lazerson, 2004: 1-2). The industrial revolution led to increased access to education. With technological advancements, more people could be educated, leading to increased health literacy and improved health outcomes. Industrialization led to greater economic growth and increased investment in education, resulting in expanded educational opportunities. Industrialization caused people to move from rural areas to urban environments resulting in creating access to schools. Industrialization brought about a greater understanding and concern for public health. The introduction of new technologies and medical advancements led to the public health movement, which emphasized preventive medicine as well as the need for sanitation and hygiene. Industrialization led to significant improvements in preventive medicine. Vaccinations for diseases like smallpox, for example, were developed, which helped reduce the spread of diseases.

Increased access to education led to greater awareness and education around health issues. This led to the development of public health campaigns, the establishment of charities, and greater awareness of public health hazards. For example in case of Britain between 1820 and 1870, literacy rates rose from 60 to 90 per cent as a result of industrialization, education reforms, and the increasing availability of cheap newspapers and books. As a result, average life expectancy in Britain increased from 40 years in 1800 to 55 years in 1850. Industrialization led to significant improvements in access to education, which in turn resulted in better health outcomes, from preventive medicine to greater public health awareness to better nutrition.

Therefore, the industrial revolution had a significant positive impact on human health. Improvements in sanitation, medicine, nutrition, working conditions, and education have positively influenced the health and well-being of people worldwide. However, it is crucial to note that the industrial revolution also had negative impacts on human health, and those must be addressed in the context of public health.

While the Industrial Revolution brought about many positive changes to society, it also had negative impacts on human health. Below are some negative impacts of industrialization on human health worldwide.

3.2.6 *Air Pollution*

With the increasing number of factories, the use of coal and other fossil fuels for energy and production caused air quality to deteriorate. Industrialization caused high air pollution levels in cities, leading to significant health problems such as cardiovascular disease, respiratory issues, and cancer. Industrialization has led to significant air pollution, causing respiratory issues, cancer, and other health problems worldwide. China, the US, and India are examples of countries that have experienced severe air pollution problems as a result of industrialization. China's rapid industrialization over the last few decades has led to significant air pollution problems, particularly in its cities. Emissions from factories, coal-fired power plants, and vehicle emissions have contributed to the country's poor air quality. Air pollution has been responsible for many health problems such as heart disease, stroke, and lung cancer. According to a study conducted in 2020 by the Global Initiative on Health and Pollution, Pollution in China was responsible for 1.8 million premature deaths in 2019.

The US has experienced issues with air pollution since the beginning of the Industrial Revolution. The country's industrialization and the reliance on oil, gas, and coal to power, the economy have led to air pollution problems in major cities. This has contributed to respiratory problems, cancer, and other health issues. In the 1970s, the United States Congress established the Clean Air Act to reduce air pollution, leading to a significant reduction in air pollution-related health problems. India's industrialization has also led to significant air pollution problems, particularly in its urban areas. The burning of fossil fuels for energy and transportation, combined with the burning of biomass for cooking, has led to high levels of air pollution. According to a report by the Lancet Commission on Pollution and Health, air pollution is responsible for approximately 2.5 million premature deaths in India each year. Industrialization has led to significant air pollution problems and health issues, including respiratory problems, cancer, and premature death in many countries worldwide. While some countries, like the US, have taken measures to address air pollution, countries such as China and India face significant challenges in reducing their air pollution levels.

Table 3.4: The Chronology of global air quality

Seventeenth century	Harmful effects of air ascribed to various components, e.g. Kenelme Digby (acids), Nehemiah Grew (lead), John Evelyn (sulfur) and John Hall (antimony or mercury)
Eighteenth century	Guillaume François Rouelle detects SO_2 by absorbing the gas in strong alkalis; Carl Wilhelm Scheele detects NH_3 via absorption with acids
1872	Robert Angus Smith publishes *Air and Rain: The Beginnings of a Chemical Climatology*, having undertaken the first multisite, multipollutant measurements
1878	The UK Royal Commission on Noxious Vapours
1894	The 'great horse manure crises' of London and New York
1905	Smoke Nuisance Acts in Bengal 1905
1952	The Great London Smog; 12,000 died in two weeks Los Angeles smog, chemistry and effects described
1956	The UK Clean Air Act
1960	Extensive local ecological damage by smelters
From 1967, air pollution problems are recognized as international issues	
1960s	Acid rain extensively described by Svante Oden
1970s	Ground-level ozone threat to ecosystems identified in North America and Europe following earlier concerns of effects of the ozone on human health
1972	United Nations Stockholm Conference confirms acid rain as an important international issue in Europe
1977	USA establishes its National Acid Deposition Programme (NADP)
1979	UNECE Convention on Long Range Transport of Air Pollution (LRTAP) established
1980s	Forest decline recognized in Europe and North America
1985	Helsinki Protocol: Commitment to reduced SO_2 emissions by 30 per cent (The 30% club)
1980s-1990s	Eutrophication of ecosystems by nitrogen deposition recognized
1991	Canada-USA Air Quality Agreement

(*Contd.*)

1993	The 'Six Cities' study in North America re-focuses attention on the human health effects of air pollution PM_{10}
1995	Launch of the first satellite for passive remote sensing atmospheric composition (GOME) for global ozone monitoring
1999	The UNECE Gothenburg Protocol adopted to tackle multipollutant multieffects (acidity, ozone and eutrophication)
2000s	Emissions of SO_2 and NO_x in Asia increasingly dominate global emissions and adverse effects
2010	Widespread evidence of recovery from effects of acid deposition in Europe and North America with the decline in emissions of SO_2 and NO_x
2012	Beijing smog, 13th January, with concentrations of PM and SO_2 similar to London 1952
2015	Global SO_2 emissions reduced by 15 per cent from the 1990 peak, while all other air pollutants still increasing
2018	Emissions of SO_2 and NO_2 declining rapidly in China
2018	Peak global NO_x emission? Global emissions of NH_3 and VOC continue to rise
2020	COVID-19: The global pandemic dramatically reduces emissions of industrial- and transport-related emissions of SO_2, NO_x, VOC and primary PM

Source: Fowler, D. *et al.*, 2020.

According to WHO, around 6.7 million deaths were attributable to air pollution worldwide in 2019. Of this total, 2.3 million were attributable to indoor air pollution. According to the Global Asthma Report 2018, approximately 339 million people worldwide have asthma. The prevalence of asthma varies across different regions due to various factors, including genetics, environmental exposures, and healthcare access.

Industrial pollution has been a significant concern in Europe, particularly in heavily industrialized regions. High levels of pollution, including air pollutants and toxic waste, have been associated with adverse health outcomes. According to a study published in *The Lancet*, outdoor air pollution was responsible for an estimated 7,90,000 premature deaths in Europe in 2015. Japan has experienced both historical and ongoing challenges related to industrial pollution. In the mid-20th century, rapid industrialization contributed to severe pollution incidents, such as the Minamata disease caused by mercury poisoning. In response to these issues, Japan has implemented strict environmental regulations and pollution control measures. However, localized pollution incidents still occur, and industrial pollution can still impact health outcomes in specific regions. Areas in South East Asia, such as India and China, often experience severe air pollution, leading to greater health risks for asthma patients. Similarly, urban areas with high pollution levels can pose significant challenges for individuals with asthma. In India, about 77 per cent of the industries contribute to water pollution while 15 per cent to air pollution and the remaining eight per cent to both air and water pollution. The industries which are dependent on natural resources are the most polluting ones and are growing rapidly. Heavy metal pollution from industries is affecting human health in a significant way (http://www.indiaenvironmentportal.org.in/). India is known to have high levels of air pollution, particularly in heavily industrialized regions and urban areas. Exposure to pollutants such as particulate matter (PM2.5), nitrogen dioxide (NO_2), sulphur dioxide (SO_2), and volatile organic compounds (VOCs) can trigger or worsen asthma symptoms. Studies indicate that air pollution is a significant contributor to the increasing prevalence of asthma in India, specifically among children. There are certain regions in India that face significant industrial pollution challenges, potentially impacting asthma rates. For example, areas around the National Capital Region (Delhi) and industrial clusters in states like Uttar Pradesh, Maharashtra, and Gujarat experience high levels of industrial pollution due to heavy industrial activity.

3.2.7 *Chemical Exposure*

Industrialization exposed workers and communities to toxic chemicals. Exposure to chemicals such as benzene, lead, and PCBs, which were used in various industrial processes, led to a range of health issues such as cancer, neurological disorders, and reproductive problems. Chemical exposure in industrial towns has had a significant impact on the health of the people living and working in these areas worldwide. In Bhopal, India, the world's worst industrial disaster happened when the Union Carbide plant released lethal gas in 1984. The disaster resulted in the immediate death of over 10,000 people, with an estimated additional 20,000 deaths occurring in the years after the disaster due to exposure to toxic chemicals. Over half a million people were exposed to the gas and suffered from respiratory issues, blindness, and cancer due to toxic exposure. Likewise, Love Canal, a neighbourhood in Niagara Falls, New York, was built on top of a toxic waste dump site created by a chemical company. Residents were exposed to toxic waste in their soil and groundwater, leading to high rates of birth defects, miscarriages, cancer, and other health issues. The situation resulted in the US Congress passing the Comprehensive Environmental Response, Compensation and Liability Act (CERCLA), also known as the Superfund, to address toxic waste sites across the country.

Table 3.5: Selected industries, exposure to type of chemicals and related health issues

Industry	Chemicals	Health issues
Chemical Manufacturing Industry	Various industrial chemicals, solvents, and reagents.	Respiratory problems, skin irritation, chemical burns, and potential long-term health effects depending on the specific chemicals used.
Oil Refining Industry	Hydrocarbons, volatile organic compounds (VOCs), benzene, toluene, and xylene.	Respiratory issues, increased cancer risk, neurological effects, and skin conditions.
Textile and Apparel Industry	Dyes, formaldehyde, chlorine-based compounds, and flame retardants.	Dermatitis, respiratory problems, allergic reactions, and potential long-term effects on endocrine systems.
Agriculture and Pesticide Industry	Pesticides (organophosphates, herbicides, insecticides), fertilizers, and fungicides.	Respiratory problems, skin disorders, neurological effects, hormonal disruption, and potential cancer risks.
Pharmaceutical Industry	Active pharmaceutical ingredients (APIs), solvents, and various synthetic compounds.	Occupational exposure risks, allergic reactions, potential reproductive concerns, and specific risks associated with individual drugs.

Source: Compiled by Author from various sources.

In 2011, over 1,000 children were found to have excessive lead levels in their blood in Zhongjin, a town in eastern China. The lead exposure was linked to a nearby battery factory, which had released toxic waste into the soil and air. The children suffered from neurological problems as a result of the exposure. Chemical exposure in industrial towns has had a severe impact on the health of the communities living in these areas worldwide. These examples demonstrate that industrial accidents or failures in managing chemical waste can cause significant harm to the environment and human health, underscoring the need for regulations and proper safety protocols in the management of hazardous chemicals.

The Bhopal gas tragedy, which occurred on December 2-3, 1984, was one of the world's worst industrial disasters. It was caused by a gas leak from the Union Carbide India Limited (UCIL) pesticide plant in Bhopal, Madhya Pradesh, India. The toxic gas released from the plant, known as methyl isocyanate (MIC), caused immense harm to the surrounding areas, leading to thousands of deaths and long-term health consequences for the survivors. While it is difficult to attribute individual deaths solely to air pollution, here are a few examples of the types of fatalities that occurred during the gas leak period:

Immediate fatalities: On the night of the gas leak, many people died due to the direct exposure to toxic gases. Their deaths were a result of severe respiratory distress, lung damage, and other complications caused by inhaling the toxic fumes.

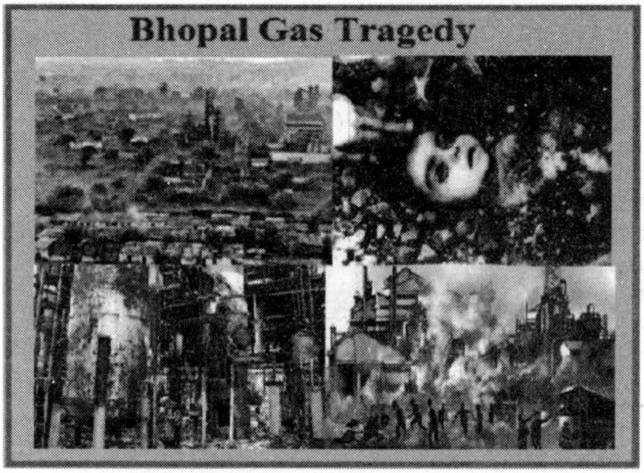

Source: Jagranjosh.com

Gas-induced injuries: Many individuals who survived the initial gas leak suffered from a range of health issues. These included respiratory ailments such as asthma, chronic bronchitis, and lung fibrosis, as well as eye infections, skin disorders, gastrointestinal problems, and neurological disorders. Prolonged exposure to the toxic gases led to these health complications, which ultimately caused some deaths among the affected population.

Long-term health effects: The gas leak also had long-term consequences for the survivors. Increased vulnerability to respiratory disorders, compromised immune systems, reproductive health issues, and higher mortality rates have been observed among the affected population. While these deaths may not be directly attributed to air pollution alone, the chronic exposure and resulting health complications stemming from the gas leak were significant contributing factors.

3.2.8 *Water Contamination*

Industrialization has led to water contamination, causing numerous health problems for people worldwide. Rapid industrialization led to untreated wastewater, which gets dumped into water bodies, leading to water contamination and soil degradation. The use of lead pipes for carrying drinking water caused lead poisoning and other diseases. The impact of water contamination on human health is often severe and long-lasting. The contaminated water passes through drains and enter river bodies. The impact of industrialization on water contamination in developing world and its impact on health are very evident like the Citarum River in Indonesia is one of the most polluted rivers in the world due to industrial waste being discharged into it. The river provides drinking water to five million people, but due to severe water contamination, people have experienced skin irritations, respiratory problems, and cancer. Similarly, the Ganges River is a source of drinking water for millions of people but has also become highly polluted due to industrial waste and agricultural run-off. Many big and small cities and industrial towns are situated on banks of the Ganga including Kanpur, Prayagraj, Varanasi etc. Most of the industries located near Ganges are of pulp, paper and chemicals. These industries together account for 60 per cent of total industries located near river Ganges. The high levels of contamination in the river have led to cholera, typhoid fever, and other water-borne diseases, making it difficult for people to access safe drinking water (Fig. 3.1). The Niger River is one of Africa's most polluted rivers, and water contamination here has been linked to numerous health issues affecting nearby communities. Due to industrialization, the river has been contaminated with heavy metals, synthetic chemicals, and other hazardous materials, leading to severe health problems like cancer, skin diseases, and birth defects.

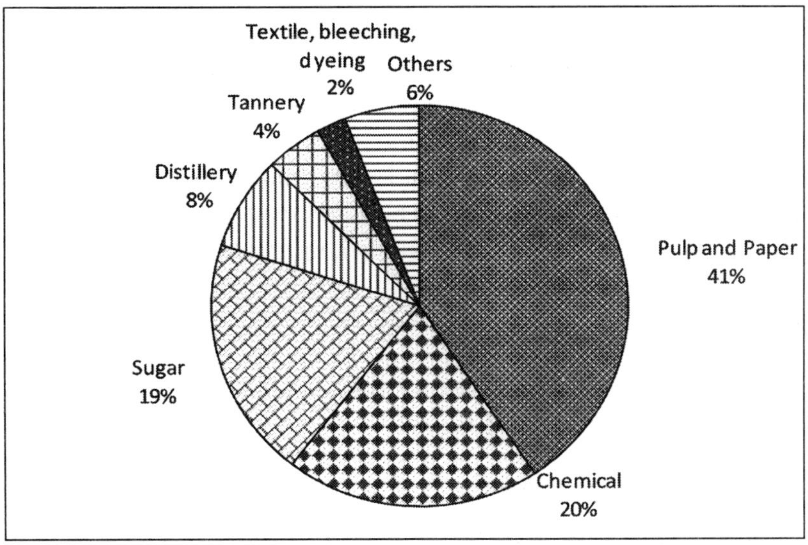

Fig. 3.1: Waste water Generation in River Ganga (contribution in per cent).

Source: Times of India, 2014.

In developing countries, water contamination is a significant public health issue arising from rapid industrialization or poor environmental policies and protections. The impact of water contamination on human health is severe and long-lasting, leading to various health problems such as infectious diseases, respiratory issues, cancer, and birth defects. The examples above demonstrate the devastating impact of industrialization on water sources in developing countries, underscoring the urgent need for proper waste management, environmental responsibility, and improved access to safe drinking water.

3.2.9 *Occupational Health Hazards*

Lack of safety regulations in the early stages of industrialization led to widespread occupational diseases and injuries, resulting in long-term health issues like black lung disease, mercury poisoning, and noise-induced hearing loss. Industrialization has led to numerous occupational health hazards, causing physical and mental health problems for workers in both developed and developing countries. For example, Asbestos, a material widely used for insulation, was linked to numerous health problems, including cancers such as mesothelioma, asbestosis, and lung cancer. Asbestos exposure is still a severe occupational hazard in developing countries, as it is sometimes still used even though it has been banned in many developed countries. Workers in the coal mining industry are exposed to various occupational hazards. This includes black lung disease from coal dust inhalation, back and joint problems from heavy lifting, and accidents such as explosions or collapses in mines. Coal mining remains a significant cause of work-related deaths worldwide, particularly in developing countries. Lead exposure leads to a significant occupational health hazard. Workers in many industries, like construction and metalworking, could be exposed to lead and suffer from the long-term health effects, including brain damage, kidney disease, and anaemia. In developing countries new industrial zones consisting of medium and large-scale industries are being set up at a rapid pace (Zhihua, 2011). Export Processing Zones (EPZs) are defined as "industrial zones with special incentives set-up to attract foreign investors, in which imported materials undergo some degree of processing before being exported again" (Cirera and Lakshman, 2017). Large number of workers especially youth are employed in these industries. Recognition of health hazards is the first step in hazard control (Arnold *et al.*, 2019). Workers in textile mills are exposed to various hazards such as long working hours, poor air quality, repetitive strain injuries, and accidents involving machinery. In developing countries, particularly in South Asia, young girls and women are often forced to work in hazardous conditions in textile mills, leading to severe health consequences.

Industrialization has led to numerous occupational health hazards in both developed and developing countries. These hazards affect workers in various industries, resulting in physical and mental health problems, and often affecting those in marginalized communities who have limited access to safety measures and healthcare.

3.2.10 *Malnutrition and Deficiencies*

With the shift towards mass-produced foods, the nutritional quality of the diet declined, leading to malnutrition and related health problems such as stunted growth in children. As industrialization leads to urbanization, people move from rural to urban areas in search of better job opportunities, leading to a decline in traditional agriculture. This, in turn, reduces the availability of nutritious food. For example, in India, as people moved from rural to urban areas due to industrialization, traditional crops like millets and pulses were replaced with crops like rice and wheat, which are less nutritious. Industrialization and urbanization have led to increasing consumption of processed and packaged foods, which are often high in calories but low in nutrients. For instance, in the United States, the consumption of processed foods has increased over the years, leading to a rise in obesity and related health problems. Industrialization has resulted in the growth of sedentary jobs, which requires less physical activity. This, coupled with an increase in the consumption of calorie-dense, nutrient-poor foods, has led to an increase in obesity and related health problems. This is evident in developed countries such as the United States and the United Kingdom. As industries expand, there is often environmental degradation, which can lead to a decrease in the availability of fresh produce. In developing countries like Nigeria, industrial growth has led to pollution, deforestation, and soil erosion, which reduces the availability of nutritious crops. One example of the negative impact of industrialization on human health was the case of the Minamata Bay disaster in Japan. In the 1950s, a factory discharged mercury into the bay, resulting in the contamination of fish and shellfish, leading to widespread mercury poisoning, and causing hundreds of deaths and birth defects.

3.2.11 *Hazardous Waste Generation*

Manufacturing resulted in massive production and higher consumption of resources leading to more waste production. The use of material like plastics, chemicals and harmful substances in various industries and households has contributed to increase in hazardous waste. Industrial products and waste carries toxics, chemicals and heavy metals that pose risk to human health. Disposal of industrial waste also has harmful effect on the health. It contaminates soil, water and air. It can lead to skin issues, gastric issues, cancers etc. Medical waste also cause disasters. Improper disposa of unused and expired Medication, injections, amputated body parts etc. have adverse impact on health. It risk disease transmission as in case of Ebola and COVID-19. In many hospitals, the dead bodies and body parts are dumped in open spaces causing bacteria and virus to spread all ones.

3.3 Impacts of Information Technology Revolution

IT revolution is a more recent economic revolution that has been taking place since the latter half of the 20th century. It is characterized by the rise of digital technologies and the widespread adoption of the internet, which has transformed the way we access and share information. Information technology has made communication faster and easier than ever before. People can now communicate using various platforms such as email, messaging apps, and social media. This has changed the way people interact and share information, whether for personal or business reasons. With the rise of the internet, people can now access information on any topic with just a few clicks. This has allowed people to work remotely, learn new skills, and become more informed on various topics, which have led to more innovation and growth. Information technology has revolutionized the way people shop online. E-commerce allows people to buy and sell goods and services online, which have made it easier for businesses to reach new customers and for consumers to access a wider range of products at competitive prices. Information technology has led to more automation in various industries, which has increased efficiency and productivity. Automated processes allow businesses to get more done in less time, leading to an increase in economic output and growth. Information technology has given people the ability to work from anywhere, anytime. This has allowed people to achieve work-life balance, reduce commuting time, and work in jobs that were once not possible.

The information technology has greatly transformed the way we live and do business, leading to significant economic growth across various industries. By enabling greater connectivity, providing access to vast amounts of information, and increasing efficiency and automation, information technology has helped to drive innovation and growth in the global economy.

The information technology revolution has brought significant positive health impacts worldwide, including:

3.3.1 *Telemedicine*

The use of telemedicine has enabled doctors in rural or remote areas to consult with specialists in urban areas, thereby increasing access to quality healthcare. For instance, in Malaysia, telemedicine has been used to provide medical services to remote areas in the country.

3.3.2 *Electronic Health Records (EHRs)*

Electronic health records have enabled healthcare providers to have immediate access to patient information, leading to better care coordination and improved patient outcomes. For example in Denmark, EHRs have reduced prescription errors and improved patient safety.

3.3.3 *Health Apps*

Mobile health apps have enabled individuals to track their health, monitor their fitness levels, and manage chronic conditions. For instance, in the United States, the MyFitnessPal app has helped people manage their weight and improve their overall health.

3.3.4 *Wearable Technology*

Wearable devices like fitness trackers have incentivized individuals to be more physically active, leading to better health outcomes. For instance, in Japan, the use of wearable technology has helped reduce the risk of lifestyle-related diseases like diabetes and cardiovascular disease.

3.3.5 *Health Information Dissemination*

Information technology has made it easier to disseminate health information to the public, leading to improved health literacy and behaviour change. For example in Australia, the Cancer Council's SunSmart programme uses social media to educate the public about skin cancer prevention.

The information technology revolution has had a significant positive impact on global healthcare, making healthcare more accessible, efficient, and patient-centred. While the information technology revolution has brought about several positive health impacts, there have also been negative health impacts associated with it, including:

3.3.6 *Sedentary Lifestyle*

Information technology has led to an increase in sedentary behaviour, with people spending more time sitting in front of screens. This has been linked to an increased risk of obesity, heart disease, and other health problems. Sedentary lifestyles and overuse of information technology can lead to several health issues, especially in children. In China, the prevalence of childhood obesity has increased over the years, and it is estimated that 1 in 5 children is overweight or obese. The use of technology, such as smartphones, has been linked to higher levels of obesity, as children spend less time being physically active. The prolonged use of computers, smartphones, or tablets can lead to poor posture, which can cause neck and back pain, headaches, and muscle strain. In Japan, the Ministry of Education has stated that the excessive use of smartphones and computers has resulted in increasing instances of postural disorders among children. In India, a study found that school children who spent more time in sedentary activities like watching television or using computers were less physically fit, with lower levels of endurance, speed, and agility. Overuse of technology has been linked to sleep problems in children. In China, a survey found that 42.6 per cent of primary school students use electronic devices everyday before going to bed, which has resulted in increased sleeplessness. Prolonged use of technology can also cause eye strain, leading to dry eyes, blurred vision, headaches, and other eye problems. In Japan, a survey found that nearly 60 per cent of junior high school students complained of eyesight problems due to the excessive use of smartphones and computers.

At the same time, sedentary lifestyles and overuse of technology can lead to several health problems in children, affecting their physical, mental, and emotional well-being. It is essential to encourage children to have a balanced usage of technology and engage in physical activities regularly to maintain good health.

3.3.7 *Digital Eye Strain (DES)*

The prolonged use of screens can cause digital eye strain, which can lead to headaches, neck and shoulder pain, and blurred vision. Digital eye strain is a growing concern due to the widespread use of digital devices. According to a survey conducted by the American Optometric Association (AOA), 58 per cent of adults in the USA have experienced symptoms of Digital Eye Strain (DES), such as dry eyes, eye strain, headaches, and blurred vision. The survey found that on average, people spend 7.5 hours per day looking at screens, which can lead to eye strain and other issues. In China, a study conducted among college students found that the prevalence of DES among students was 63.2 per cent, with dry eyes being the most commonly reported symptom. Another study conducted among IT professionals in China found that the prevalence of DES was higher in those who spent more time using computers. In the US, Digital Eye Strain is impacting productivity. People suffering from DES report that they take more breaks, suffer work performance or functionality limitations, and have difficulty staying focused on tasks. One study found that digital eye strain costs U.S. companies an estimated $2.8 billion a year in lost productivity.

3.3.8 *Sleep Disturbances*

The use of screens before bed can disrupt sleep patterns due to the impact of blue light on melatonin levels. This can lead to poor sleep quality, which is associated with a range of health problems like obesity, diabetes, and depression. Blue light, emitted from digital screens, has been shown to inhibit melatonin production, which can prevent sleep. One study found that 90 per cent of Americans used electronic devices within an hour of bedtime, which can negatively impact sleep quality.

3.3.9 *Cyber Bullying*

The internet has created new avenues for cyber bullying, which can have significant negative impacts on mental health, leading to depression, anxiety, and even suicide. Cyber bullying is a form of bullying that happens through digital technologies like social media, text messages, online forums, and chat rooms. It can lead to several mental health issues. Cyber bullying can cause feelings of anxiety, depression, and low self-esteem. In the UK, a study found that a significant proportion of children who experienced cyber bullying had symptoms of anxiety and depression. According to a study in the US, adolescents who experienced cyber bullying were twice more likely to report symptoms of depression than those who have not. Cyber bullying can also cause suicidal ideation and behaviour. In India, a study found that students who experienced cyber bullying were more likely to have suicidal thoughts. Similarly, in the US, a study found that youth who were victims of cyber bullying were three times more likely to attempt suicide than those who have not experienced cyber bullying. Cyber bullying has also been linked to eating disorders. A study in South Korea found that female students who experienced cyber bullying were more likely to have disordered eating behaviours.

Cyber bullying can also have an impact on physical health, with higher levels of stress, headaches, and other physical health problems. In Australia, a study found that children who experienced cyber bullying had higher levels of stress and headaches than those who had not experienced cyber bullying.

3.3.10 *24 × 7 and Overload Information*

The abundance of health information available on the internet can lead to information overload, which can be overwhelming and lead to confusion about health choices, making it difficult to make informed decisions. Information overload and untimely mails can lead to several health issues. Constantly checking emails, social media sites and being bombarded with large amounts of information can lead to increased stress levels. Studies have shown that information overload can cause feelings of overwhelm, frustration, and burnout, which can lead to chronic stress. Overuse of technology and being constantly 'plugged in' often leads to sleep disruption. For example, if someone has the habit of checking their emails or working late into the night, it can lead to insomnia. A person may struggle to fall asleep, sleep lightly, or wake up frequently throughout the night, which can cause fatigue. Regularly using electronic devices like computers, smartphones, and tablets, can cause headaches, and eye strain, a condition known as computer vision syndrome (CVS).

Constant notifications, emails, and messages can be distracting and can lead to poor time management. It can disrupt productivity, decrease focus and can lead to people feeling overwhelmed or consistently underperforming. Information overload can also lead to other physical health concerns like back pains, neck pains, and carpal tunnel syndrome, if poor ergonomics are not taken into account.

It is imperative to be mindful of the time spent on technology and look for strategies to reduce overload, like scheduling specific times and notifications to stay focused and lessen burn-out. Therefore, while information technology can provide many benefits, it is essential to balance its use with other healthy habits to address the negative health impacts associated with it.

3.4 Impact of Globalization

This is an ongoing economic revolution that has been occurring since the late 20th century. It is characterized by the increasing interconnectedness of the world's economies, the rise of multinational corporations, and the growth of international trade. It has had significant impacts on both the global economy and individual countries. Globalization has made it easier for countries to trade goods and services with each other. This has led to the creation of new markets, increased competition, and the exchange of expertise and technology. Free trade agreements, such as NAFTA and the EU, have removed barriers to trade and made it easier for businesses to operate across borders. Globalization has also led to investment in emerging markets, such as China and India, which have become major players in the global economy. Multinational corporations have set up operations in these countries, creating jobs and contributing to their economic growth. This has also led to the growth of manufacturing industries in these countries. Globalization has made it easier for countries and businesses to share ideas and technology with each other. This has led to the adoption of new technologies and innovative practices, which has helped to increase productivity and generate economic growth. It has led to the outsourcing of jobs and production to countries with lower labour costs. While controversial, this has led to increased efficiencies and cost-savings for businesses, which has contributed to economic growth. Globalization has also led to increased tourism between countries, as people travel more and are exposed to new cultures and experiences. This has created new jobs and businesses in the tourism industry, which is an important source of economic growth for many countries. There are several positive health impacts of Globalization:

3.4.1 *Increased Access to Healthcare*

Globalization has increased access to healthcare in developing countries by improving the distribution of medical supplies and equipment, and providing access to healthcare training and facilities. For instance, in Ghana, public-private partnerships facilitated by global health organizations have enabled better access to essential medication to fight infectious diseases like malaria. Partnerships with global health organizations have enabled better access to healthcare and medical supplies in developing countries. For instance, in Uganda, the Partnership for Transforming Health Systems II project, funded by USAID, has enabled better distribution of antiretroviral drugs and improved healthcare for HIV patients. Telemedicine has enabled better access to healthcare for people in remote areas. For example, in Ethiopia, the USAID-funded Ethiopia Network for HIV/AIDS Treatment, Care and Support project has provided telemedicine services to rural and remote areas, enabling patients to receive medical consultations and support remotely.

3.4.2 *Improved Health Outcomes*

The sharing of knowledge and expertise between countries has led to improved health outcomes globally. Developed countries such as Japan have provided valuable medical expertise and resources to poorer countries to improve health and healthcare outcomes. For instance, Japan has supported emergency care training programmes for health workers in Cambodia, resulting in better emergency care practices and improved response to emergencies. Malllaye and Yogo (2012) reported that due to foreign aid Sub Saharan Africa contributed to improvement in health outcomes. They mentioned an increase in health aid by one will increase the life expectancy by 0.14, decreasimg HIV prevalence and infant mortality by 0.05 and 0.17 respectively.

3.4.3 *Increase in Awareness of Health Issues*

Globalization has led to better dissemination of health information and knowledge, improving awareness of health issues and healthy practices. For instance, in the United States, global health initiatives have led to increased awareness of diseases like HIV/AIDS, leading to increased prevention measures and better treatment outcomes. International cross-border knowledge sharing has enabled developing countries to access expertise in medicine and healthcare. For instance, the Global Health Equity Scholars fellowship programme, sponsored by UC Berkeley and the Fogarty International Centre, trains participants from developing countries to conduct research in a variety of health fields, including medicine, public health and nutrition.

3.4.4 *Improving Food Security*

Globalization has enabled greater access to food and improved agricultural production methods, improving food security and nutrition globally. In India, the Green Revolution, which relied on cross-border knowledge transfer, led to a significant increase in food production, resulting in improved nutrition levels and decreased malnutrition. Israel has shared its advanced agricultural irrigation technology with several African countries, resulting in increased agricultural productivity and food security. Global trade has enabled countries to access a wider range of food and agricultural products, improving food security. For instance, in India, the liberalization of trade policies in the 1990s led to increased agricultural trade and greater access to food imports, increasing food security and reducing malnutrition. Globalization has facilitated investment in agriculture, leading to improvements in food security. In Brazil, foreign investment in agriculture has helped to increase productivity, expanding agricultural production, and improving food security. Globalization has led to increased research and development in agriculture, resulting in new technologies and improved crop varieties. For example, in the Philippines, the International Rice Research Institute (IRRI), a global research centre for rice, has developed high-yielding rice varieties that have significantly increased rice production and improved food security in the country. Globalization has facilitated collaborations between organizations in different sectors, benefiting agriculture and food security. For example, the partnership between the International Fund for Agricultural Development (IFAD) and the Global Environment Facility (GEF) has led to the development of sustainable agricultural practices, conserving the environment and boosting agricultural productivity.

3.4.5 *Development of New Medical Technologies and Infrastructure*

Globalization has led to the rapid development and sharing of medical technologies globally. For example, globalized collaborative research efforts, such as those involving the development of vaccines for infectious diseases like COVID-19, are crucial for developing new medical treatments and vaccines quickly. Infrastructure development in healthcare facilities has been made possible through foreign aid. For example, in Kenya, the China Communications Construction Company has partnered with the Kenyan government to develop infrastructure at the national hospital level, which includes construction and expansion of several critical healthcare facilities. Medical technology and globalization have worked together to bring about significant health benefits worldwide. Globalization has enabled the distribution of medical equipment, including diagnostic testing and hospital supplies, both regionally and internationally. In particular,

India and China have emerged as major manufacturers and exporters of high-quality medical equipment and devices, making them more accessible and affordable for developing countries. Collaboration and cross-border sharing of medical research, data, and knowledge have led to the development of new medical treatments and solutions to global health challenges. For instance, the Human Genome Project, a global research initiative to map and analyze the human genome, has improved diagnosis and treatment of several diseases. The globalization of telehealth and telemedicine has enhanced medical care accessibility, enabling patients to receive medical consultations and treatment remotely through digital technology. This has been particularly beneficial in rural areas and developing countries where there are inadequate medical facilities. For example, in Africa, the use of mobile phone technology has significantly improved access to healthcare, enabling patients to have virtual consultations with medical practitioners and seek medical advice. Globalization has led to the distribution of medical staff across international borders, helping to address shortages in healthcare personnel in different countries. For example, nurses and medical professionals from the Philippines have migrated to other countries, including the US and the UK, to work and assist with medical facilities' staffing. It has led to the global coordination and mobilization of medical personnel and resources to assist in disaster response and relief efforts. For example, following the 2010 earthquake in Haiti, international organizations, including Doctors Without Borders (DWB), deployed medical teams and supplies to provide critical medical care to people impacted by the disaster.

Overall, the globalization of medical technology has led to significant health benefits, improving access to medical equipment, advancing medical research and treatments, improving healthcare accessibility remotely, and providing relief efforts in times of crises. Thus, globalization has had a positive impact on health, leading to improved health outcomes, better access to healthcare, increased awareness of health issues, improved food security, and the development of new medical technologies. It is important to continue supporting these efforts to improve global health outcomes.

While globalization has brought many benefits, it has also had some negative health impacts, particularly in low and middle-income countries. Here are some examples of negative health impacts of globalization:

3.4.6 *Spread of Diseases*

Globalization has led to the rapid spread of infectious diseases across borders. Globalization has dramatically impacted the spread of diseases worldwide. Increased travel and trade make it easier for diseases to transmit across borders. The Spanish Flu (1918-1919) pandemic was one of the deadliest outbreaks in history, killing an estimated 50 million people worldwide. Globalization made it easier for the virus to spread, as soldiers returning from World War I and increased travel contributed to its transmission. The virus likely originated in the United States and then spread throughout the world. SARS (Severe Acute Respiratory Syndrome) (2002-03) was a viral respiratory illness that first emerged in China and quickly spread to several other countries, including Canada and the United States. Globalization allowed the virus to spread through international travel, and the World Health Organization (WHO) declared it a global health threat in March 2003. Zika Virus (2015-16) outbreak occurred in Brazil in 2015 before spreading quickly to other countries, including the United States, globalization facilitated the virus's spread. The virus was likely introduced into Brazil during the 2014 World Cup, during which thousands of people travelled to Brazil. COVID-19 (2019-20) pandemic has had an unprecedented impact worldwide, infecting millions and causing death on a massive scale. Globalization and international travel have led to the rapid spread of the virus around the world, reaching pandemic levels in early 2020. These examples demonstrate how globalization has impacted the spread of diseases worldwide. As trade and travel continue to increase globally, it is essential to prioritize healthcare and disease prevention measures to address the risks posed by easily transmittable diseases.

3.4.7 *Increase in Non-communicable Diseases*

Globalization has also led to an increase in non-communicable diseases (NCDs) in developing countries. Changes in lifestyle and diet, driven in part by global food trade and extensive marketing of processed foods, have contributed to the prevalence of NCDs such as obesity, Type 2 diabetes, and cardiovascular disease. This trend has been evident in developing countries such as China, where an increasing number of people now experience NCDs. Globalization has allowed for the easy transfer of processed and packaged foods worldwide. The rise of fast food chains and other western-style restaurants has encouraged people to consume high-calorie and high-fat diets that are low in nutritional value. This has contributed to the increase of obesity, diabetes, and heart disease in many countries. Globalization has stimulated the process of urbanization, leading to more people living in cities than ever before. Urban areas are more likely to have easy access to processed and unhealthy foods compared to rural areas. This leads to less physical activity and contributes to an increased risk of lifestyle-related diseases like obesity. Globalization has increased the adoption of sedentary lifestyles that include less physical activity. This is because modern means of transportation like cars and airplanes make it unnecessary to walk long distances. Technology advancements such as smartphones, computers, and other electronic devices have increased the time spent on screens, which has led to a reduction in physical activity. This unhealthy lifestyle-related choices lead to NCDs such as obesity and diabetes. It has allowed for widespread marketing and advertising of unhealthy food and drink products. The aggressive marketing of unhealthy food and drinks to vulnerable populations, especially children, has contributed to the increase in NCDs like obesity and diabetes. Mainly due to lifestyle choices and easily available affordable unhealthy diets NCD have been increasing worldwide. It is important to raise awareness about the health consequences of these factors and promote healthy behaviour and nutritional practices through health education and lifestyle modifications.

3.4.8 *Environmental Pollution and Health Hazards*

Globalization has led to an increase in environmental pollution in many countries. In India, pollution in heavily industrialized areas such as Delhi has resulted in significant health hazards, including respiratory illness. Globalization has led to an increase in economic activity and international trade, which has had negative impacts on the environment and public health. Globalization has led to increased demand for paper, wood products, and agricultural land, resulting in deforestation. This has led to a loss of biodiversity, soil erosion, and increased greenhouse gas emissions. The transportation of goods across the globe emits significant amounts of air pollutants, such as nitrogen oxides and particulate matter. Industrialization in developing countries has also led to increased emissions of pollutants and contributes to climate change. The production of goods and services often requires large amounts of water, which can lead to water scarcity and pollution. Large-scale agriculture and industrial practices often cause water pollution, leading to the spread of water-borne diseases and reduced access to clean drinking water. Global trade has increased the use of chemicals in many countries. Certain chemicals used in agricultural production, manufacturing, and mining can be harmful to human health and the environment. For example, pesticides used in agriculture can accumulate in the environment and harm wildlife and humans. Many manufacturing facilities have moved to countries where labour and resources are cheaper. These facilities often produce goods that require large amounts of water, and also release pollutants into the surrounding waterways. For example, the leather industry in India is a significant source of water pollution, as the chemicals used in the production process are often dumped directly into nearby rivers and streams. The global transport of hazardous materials, such as oil and chemicals, poses a significant risk to water quality and human health. Spills and accidents during transport can contaminate water sources and cause acute health effects for local populations. For example, the Exxon Valdez oil spill in Alaska in 1989 caused significant environmental damage and long-term health impacts for local communities.

3.4.9 *Poor Working Conditions*

Globalization has led to the expansion of global supply chains, which often involve low wages, long working hours, and poor working conditions. Globalization has led to the creation of sweatshops, which are factories that have poor working conditions, low wages, and long hours. Workers in sweatshops are often subjected to verbal and physical abuse, and may not have access to adequate safety equipment or training. For example, in many clothing factories in Bangladesh, workers are paid low wages and work long hours in unsafe conditions. In countries such as Bangladesh, workers in the garment industry have reported exposure to hazards such as fire and accidental injury, resulting in negative health impacts. Globalization has also led to the use of child labour in some industries, particularly in developing countries. Children may be forced to work in harsh conditions and for long hours, which can have a negative impact on their health and education. For example, in the cocoa industry in West Africa, children as young as six may be forced to work on cocoa farms for long hours, often without pay. Such children go through various physical and mental stresses. They are deprived of education and good health facilities and nutritious food that hamper their growth. Globalization has also led to an increase in the number of migrant workers who are vulnerable to exploitation. These workers may be brought to countries under false pretences, and may be subjected to low wages, long hours, and poor working conditions. For example, in the construction industry in Qatar, many migrant workers have been subjected to poor living conditions, low wages, and limited access to healthcare.

3.4.10 *Diaspora and Health*

Diaspora is the dispersion of people from their original homeland to other parts of the world. While diaspora has many advantages, such as economic and cultural exchange, it can also lead to health hazards. When people from different parts of the world come together, exposure to different diseases can occur, increasing the spread of infectious diseases. Refugees and immigrants who settle in new countries may bring with them diseases, such as tuberculosis and

HIV/AIDS, that were prevalent in their home countries but are not common in the new country. For example, in Canada, tuberculosis rates among immigrant communities are significantly higher than among the general population. Diaspora can also have negative impacts on mental health. Immigration can be stressful and traumatic, and feelings of isolation and discrimination can lead to mental health problems. For example, among the South Asian diaspora in Canada, there are high rates of mental health issues related to the stress of adjusting to a new country, as well as the challenges of dealing with cultural barriers and discrimination. Diaspora communities often have specific dietary preferences and requirements that may not be available in their new country. This can lead to food insecurity and nutritional deficiencies. For example, in the USA, many refugees have limited access to traditional foods and may struggle to maintain their cultural food practices. This can have negative impacts on their health, such as an increased risk of obesity and Type 2 diabetes. It is important for governments, healthcare providers, and communities to work together to support the health needs of diaspora communities, including access to healthcare, mental health services, and culturally appropriate food options. Globalization can also lead to social and cultural disruption, which can impact mental health and well-being. For immigrants to industrialized countries, for example, feelings of isolation and discrimination can have detrimental mental health effects.

3.5 Impacts of Urbanization

Urbanization is the process of people migrating from rural areas to cities in search of better economic opportunities, improved living standards, and access to healthcare and other services. While urbanization can also have negative impacts on health, such as increased air pollution and sedentary lifestyles, it can also have positive impacts. Here are some of the positive impacts of urbanization on health:

3.5.1 *Access to Healthcare*

Urban areas typically have better healthcare infrastructure, with more hospitals, clinics, and healthcare professionals per capita. This means that people living in cities have better access to healthcare services, including preventative care, diagnosis, and treatment of illnesses. In Bangladesh, the government has made efforts to improve healthcare access in urban areas by increasing the number of public hospitals and clinics, as well as providing relocation packages for healthcare professionals. As a result, urban areas such as Dhaka have better access to healthcare services than rural areas. In China, many rural areas are underserved by healthcare providers, and people often need to travel significant distances to access healthcare. In contrast, urban areas have better healthcare infrastructure, with more hospitals and healthcare professionals per capita. This has led to a significant disparity in healthcare access between rural and urban areas. In the US, rural areas often have lower access to healthcare than urban areas, particularly in terms of speciality care. There are fewer healthcare providers per capita in rural areas, and transportation can be a significant barrier to accessing healthcare services. As a result, rural residents often have poorer health outcomes than their urban counterparts. In South Africa, there is a significant disparity in healthcare access between urban and rural areas. Rural areas have fewer healthcare providers and services, and many people lack access to basic healthcare services such as prenatal care and immunizations. In contrast, urban areas have better healthcare infrastructure, with more hospitals and clinics, as well as greater availability of specialized care. World over the disparities in healthcare access between urban and rural areas are a global issue, and efforts are being made to improve healthcare services in rural areas, such as through telemedicine and mobile health services. However, more investment is needed to bridge the gap in healthcare access and improve health outcomes for people living in rural areas.

3.5.2 *Food Security and Improved Nutrition*

Urbanization can also lead to improved nutrition. Cities often have greater access to fresh fruits and vegetables, as well as a variety of other foods that may not be available in rural areas. Urban dwellers may also have greater access to education about healthy eating, which can lead to better dietary habits. Urban areas tend to have a greater variety of food options due to their diverse population and access to global markets. This means that people in urban areas have access to a wider range of fresh, healthy foods, as well as culturally specific foods that may not be available in rural areas. Urban areas have a greater number of grocery stores and supermarkets per capita than rural areas, making it easier to access fresh produce, meat, and dairy products. Urban areas also tend to have more speciality food stores, such as health food stores and ethnic grocers, which can be more difficult to find in rural areas. In urban areas, there are more options for food delivery services, such as meal kit delivery and grocery delivery services. This can make it easier for people to access healthy foods and ingredients, particularly for those who may not have easy access to transportation. Urban areas may have more farmers' markets, which provide fresh, local produce and other food products. These markets often attract a diverse group of vendors and consumers, which can contribute to community building and support for local agriculture.

3.5.3 *Increased Physical Activity*

While urbanization can also lead to sedentary lifestyles, it can also increase physical activity levels. Many cities tend to have more opportunities for physical activity, such as sidewalks for walking and biking, public parks, and recreation centres. This can lead to a decrease in chronic diseases such as obesity and diabetes. Amsterdam is known as one of the most bike-friendly cities in the world, with a network of bike lanes and paths that make cycling a safe and convenient option. In fact, more than 60 per cent of trips in Amsterdam are made by bike, which has helped to reduce traffic congestion and improve air quality. Copenhagen is another city with a strong cycling culture. The city has invested in dedicated bike lanes and paths, and more than 50 per cent of resident's bike to work or school. In addition to reducing congestion and emissions, cycling has also had positive impacts on public health, with lower rates of obesity and chronic diseases. Tokyo has a dense urban core with narrow streets, which makes walking and cycling a practical option for many residents. The city has also invested in pedestrian plazas and bike parking facilities to encourage active transportation, which has helped to reduce traffic congestion and improve air quality. The workplaces or educational institutes are at far distance from homes so people prefer moving in public transport like buses, metro trains etc. so they happen to walk long distances.

3.5.4 *Safer Living Conditions*

Urbanization can lead to improved living conditions, including better housing, sanitation, and access to clean water. This can lead to a decrease in infectious diseases such as cholera and typhoid fever. Urban areas typically have better access to healthcare facilities, including hospitals, clinics, and pharmacies. This means that residents of urban areas are more likely to receive prompt and effective healthcare when they need it. In addition, urban areas are often home to more specialized healthcare providers, which can lead to better health outcomes for people with chronic or complex health issues. Urban areas often have better sanitation infrastructure, such as waste management systems and sewage treatment plants. This can lead to lower rates of infectious diseases and other types of illnesses that thrive in unsanitary conditions. Additionally, cities may be able to provide clean drinking water and improved access to sanitation facilities, such as public restrooms and handwashing stations. Urban areas typically offer more job and economic opportunities, which can help to improve living conditions. This can lead to higher wages, better living conditions, and access to consumer goods and services that may not be available in rural areas. Improved economic conditions can also lower stress levels, which has been linked to better overall health. Urban areas can also offer access to green spaces, such as parks and other recreational areas. These spaces can promote physical activity, which can lead to better physical and mental health. Exposure to nature has also been linked to improved stress levels and a sense of well-being.

Thus, urbanization can have positive impacts on health, including improved access to healthcare, better nutrition, increased physical activity, and safer living conditions. However, it is important for policymakers and urban planners to be mindful of potential negative impact.

3.5.6 *Air Pollution*

The prevalence of asthma in cities around the world is often associated with air pollution levels. According to the World Health Organization (WHO), 91 per cent of the world's population lives in areas with air pollution levels that exceed the WHO's recommended limits. According to a study published in Lancet, subjects exposed to high levels of air pollution in Beijing had a 69 per cent increase in the likelihood of developing asthma. With PM2.5 particulates consistently exceeding safe levels, air pollution in Mexico City has been linked to a higher rate of asthma hospitalizations and exacerbations. Home to over 3,30,000 asthmatics and identified as having some of the worst air quality, has consistently high levels of PM2.5, nitrogen dioxide and carbon monoxide, creating severe respiratory problems. Delhi has been rated as the world's most polluted city, with the average annual PM2.5 level exceeding the recommended limit by 14.3 times, leading to a significant increase in the rate of asthma among children and adults. In 2019, asthma hospital admissions in London came to an average weekly total of 192, arising from the city's polluted air with nitrogen dioxide concentrations exceeding EU benchmarks and causing asthma exacerbations. Ensuring clean air in cities is vital for preventing asthma exacerbations, and it requires strategies like public awareness campaigns, regulation of emissions, better public transportation, and creation of green spaces.

3.5.7 *Water Pollution*

Urbanization can lead to increased sewage and waste discharge into waterways, which can lead to higher rates of water-borne diseases such as cholera, typhoid fever, and Hepatitis A. According to the World Health Organization, water-borne diseases are responsible for an estimated 4,85,000 deaths each year. It can also lead to chemical contamination of waterways, particularly from industrial activities and mining. Exposure to chemicals such as lead, mercury, and arsenic can lead to a range of health issues, including neurological damage, developmental delays in children, and cancer. Urbanization can contribute to nutrient pollution of waterways, which can lead to harmful algal blooms. These blooms can produce toxins that can cause illness or death in humans and animals, as well as disrupt aquatic ecosystems. Algal blooms have been linked to health issues such as liver damage, respiratory problems, and neurological disorders. Urbanization and water pollution can also lead to the loss of aquatic biodiversity, which can have negative impacts on public health. Healthy aquatic ecosystems can help to purify water and support local food systems, which can contribute to better overall health. Loss of aquatic biodiversity can also lead to negative impacts on mental health and well-being. It is important for cities and urban planners to prioritize sustainable development practices, such as reducing industrial pollution and improving wastewater management, to protect public health and preserve valuable natural resources.

3.5.8 *Noise Pollution*

Loud and constant noise can disturb a person's sleep pattern leading to insomnia and related issues. It can increase the stress levels in individuals leading to mental health disorders like anxiety, depression, irritability, and aggressive behaviour. Prolonged exposure to high-intensity noise can lead to an increase in blood pressure and heart rate, which in turn can cause heart diseases and stroke. *Hearing impairment*: Continuous exposure to loud noises can result in hearing impairment and tinnitus, which is an irreversible condition. Noise pollution can have a significant impact on the mental well-being of people, especially in children and elderly people, leading to learning difficulties, concentration problems, and cognitive impairment. Mumbai is one of the busiest cities in the world with a population of about 20 million people. According to a study by the World Health Organization (WHO), about 60 per cent of the city's population is exposed to noise levels greater than 70 decibels (dB) during the day time, which can cause noise-induced hearing loss and other health issues. New York City is another bustling city with a population of over 8 million people. According to the New York City Department of Health, about 90 per cent of the city's population is exposed to noise levels greater than 50 dB. The high noise levels can cause sleep disturbance, hearing impairment, and stress-related disorders. Tokyo is known to be the busiest city in the world with a population of about 37 million people. According to a report by the Tokyo Metropolitan Government, noise levels in Tokyo are often above 70 dB and can lead to heart diseases, hypertension, and other stress-related disorders.

3.5.9 *Sedentary Lifestyles*

Urbanization can also encourage sedentary lifestyles, particularly if residents are dependent on cars for transportation. Lack of physical activity has been linked to a range of health issues, including obesity, heart disease, diabetes, and mental health problems. A study published in *PLoS Medicine* found that lack of physical activity accounted for 6 per cent of the global burden of disease. People who have a sedentary lifestyle tend to burn fewer calories than those who are physically active. Over time, the lack of physical activity can contribute to an accumulation of body fat and lead to obesity.

3.5.10 *Consumerism and Packaged Food*

In urban areas, consumerism, i.e., the idea that increasing the consumption of goods and services purchased in the market is always a desirable goal, and that a person's well-being and happiness depend fundamentally on obtaining consumer goods and material possessions. Consumerism often leads to over-consumption of packaged foods, which are typically high in calories, sugar, salt, and unhealthy fats. These foods can contribute to obesity, diabetes, and other chronic diseases. Consumerism contributes to food waste, deforestation, and other environmental issues that can harm human health, including exposure to toxins and pollutants. Packaged foods available in grocery shops in cities and towns often lack essential nutrients such as vitamins, minerals, and fibre, leading to nutrient deficiencies and related health problems. Packaged foods often contain chemical additives such as preservatives, artificial flavours, and colours, which can have adverse effects on health, including allergic reactions, digestive problems, and neurological disorders. The promotion and consumption of packaged foods may displace healthier, locally sourced, and traditional foods, which can have significant health benefits but may be neglected due to increased demand for packaged, processed food alternatives. Over-consumption, nutrient deficiencies, chemical additives and the environmental impact of production and consumption can lead to various negative health outcomes, making it essential for individuals and communities to prioritize healthier and sustainable food choices.

3.5.11 *Urban Housing and Slums*

Urban areas in the world have more density of population and compact settlements. These areas also have slums which are characterized by densely packed housing units of weak build quality and often associated with poverty. These areas lack infrastructure facilities and have poor ventilated compact houses. The residents of these units are exposed to poor sanitation facilities, unsafe drinking water and are located in risk prone areas. They also use unsafe fuel for cooking and heating. People in such areas are exposed to household air pollution and unsafe drinking water facilities. Children living in slums are more at risk of diarrheal disease (loose watery stools), due to their exposure to contaminated water and improper sanitation. Crowding also exacerbates risks of airborne disease transmission, particularly of tuberculosis (www.who.int). The elderly population and children are also exposed to extreme cold and hot weather conditions causing sickness and discomfort. Home injuries can be an outcome of poor housing conditions, although global statistics on domestic injuries are lacking. Domestic environments are linked to the majority of childhood burns, falls, drowning, and poisonings etc.

Housing in urban areas contains polluted air in combination with poor ventilation causes dry throat and eyes, concentration disorders, fatigue, headaches, shortness of breath, poor sleep, drowsiness, dizziness. Household poisons are substances used in home that can cause harm when swallowed, inhaled or touched. They include medicines, detergents, cleaning products, paints, toiletries, garden chemicals and other common household products. Poisoning occurs most often in children under five years of age. Molds are very common in buildings and homes. Mold will grow in places with a lot of moisture, such as around leaks in roofs, windows, or pipes, or where there has been flooding. Mold grows well on paper products, cardboard, ceiling tiles, and wood products. Mold can also grow in dust, paints, wallpaper, insulation, drywall, carpet, fabric, etc. Exposure to damp and moldy environments may cause a variety of health effects, or none at all. Some people are sensitive to molds. For these people, exposure to molds can lead to symptoms such as stuffy nose, wheezing, and red or itchy eyes, or skin. Some people, such as those with allergies to molds or with asthma, may have more intense reactions.

Domestic waste generated by urban houses in day to day activities also poses risk to health. According to NITI Ayog, it is estimated that urban India generates between 1,30,000 to 1,50,000 metric tonne (MT) of municipal solid waste every day—some 330-550 gram per urban inhabitant a day. This adds up to roughly 50 million MT per year; at current rates, this will jump to some 125 million MT a year by 2031. The composition of waste is changing from high percentage of biodegradable waste to non-biodegradable waste. The waste characterization determines the strategy for its management. And then there is the problem of legacy waste lying in dumpyards scattered across cities. It is estimated that some 800 million MT has been 'disposed of' in the 3,159 dumpsites across the country, according to data from the Central Pollution Control Board (CPCB). Health hazards associated with poor municipal solid waste management are real and pose serious public health threats ranging from the transmission of endemic zoonoses to the emergence and re-emergence of new zoonoses arising either from direct or indirect effects of poor waste management. It is pertinent that all human settlements regardless of their sizes and locations develop sustainable and efficient methods for proper waste management which will preserve the environment and promote the health of the residents.

3.5.12 *Mental Health*

Living in urban areas can also have negative impacts on mental health, such as increased stress levels and higher rates of depression and anxiety. A study published in *JAMA Psychiatry* found that people living in urban areas had a 39 per cent higher risk of mood disorders than those in rural areas. According to a study by Harvard School of Public Health, the prevalence of anxiety disorders is higher in urban areas than rural areas. The study found that residents of cities were 21 per cent more likely to experience anxiety disorders than those in rural areas. Depression is a common mental health problem in urban areas. According to the World Health Organization (WHO), major depressive disorders are expected to be the leading cause of disability by the year 2030. Urbanites often have limited social support networks, high levels of stress, and poor access to nature, all of which can contribute to higher rates of depression. Urban residents are at higher risk of substance abuse and addiction than those in rural areas. According to the Substance Abuse and Mental Health Services Administration (SAMHSA), illicit drug use was highest among people living in large metropolitan areas in the US. Cities have higher rates of suicide than rural areas. According to the World Health Organization, suicide rates are higher in urban areas in low- and middle-income countries. Post-Traumatic Stress Disorder (PTSD) is common in urban residents due to higher exposure to violence and traumatic events. Thus, mental health problems are a significant issue in cities, and they can have long-lasting and significant impacts on a person's health and well-being. Factors such as stress, isolation, substance abuse and a lack of access to natural environments and social support can contribute to the high rates of these issues in urban areas.

3.5.13 *Chronic Diseases*

Urbanization can also lead to higher rates of chronic diseases such as diabetes and hypertension. According to the International Diabetes Federation, the prevalence of diabetes in urban areas is expected to increase by 54 per cent between 2019 and 2045. This is due to factors such as sedentary lifestyles, unhealthy diets, and stress. People who have a sedentary lifestyle tend to burn fewer calories than those who are physically active. Over time, the lack of physical activity can contribute to an accumulation of body fat and lead to obesity. Lack of physical activity can also contribute to the onset of type 2 diabetes. Physical activity helps to regulate blood sugar levels, and a sedentary lifestyle reduces the body's ability to do so. Sedentary lifestyle is a risk factor for cardiovascular diseases such as heart attack, stroke and hypertension. Being inactive can lead to increased cholesterol and blood pressure levels, which can put a strain on the heart and blood vessels. Prolonged sitting in a poor posture is a common cause of musculoskeletal problems such as back pain, neck pain, and joint problems. A sedentary lifestyle can also contribute to mental health problems such as increased feelings of anxiety and depression. According to the Centres for Disease Control and Prevention (CDC), an estimated 10.5 per cent of adults in the US have diabetes. In some cities, such as Detroit, the prevalence is much higher, with an estimated 18 per cent of adults living with diabetes. Diabetes is a growing concern in India, with an estimated 77 million people living with the condition. According to a study published in the *Indian Journal of Endocrinology and Metabolism*, the prevalence of diabetes in urban areas of India ranges from 7 per cent to 16 per cent. Obesity is a significant public health concern in the US and contributes to many chronic diseases, including type 2 diabetes, heart disease, and cancer. According to the CDC, the prevalence of obesity in the US is approximately 42 per cent, with even higher rates in some cities, such as Houston and Cleveland. Obesity is also on the rise in urban India, with approximately 14.4 million people living with the condition. According to a study published in the *Journal of Clinical and Diagnostic Research*, the prevalence of obesity in urban areas of India ranges from 21 per cent to 37 per cent.

3.5.14 *Infectious Diseases*

Cities are vulnerable to becoming a hub for infectious diseases due to several factors. Cities have a high density of population, which means that people live in close proximity to each other, facilitating the spread of infectious diseases. For example, respiratory infections like COVID-19 can spread rapidly through cities due to the ease of human-to-human transmission. Cities are often well-connected through various modes of transportation, such as air, road, and rail, which allows people and goods to travel easily, facilitating the spread of infectious diseases across regions and countries. Moreover, cities often have a significant population of people living in poverty and overcrowded conditions, which makes them more vulnerable to infection and disease. These conditions are perfect breeding grounds for disease spread.

In some cities especially in developing countries urban planning practices that do not prioritize public health can lead to poor sanitation, inadequate health facilities, lack of access to clean water and safe food. This can make the city more vulnerable to infectious diseases. Climate change has a substantial impact on vector-borne infectious diseases spread in urban areas. For example, warmer temperatures and increased precipitation can make the environment favourable for mosquitoes that spread dengue fever, malaria and other vector-borne diseases. Cities are vulnerable to becoming hubs of infectious diseases due to high population density, interconnectedness, poverty and inequality, poor urban planning etc. For example Wuhan, the capital of Hubei Province, China, is where the COVID-19 pandemic was first identified in December 2019. The rapid spread of this infectious disease in Wuhan is attributable to factors such as a high population density, a large number of tourists, and the Chinese New Year festivities that involved a massive movement of people. The COVID-19 pandemic quickly became a global health crisis and has affected millions of people worldwide. Similarly, a large-scale measles outbreak took place in the DRC (Democratic Republic of Congo) in 2019, affecting over 3,00,000 people. The spread of the disease was attributed to the high population density in cities, poor vaccination coverage, and a lack of access to healthcare facilities. The outbreak led to the loss of thousands of lives, including many children.

While urbanization can have positive effects on health, it can also lead to a range of health issues such as air pollution, sedentary lifestyles, mental health problems, and chronic diseases. These issues highlight the importance of addressing the negative impacts of urbanization, while also emphasizing the need for sustainable urban planning that prioritizes public health.

REFERENCES

Arnold, S.M., Wickrematilake, M.S.K., Fernando, R.M.S.D., Sampath, H.M.R.C., Karunapema, R.P.P., Mahesh, P.K.B., Munasinghe, P.M., Denawaka, C.J. (2019 Nov.). Occupational hazards in medium and large scale industrial sectors in Sri Lanka: experience of a developing country. *BMC Res Notes.,* 20: 12(1): 755. doi: 10.1186/s13104-019-4790-2. PMID: 31747965; PMCID: PMC6865055.

Bailey, J. (2022). Drawbacks with Industrialization. Sanitary Revolution Offering Technologies to Improve Public Health. In: *Inventive Geniuses Who Changed the World.* Springer, Cham. https: //doi. org/10.1007/978-3-030-81381-9_5

Bloch, M. (1963). *Feudal Society.* (L.A. Manyon, Trans.). Chicago: University of Chicago Press.

Bob Savoie and Jamie Bartram. *Protecting Groundwater for Health.* World Health Organization (WHO). Available at: https: //www.who.int/water_sanitation_health/publications/protecting_groundwater_rev.pdf

Christopher Barrett and Marc F. Bellemare. "Agricultural Technology, Productivity, and Human Health." In *Handbook of Agricultural Economics,* Volume 4, edited by Bruce L. Gardner and Gordon C. Rausser, 2010, Pages 2663-2717. Available at: https: //doi.org/10.1016/S1574-0072(10)04011-8

Cirera, X., Lakshman, R.W.D. (2017). The impact of export processing zones on employment, wages and labour conditions in developing countries: systematic review. *J Dev Eff.* 9(3): 344-360. doi: 10.1080/19439342.2017.1309448

Corbridge, S. (ed.) (1995). *Development Studies a Reader.* London: Arnold.

David Molden and John P. McCornick (2007). *Water for Food, Water for Life: A Comprehensive Assessment of Water Management in Agriculture.* International Water Management Institute (IWMI). Available at: https: //www.iwmi.cgiar.org/Publications/IWMI_Research_Reports/PDF/PUB029/RR2.pdf

Deane, P. (1965). *The First Industrial Revolution.* Cambridge: Cambridge University Press.

Fowler David *et al.,* (2020). A chronology of global air quality in Phil. Trans. R. Soc. A.3782019031420190314 http: //doi.org/10.1098/rsta.2019.0314

Grubb, W. & Lazerson, M. (2004). *The education gospel: The economic power of schooling.* Cambridge, MA: Harvard University Press.

https: //eands.dacnet.nic.in accessed on 13 November, 2019.https: //pib.gov.in/Press Release I frame Page. aspx?PRID=1582362, 4th advance estimates August 19, 2019, accessed on 20 January, 2020.

Hueston, W. and Mcleod, A. (2012). *Overview of the global food system: changes over time/space and lessons for future food safety in Improving Food Safety Through a One Health Approach: Workshop Summary,* Institute of Medicine (US). Washington (DC): National Academies Press.

Kpoda, N.W. *et al.* (2022). "Risk of Waterborne Parasitic Infection among Vegetables Producers in the City of Ouagadougou, Burkina Faso: An Attempt to Quantify Them Using the Quantitative Microbiological Risk Assessment Method" in *Agricultural Sciences,* Vol.13, No.1, January, doi: 10.4236/as.2022.131002

Madrick, J. (2002). *Why economies grow: The forces that shape productivity and how we can get them working again.* New York: Basic Books.

Mallaye, D. and Yogo (2012). *Health aid and Health Improvement in Sub Saharan Africa. MPRA Paper No. 44938.* http: //mpra.ub.unimuenchen.de/44938

McMichael, Philip (2012). *Development and Social Change: A Global Perspective.* SAGE Publications, Inc.

O. Ecker, C. Breisinger, K. Pauw (2011). *Growth Is Good, but Not Good Enough to Improve Nutrition,* International Food Policy Research Institute, New Delhi.

P. Hazell, *Proven Successes in Agricultural Development* (eds.) D. Spielman, R. Pandya-Lorch (International Food Policy Research Institute, Washington, DC), pp. 67-97 (2010).

Pingali, P.L. Green Revolution: Impacts, limits and the path ahead. *Proc Natl Acad Sci,* USA 2012, Jul 31; 109(31) 12302-8. doi: 10.1073/pnas.0912953109. Epub 2012 Jul 23. PMID: 22826253; PMCID: PMC3411969.

P.J.R. Webb (2009). *Fiat Panis: For a World Without Hunger* (ed.) H. Eiselen (Hampp Media/Balance Publications, Stuttgart), pp. 410-434.

Srinivasan, Jeena & Reddy, V. (2009). "Impact of irrigation water quality on human health: A case study in India". *Ecological Economics,* 68, 2800-2807. 10.1016/j.ecolecon.2009.04.019

Susanne Scheierling *et al.* (2012). "Water and Health: Where Science Meets Policy." World Bank Policy Research Working Paper No. 6050. Available at: https: //openknowledge.worldbank.org/handle/10986/14923

Wale, Animashaun & Fabunmi, John & Akanmu, Diekola. (2019). Health impact of irrigation scheme on its immediate environment. *International Journal of Research in Marketing Management and Sales,* 1, 40-50. 10.33545/26633329.2019.v1.i1a.8.

Zeng Douglas Zhihua. (2011). *How do special economic zones and industrial clusters drive China's rapid development?*

Chapter 4

Communicable and Infectious Diseases

Trends and Patterns

Communicable diseases, also known as infectious diseases, are diseases caused by microorganisms that can spread from one person to another through various modes of transmission. Communicable diseases are illnesses caused by viruses or bacteria that people spread to one another through contact with contaminated surfaces, bodily fluids, blood products, insect bites, or through the air (Edemekong and Huang, 2022). These diseases can spread easily in environments with high population density, poor sanitation, malnutrition, and inadequate healthcare facilities.

How these diseases spread depends on the specific disease or infectious agent. Some ways in which communicable diseases spread are by:

1. Physical contact with an infected person, such as through touch (staphylococcus), sexual intercourse (gonorrhea, HIV), fecal/oral transmission (Hepatitis A), or droplets (influenza, TB);
2. Contact with a contaminated surface or object (Norwalk virus), food (salmonella, E. coli), blood (HIV, Hepatitis B), or water (cholera);
3. Bites from insects or animals capable of transmitting the disease (mosquito: malaria and yellow fever, flea, plague);
4. Respiratory infections that travel through the air, such as tuberculosis or measles (acphd.org); and
5. Zoonotics diseases, i.e., the ones that travel from animals to humans like rabies.

4.1 Chronology of Communicable Diseases in the World

Throughout history, communicable diseases have impacted humanity; however, these diseases became more threatening as society made the shift to agrarian life around 10,000 years ago. The creation of more closely connected communities gave infectious diseases the chance to grow into epidemics. Diseases like influenza, smallpox, leprosy, malaria, and tuberculosis were among those that have thrived since this shift (www.news-medical.net). The first recorded pandemic occurred during the Peloponnesian War in Athens, Greece in 430 B.C. The disease was carried across the Athenian walls during the siege. Historians estimate around two-thirds of the population died from contracting the disease (www.news-medical.net).

Table 4.1: History of infectious diseases in the World

Year	Infectious diseases
429 BC	**Plague of Athens:** Epidemic in Athens during the Peloponnesian War (431-404 BC), the city of Athens was under siege by Sparta when the plague struck. Most of the population became sick over the course of the following three years, and up to 75,000-1,00,000 people—or 25 per cent of the city's population—may have perished.
165 AD	**Antonine Plague:** The first recorded pandemic to affect the Roman Empire, the Antonine Plague (also known as the Plague of Galen after the Greek physician who first described it) that lasted from 165 to 180 AD, was presumably infected and spread by troops who were coming home from a campaign in the Near East. Although measles has also been considered, most scholars believe that smallpox was the cause of the epidemic.
541 AD	**Plague of Justinian:** The Justinian or Justinianic Plague (541-549 AD) was the first significant epidemic of the first plague pandemic, the infectious illness brought on by the bacterium Yersinia pestis in the Old World. The plague devastated the Sasanian Empire, the Byzantine Empire, and particularly Constantinople as it spread throughout the Mediterranean Basin, Europe, and the Near East.
1347	**Black Death:** The bubonic plague epidemic known as the Black Death, often referred to as the Pestilence, the Great Mortality, or the Plague, struck Western Eurasia and North Africa between 1346 and 1353. The height of the pandemic, which claimed 75-200 million lives and peaked in Europe between 1347 and 1351, is considered to be the deadliest in recorded human history. The bacterium Yersinia pestis, which causes bubonic plague and is spread by fleas, also likely caused pneumonic plague during the Black Death by spreading *via* aerosols from person to person.
1494	**Syphilis:** Syphilis can spread through blood transfusions, oral, vaginal, and anal intercourse, as well as during pregnancy. Pregnancy-related syphilis increases the risk of stillbirth, neonatal death, and congenital syphilis in newborns. Ruy Diaz de Isla accepts syphilis as a "unknown disease, so far not seen and never described" that began in Barcelona in 1493 and originated at Espaola Island (Spanish: Isla Espaola), a part of the Galápagos Islands. Syphilis was first discovered on Espaola Island in the Galápagos Islands. Additionally, Pinzon de Palos, Columbus' pilot, and other crew members were already suffering from syphilis when they returned from the New World, according to a manuscript by Ruy Diaz de Isla.
1798	**Smallpox:** Between fifth and seventh centuries saw the introduction of smallpox to Europe, and the Middle Ages saw repeated epidemics of the disease. The Spanish and Portuguese conquistadors imported smallpox, which was unknown in the New World. Bishop Marius of Avenches (located close to Lausanne, Switzerland) first used the term "variola" to describe smallpox in 570 AD. Its origins are in the Latin words varius, which means "stained", or varus, which means "mark on the skin". In order to distinguish the illness from syphilis, which was then known as the large pockes, the word "small pockes" (pocke meaning "sac") was first used in England around the end of the 15th century.
1817	**Cholera:** The first cholera pandemic, also known as the first Asiatic cholera pandemic or Asiatic cholera, originated close to the city of Calcutta and spread over South and Southeast Asia to the Middle East, Eastern Africa, and the Mediterranean coast. It lasted from 1817 to 1824. In centuries past, infections including nausea and vomiting were referred to as cholera. Today, the term "cholera" refers particularly to a disease brought on by the Vibrio cholerae bacteria.

Year	Infectious diseases
1918-1920	**Influenza (Spanish flu):** The influenza virus, which spreads by respiratory droplets generated when an infected person coughs, sneezes, or talks, is responsible for influenza, a contagious respiratory illness. The 1918 flu pandemic, sometimes referred to as the Great Influenza epidemic or the Spanish flu because to its widespread misconception, was a particularly lethal worldwide influenza pandemic brought on by the H1N1 influenza A virus. The United States' state of Kansas reported the first case in March 1918. In April, cases were also reported in France, Germany, and the United Kingdom. Two years later, four subsequent waves of infection had affected over 500 million people worldwide, or close to one-third of the world's population. Death toll estimates range from 17 million to 50 million.
1981	**AIDS:** Beginning in January 1981, medical professionals in Los Angeles, New York, and San Francisco all reported that some of their gay male patients had odd symptoms. Immune system health was affected in all of the individuals. Since the bizarre new illness mainly affected gay males, it was initially called "gay cancer". Researchers identified the disease-causing virus, known as the Human Immunodeficiency Virus (HIV), two years into the epidemic, but it took another two years for the first HIV test to be approved for use in the United States. By that time, the illness had claimed the lives of nearly 9,000 people, with half of them already deceased. LGBT and bisexual men made almost 70 per cent of the cases that were officially reported, and the epidemic wreaked havoc on the LGBT community.
2019	**COVID-19:** Since its breakout in 2019, COVID-19, a respiratory infectious disease brought on by the SARS-CoV-2 virus, has expanded quickly throughout the world. Respiratory droplets, surfaces, and close contact with sick people are all routes by which the disease is spread. Johns Hopkins University & Medicine reports that there have been 3.8 million fatalities and 177 million documented cases worldwide.

Source: Compiled by author from various sources.

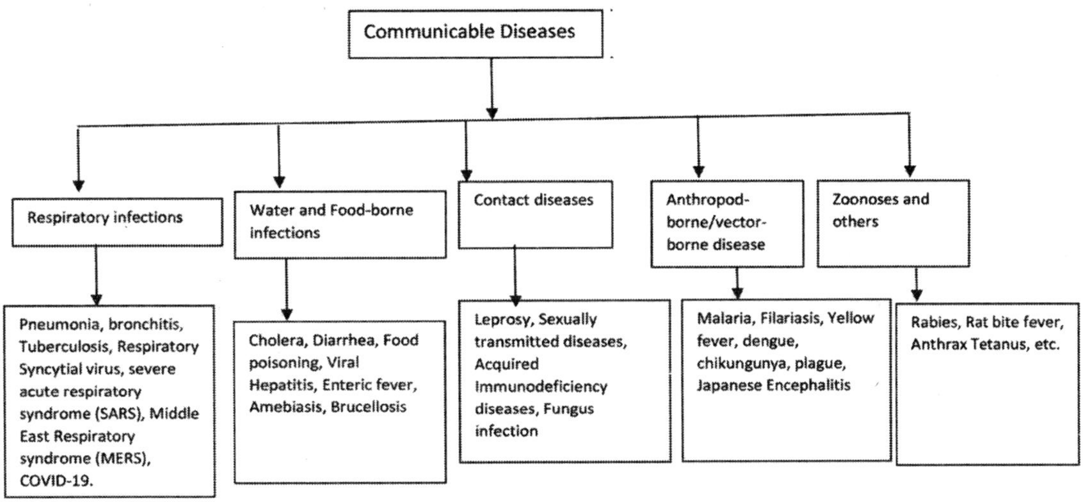

Fig. 4.1: Classification of Communicable Diseases.

Source: Compiled by Author.

4.2 Spatial Epidemiology of Infectious Diseases

Spatial epidemiology is the study that deals with distribution of health outcomes and diseases. It deals with disease mapping, geographic correlation studies and surveillance and clustering.

It encompasses collection, handling and management of data and its analysis linked to various health parameters. It is considered to be the core of health geography. Spatial epidemiology is the description and analysis of geographic variations in disease with respect to demographic, environmental, behavioural, socio-economic, genetic, and infectious risk factors (Elliot and Warternberg, 2004). Spatial epidemiology extends the rich tradition of ecologic studies that use explanations of the distribution of diseases in different places to better understand the etiology of disease (Doll, 1980; Keys, 1980). Spatial epidemiology is increasingly being used to assess health risks associated with environmental hazards. Risk patterns tend to have both a temporal and a spatial component; thus, spatial epidemiology must combine methods from epidemiology, statistics, and geographic information science. Recent statistical advances in spatial epidemiology include the use of smoothing in risk maps to create an interpretable risk surface, the extension of spatial models to incorporate the time dimension, and the combination of individual- and area-level information. Advances in geographic information systems and the growing availability of modelling packages have led to an improvement in exposure assessment (Beale *et al.*, 2008). The spatial component of health data can play a crucial part in helping explain variability in risk because health status, environmental hazards, population numbers, demographic and socio-economic profiles, and other relevant characteristics (e.g. susceptibility and exposures) all vary across space. In this sense, geographic space varies uniquely in different locations and at different times and creates unique places in which people live and work. Geography defines the spatial context and character in which health risks occur. Any movement between places is significant (Wakefield *et al.*, 2001); pollution and other hazards that form concentrations can be modified as they move through the environment and affect different places in different ways, whereas spatial patterns in risk will be complicated by differences in susceptibility and by variations that arise simply because populations are unique to particular places (Beale *et al.*, 2008). This chapter discusses only selected diseases.

Anthropod/Vector Borne Diseases

Vector-borne diseases refer to infectious diseases that are transmitted from an infected organism to a human host by a vector such as mosquito, flies, ticks, or rodents. Here is a brief chronological history of the occurrence of vector-borne diseases:

(a) **Malaria (2700 BC to present):** Malaria is one of the oldest infectious diseases and has been present for thousands of years, recorded in ancient Chinese medical texts and hieroglyphics in ancient Egypt. This disease is transmitted by the Anopheles mosquito and continues to be a significant health burden, especially in Africa.

(b) **Yellow Fever (1648-ongoing):** Yellow fever emerged as a significant infectious disease in the 17th century during the slave trade from Africa to the Americas. The virus is transmitted by Aedes or Haemagogus mosquitoes that bite humans and non-human primates. A vaccine against yellow fever became available in the 1930s.

(c) **Plague (1855-ongoing):** Plague, caused by the bacterium Yersinia pestis, is transmitted by fleas that feed on infected rodents. The disease caused three major pandemics throughout history: the Justinian Plague, the Black Death, and the Third Pandemic. The disease is still present in some parts of the world and is treatable with antibiotics.

(d) **Zika Virus Disease (1947-ongoing):** The Zika virus causes a mosquito-borne illness that emerged in the Zika Forest of Uganda. In 2015, an outbreak occurred in Brazil and eventually spread to other countries worldwide. The virus is transmitted by Aedes mosquitoes, which also transmit dengue and chikungunya viruses.

(e) **West Nile Virus (1999-ongoing):** West Nile virus is transmitted to humans through the bites of infected mosquitoes. It was first detected in Uganda in 1937 but was identified in the United States in 1999. The virus has since been reported in many countries and can cause neurological diseases in humans.

Vector-borne diseases have been prevalent throughout history, and they continue to be a significant global public health concern. As the world becomes more interconnected, early detection, preparation, prevention, and treatment of vector-borne diseases will be critical for global health security measures.

4.2.1 *Plague*

The Plague is a highly infectious disease caused by the bacterium Yersinia pestis. The germs mostly live in small rodents and their fleas. The Bubonic plague is the most common and is caused by the bite of an infected flea. It is a rare disease. Plague usually can be treated with antibiotics. If not treated, the illness is often deadly. People infected with plague usually develop influenza-like symptoms after an incubation period of 3-7 days. Symptoms include fever, chills, aches, weakness, vomiting and nausea (who.int).

Three ways in which humans can be infected for plague are:

- the bite of infected vector fleas,
- unprotected contact with infectious bodily fluids or contaminated materials, and
- the inhalation of respiratory droplets/small particles from a patient with pneumonic plague.

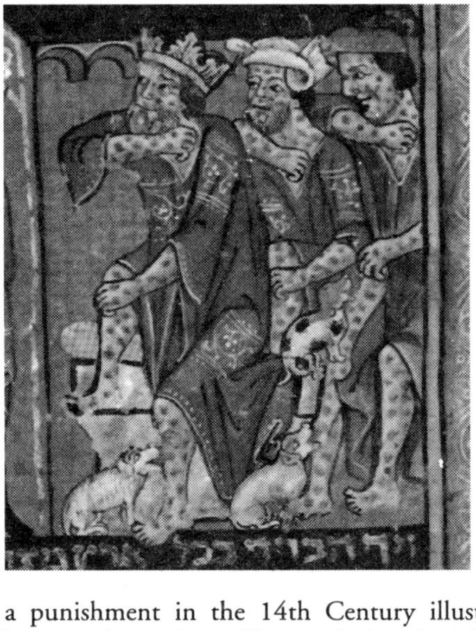

Fig. 4.2: Plague is portrayed as a punishment in the 14th Century illustration (Credit: Rylands Library, University of Manchester) retrieved from/www.bbc.com/culture/article/20200514-how-art-has-depicted-plagues.

(a) *First recorded outbreak (541-542 AD):* The first recorded outbreak of the Plague, known as the Justinian Plague, occurred in the Eastern Roman Empire affecting Constantinople and other cities (Brazilian empire). The disease reportedly killed about 5,000 people a day. It spread to various countries of Europe, Asia and Africa. An estimated 25 million people or more died during this outbreak.

(b) *The Black Death (1347-1353):* The most infamous plague outbreak occurred in Europe in the 14th century, known as the Black Death. This epidemic originated in Asia, and the bacteria travelled along trading routes to the Mediterranean ports, where it rapidly spread across Europe. Ships from the East arrived Italy with their crews dying of a strange illness. The disease spread from the ships to the port towns and further. Within few months, the disease spread to France, Italy and Iberian peninsula. The literature shows the impact was so bad that healthy people were found dead next morning in their beds and the wild wolves especially in Dubrovnik were found on streets feeding on deads. Doctors were unable to help as the disease was untreatable. It is estimated that the Black Death killed around 25 million people, which amounted to one-third of Europe's population. This second pandemic, which lasted more than 130 years, had major political, economic, cultural, and religious ramifications.

(c) *Third Pandemic (1855-1959):* This pandemic began in China and spread across the world *via* global trade and transportation during the nineteenth century. It hit Canton in 1894, where it caused 70,000 deaths, and then appeared in Hong Kong. Ships carried it to Japan, India, Australia, and North and South America between 1910 and 1920.The third pandemic is estimated to have caused 15 million deaths globally, with significant outbreaks reported in India, China, and California. Plague spread rapidly throughout the world through all inhabited continents, except Australia. Rats aboard the faster steamships that had replaced slow-moving sailing vessels in merchant fleets carried the disease. Between the years 1894 and 1903, plague had entered 77 ports on 5 continents. Since then, smaller outbreaks have occurred around the world. During the early years of this third pandemic, the ultimate death toll in India and China alone was 12 million. In 1900, plague was introduced into North America (San Francisco), and between 1900 and 1924 most plague cases in the USA occurred in port cities along the Pacific and Gulf coasts (Link, 1955).

(d) *Modern Plague Outbreaks:* Since then, there have been isolated outbreaks of plague across the world, including in Africa, Asia, and the Americas. Madagascar experienced a large outbreak in 2017 and 2018, which resulted in more than 2,300 cases and over 200 deaths. Three endemic countries since 1990s—Democratic Republic of Congo, Madagascar and Peru—are the three most endemic countries.

Throughout history, the plague has been a highly infectious disease that has caused significant destruction and loss of life. Although modern medicine and public health initiatives have greatly reduced the severity of plague outbreaks, preventative measures such as identifying and isolating people with the disease, targeted use of antibiotics, and public health education is crucial for dealing with the threat of the plague.

In India, the bubonic and pneumonic plagues were first reported in Bombay (now Mumbai) in 1896. Bombay was one of the most important ports and commercial centres in India during colonial times. The city was inhabited by 8 lakh people. The municipal committee, at that time instigated a policy of isolating plague victims, disinfecting or destroying infected dwellings, and inspecting travellers. However, these measures not only failed to stem the spread of the disease, but also proved unpopular and exacerbated the mass exodus from the city which had been caused by the outbreak. By March 1897, hundreds of thousands of people had fled and the plague's death toll stood at around 20,000. It had also begun to spread inland and would eventually afflict many parts of the country (www.nam.ac.uk) leading to thousands of deaths and widespread fear and panic. Plague is a rare disease in India. In September 1994, the city of Surat, in the state of Gujarat in western India, witnessed a plague. It was a pneumonic preceding a bubonic plague. Around 2 lakh people fled from the city. It got spread to five states, namely Maharashtra (488 cases), Gujarat (77 cases), Karnataka (46 cases), Uttar Pradesh (10 cases), Madhya Pradesh (4 cases) and New Delhi (68 cases). According to the studies, the ultimate cause as the 1993 Latur earthquake, which caused a large number of homes to be abandoned with food grains inside. This destabilized the population of domestic and wild rats (in which the plague is endemic), allowing transmission of the plague from wild rats to domestic rats to people (Basu and Mohana, 2020). The flood in Surat led to spread of dead rats in open streets and later the people came in contact with these rats leading to spread of disease. Almost 80 per cent of the infectants belonged to slum areas.

According to National Health Profile 2019, the cases of plague are less than 20-25 in entire India mainly concentrated in Himachal Pradesh, Karnataka and Maharashtra. Maximum number of deaths occurred in Mumbai followed by Punjab, Bengal and United Provinces respectively (1896-1904). Western India was severely affectd in 1994 plague. Around 693 suspected cases and 56 deaths were reported from the five affected Indian states as well as the Union Territory of Delhi. These cases were from Maharashtra (488 cases), Gujarat (77 cases), Karnataka (46 cases), Uttar Pradesh (10 cases), Madhya Pradesh (4 cases) and New Delhi (68 cases). There are no report of cases being exported to other countries (CDC, 2015).

4.2.2 *Malaria*

Malaria is the disease often associated with marshy regions and was once considered to be caused by bad air or "miasma". The Roman writer, Celsus, later called it "quartan fever" due to its recurring pattern every fourth day. Scientists at the University of Rome have found evidence showing that falciparum malaria came from Africa, underwent mutations in Sardinia and was introduced in the marshy, mosquito-infested Tiber River basin by the fifth century. Dr. Frank Romer, a Roman historian at Arizona, noted accounts of pestilence spreading through the countryside at this time and causing "sweats and chills", symptoms typical of malaria. It was in 452, a year or two after the infant burials, that Attila, marching towards Rome, suddenly decided against entering the city (nytimes.com).

The true cause of malaria was not known until the late 19th century when the link between the disease and mosquito bites was discovered. In 1880, French army surgeon Charles Louis Alphonse Laveran identified the malaria parasite in red blood cells. In 1897, Ronald Ross, a British physician, demonstrated that malaria is transmitted through the bites of infected mosquitoes. Malaria has had a significant impact on human history and continues to be a major public health concern today. It has influenced the outcome of wars and shaped the socio-economic development of affected regions. Malaria's prevalence has limited settlement in certain areas and hindered economic progress, especially in tropical and subtropical regions where the disease is endemic.

Malaria is prevalent in Sub-Saharan Africa, but is also found in parts of Asia, Latin America, and the Middle East. Nearly forty per cent of the population of South East Asian region resides in malaria prone region. This is due, in part, to the presence of mosquitoes that can spread the disease in these regions. Although malaria was once present in many parts of the world, it has been largely eradicated in North America and Europe. Globally, the total number of malaria cases increased to an estimated 241 million (UI 218-269 million) in 2020, up from 227 million (UI 208 to 248 million) in 2019. The WHO African Region accounted for most of the 14 million increase. About 96 per cent of malaria deaths globally were in 29 countries. Six countries—Nigeria (27%), the Democratic Republic of the Congo (12%), Uganda (5%), Mozambique (4%), Angola (3%) and Burkina Faso (3%)—accounted for just over half of all malaria deaths globally in 2020. The WHO Western Pacific Region had an estimated 1.7 million cases in 2020, a decrease of 39 per cent from the 3 million cases in 2000. Over the same period, malaria case incidence reduced from four to two cases per 1000 population at risk. Papua New Guinea accounted for nearly 86 per cent of all cases in this region in 2020. China was certified malaria free in 2021 and Malaysia had no cases of non-zoonotic malaria for 3 consecutive years. In the WHO Region of the America, malaria cases reduced by 58 per cent (from 1.5 million to 0.65 million) and case incidences by 67 per cent (from 14 to 5) between 2000 and 2020. The region's progress in recent years has suffered from the major increase in malaria in the Bolivarian Republic of Venezuela, which had about 35,500 cases in 2000 and more than 4,67,000 cases by 2019. In 2020, cases reduced by more than half compared with 2019, to 2,32,000, owing to restrictions on movement during the COVID-19 pandemic and a shortage of fuel that affected the mining industry, which is the main contributor to the recent increase in malaria in the country. These restrictions may also have affected access to care, reducing cases reported from health facilities (World Malaria Report, 2021).

It can be seen from Fig. 4.3 no ongoing malaria transmission has happened in North America, Canada, Russia and Europe. According to World Malaria Report, 2022, the African Region continues to shoulder the heaviest burden of malaria. Globally in 2021, the Region accounted for 95 per cent of all malaria cases (234 million cases); 96 per cent of all malaria deaths (5,93,000 deaths) and nearly 80 per cent of all malaria deaths were among children under the age of 5. The case incidence and mortality rates in the Region increased in the first year of the pandemic, between 2019 and 2020, and then declined from 2020 to 2021 (World Malaria Report, 2022). Nearly four countries also accounted for just over half of all malaria deaths globally are Nigeria (31.3%), the Democratic Republic of the Congo (12.6%), the United Republic of Tanzania (4.1%) and Niger (3.9%). In South East Asia, by 2021, seven of the nine endemic countries in the region saw reductions in case incidence of 40 per cent or more compared to a 2015 baseline: Bangladesh, Bhutan, the Democratic People's Republic of Korea, India, Nepal, Thailand and Timor-Leste (World Malaria Report, 2022).

In India, nine Anopheline vectors are involved in transmitting malaria in diverse geo-ecological paradigms. About 2 million confirmed malaria cases and 1,000 deaths are reported annually, although 15 million cases and 20,000 deaths are estimated by WHO, South East Asia

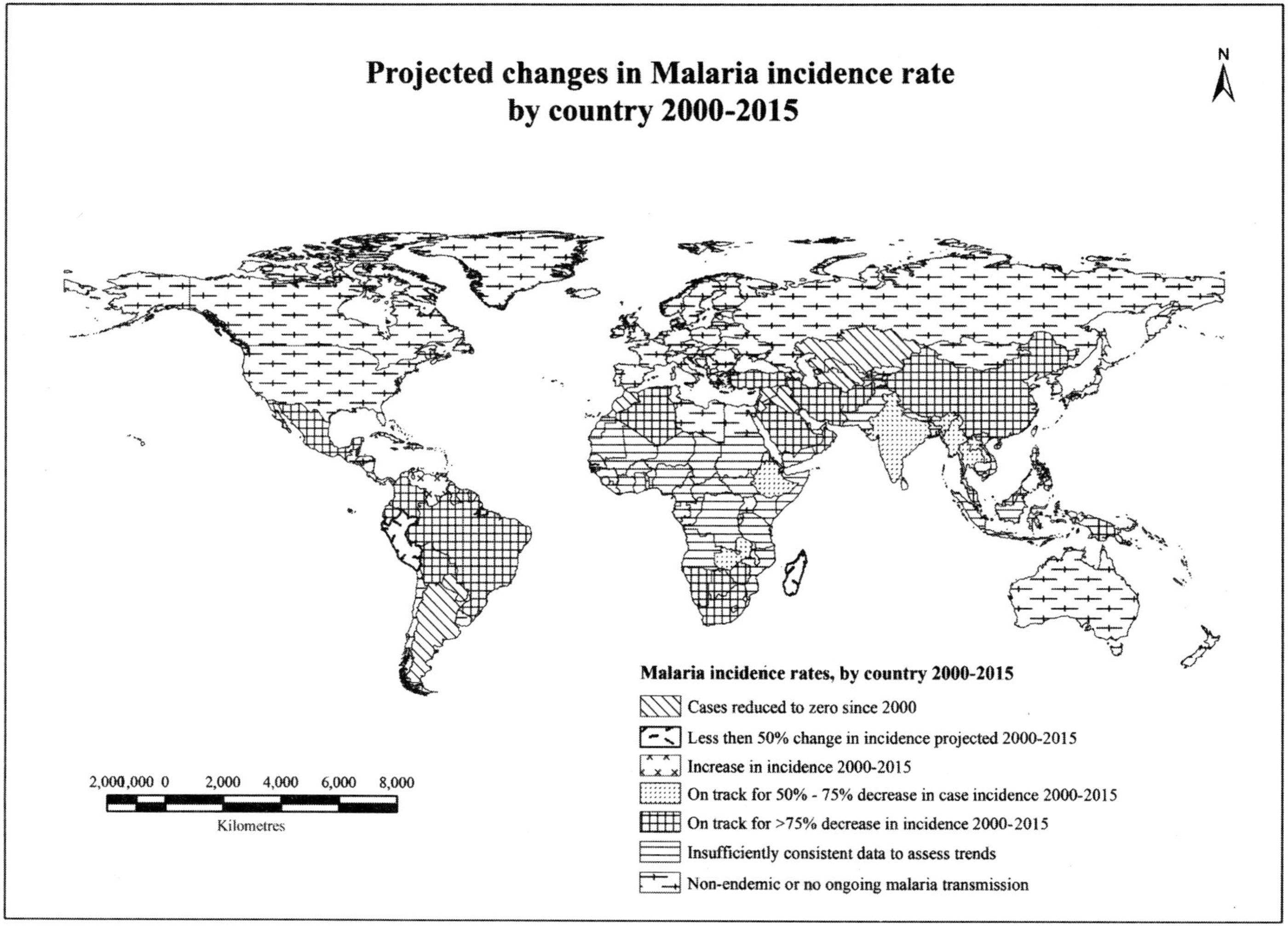

Fig. 4.3: Projected changes in Malaria incidence rate by country—2000-2015.

Source: Adopted from WHO, 2018.

Regional Office. India contributes 77 per cent of the total malaria in Southeast Asia (Kumar *et al.*, 2007). In India, the epidemiology of malaria is complex because of geo-ecological diversity, multi-ethnicity, and wide distribution of nine anopheline vectors transmitting three Plasmodial species: *P. falciparum, P. vivax,* and *P. malariae. Anopheles culicifacies* is widely distributed and is the principal vector of rural malaria, *An. stephensi* is the primary urban vector, *An. fluviatilis* is a vector in the hills and foothills, and *An. minimus, An. nivipes, An. philippinensis,* and *An. dirus* are vectors in the northeast and *An. sun-daicus* is restricted to Andaman and Car Nicobar islands. *An. annularis* and *An. varuna* are secondary vectors with wide distribution (Kumar *et al.*, 2007). Before 1953, the incidences of malaria in India were as high as around 75 million per year. In 2003, about 1.65 million cases and 933 deaths due to malaria were reported. During 2008, about 88 per cent of malaria cases and 97 per cent of death cases due to malaria in India were reported from high disease burden states, namely NE states, Odisha, Andhra Pradesh, Maharashtra, Gujarat, Rajasthan, West Bengal and Karnataka. At state level, Odisha contributes around 25 per cent of Malaria cases followed by Chhattisgarh, West Bengal, Jharkhand, and Karnataka respectively. Together these states contribute around 90 per cent of malaria cases of India.

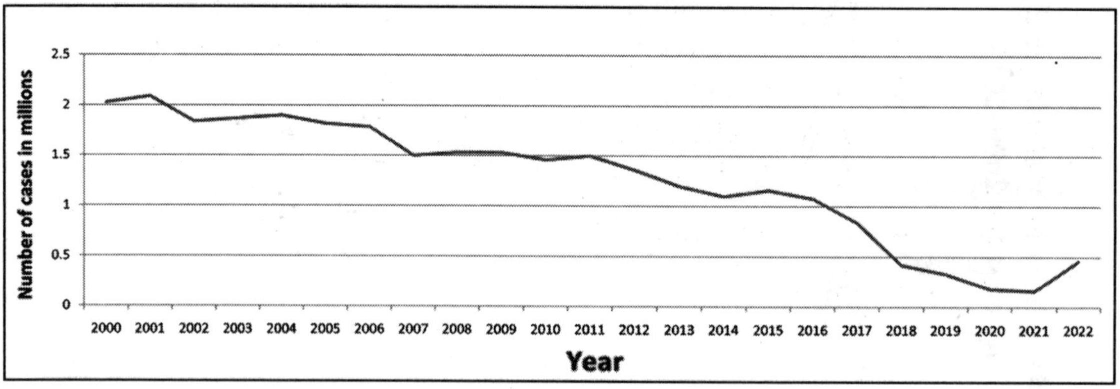

Fig. 4.4: Cases of Malaria in India (2000-2022).

Source: www.statista.com and World Malaria Report, 2008.

4.2.3 *Dengue Fever*

Dengue fever is caused by bite of female *A. aegypti*, a domestic mosquito which is the most common vector. The incubation period is 8 to 10 days during which the transmitted virus multiplies in salivary glands. Two severe manifestions of Dengue fever are: (a) Dengue Haemorrhagic Fever (DHF), and (b) Dengue Shock Syndrome (DSS). Dengue is an acute viral infection with potential fatal complications. Dengue fever was first referred as "water poison" associated with flying insects in a Chinese Medical Encyclopedia in 992 from the Jin Dynasty (265-420 AD). The word "dengue" is derived from the Swahili phrase Ka-dinga pepo, meaning "cramp-like seizure". The first clinically recognized dengue epidemics occurred almost simultaneously in Asia, Africa, and North America in the 1780s. The first clinical case report dates from 1789 of 1780 epidemic in Philadelphia is by Benjamin Rush, who coined the term "break bone fever" because of the symptoms of myalgia and arthralgia (quoted from www.globalmedicine.nl/index.php/dengue-fever). DHF was first identified in Malina, Phillipines in

1954. Dengue has become a global problem since the Second World War and is common in more than 120 countries, mainly in Southeast Asia, South Asia and South America (www.who.int).

Dengue fever is prevalent in tropical and subtropical regions around the world, including Southeast Asia, Latin America, and the Caribbean. This is due to the presence of mosquitoes that can spread the disease. While dengue is not common in the United States, the mosquito that spreads the disease has been found in some southern states, such as Florida and Texas. The disease is now endemic in more than 100 countries in the WHO Regions of Africa, the Americas, the Eastern Mediterranean, South-East Asia and the Western Pacific. The Americas, South-East Asia and Western Pacific regions are the most seriously affected, with Asia representing around 70 per cent of the global disease burden. Dengue is spreading to new areas including Europe, and explosive outbreaks are occurring. Local transmission was reported for the first time in France and Croatia in 2010 and imported cases were detected in 3 other European countries. The largest number of dengue cases ever reported globally was in 2019. All regions were affected, and dengue transmission was recorded in Afghanistan for the first time. In the American Region reported 3.1 million cases, with more than 25,000 classified as severe. A high number of cases were reported in Bangladesh (1,01,000), Malaysia (1,31,000), Philippines (4,20,000), Vietnam (3,20,000) in Asia. Dengue continues to affect Brazil, Colombia, the Cook Islands, Fiji, India, Kenya, Paraguay, Peru, the Philippines, the Reunion Islands and Vietnam as of 2021 (WHO, 2020). Almost half of the world's population, about 4 billion people, live in areas with a risk of dengue. Each year, up to 400 million people get infected with dengue. Approximately, 100 million people get sick from infection, and 40,000 die from severe dengue (who.int).

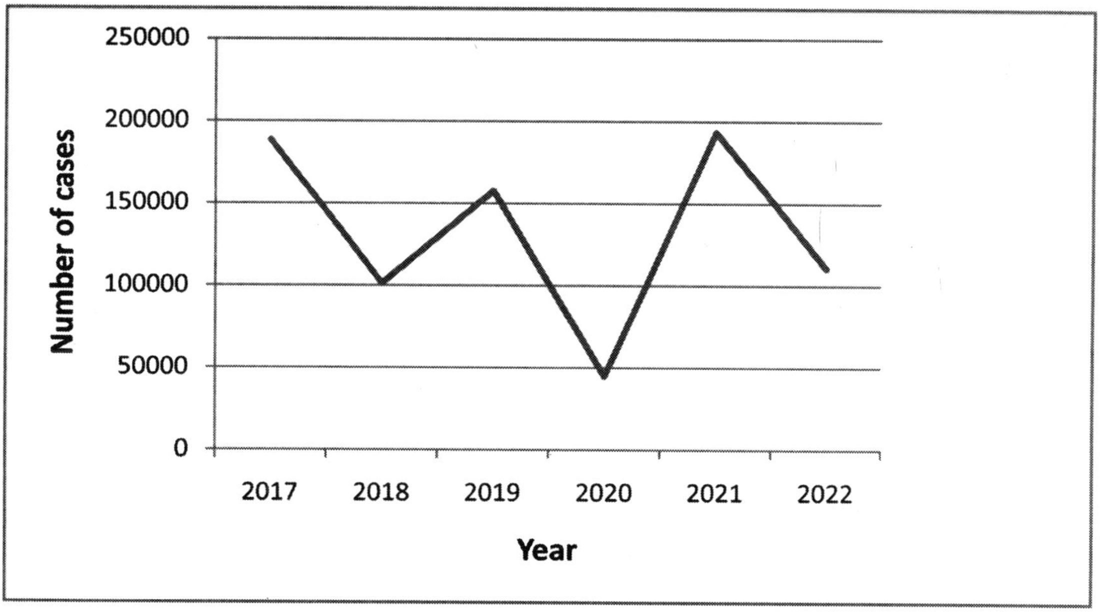

Fig. 4.5: Dengue cases in India.

Source: ncvbdc.mohfw.gov.in

In India, the first epidemic of clinical dengue-like illness was recorded in Madras (now Chennai) in 1780 and the first virologically proved epidemic of dengue fever (DF) occurred in

Calcutta (now Kolkata) and Eastern Coast of India in 1963-64 (Gupta *et al.*, 2012). In India, dengue has occurred in Kokatta (1963), Vishakapatnam and Chennai (1964), Jabalpur (1966), Pondicherry (1968) and various places in North India (1988) and Delhi (1996) (Roy and Saha, 2013). Fig. 4.5 shows that the cases of dengue have fluctuated in last six years. In 2020, during COVID period, the dengue cases fell but it rose in 2021 and declined thereafter. The data of 2013 shows that around 6608 cases of dengue were found in Kerala with 31 deaths. Kerala was followed by Karnataka (4805 cases), Sikkim (3309), Maharashtra (3164), Andhra Pradesh (2718) and Assam (1756) respectively. In 2018, the dengue cases were extremely high in Punjab, Maharashtra, Gujarat and Delhi.

Food and Water-borne Diseases

4.2.4 *Cholera*

Cholera is an infectious disease that affects the small intestine, caused by the bacterium Vibrio cholerae. It is an acute diarrhoeal infection caused by ingestion of contaminated food or water with the bacterium *Vibrio cholerae.*

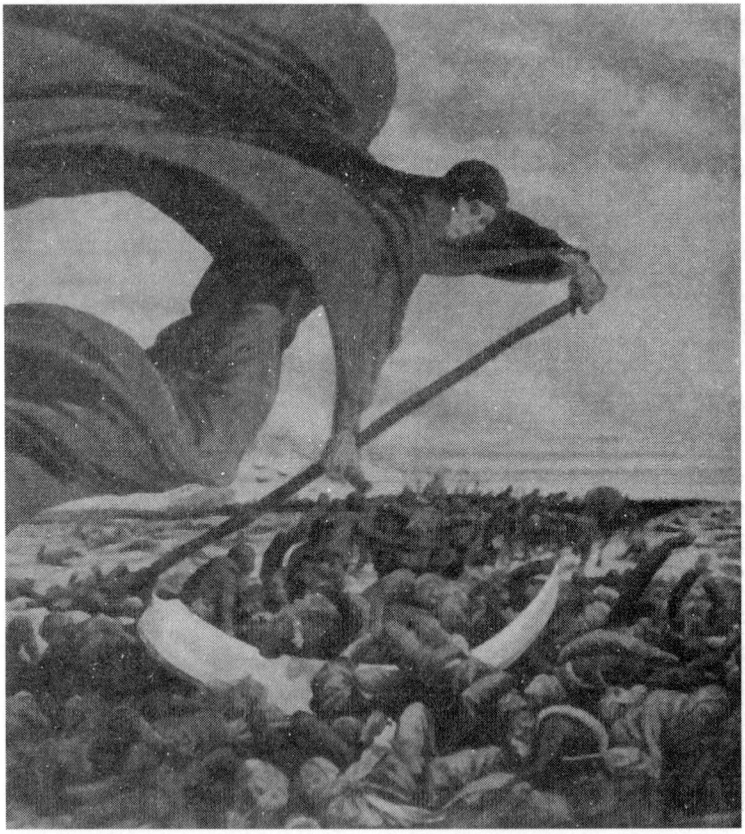

Fig. 4.6: Artwork of Death and troops with cholera, Credit Jean-loup Charmet/science photo library, retrieved from www.sciencephoto.com

(a) *First Cholera Pandemic (1817-1824):* The earliest known pandemic of cholera began in 1817 in India and then spread to South-East Asia, the Middle East, and Africa. It claimed millions of lives and ultimately reached as far as Europe, North America, and South America by 1832.

(b) *Second Cholera Pandemic (1829-1851):* The second pandemic started in India, then spread to Europe, the Middle East, and Africa. The outbreak claimed millions of lives, including prominent people, such as the infant son of Queen Victoria in Britain.

(c) *Third Cholera Pandemic (1852-1860):* The third pandemic started in India and then spread through trade routes to the rest of Asia, the Middle East, Africa, Europe, and the Americas. This pandemic reached its peak between 1852 and 1855 and claimed over one million lives in India alone.

(d) *Fourth Cholera Pandemic (1863-1875):* The fourth pandemic began in the Ganges delta near Calcutta and quickly spread to other parts of Asia, the Middle East, Africa, Europe, and the Americas. The pandemic claimed the lives of approximately 2,00,000 people in Spain and 90,000 in Japan.

(e) *Fifth Cholera Pandemic (1881-1896):* This pandemic began in Bengal, India, and then spread to South-east Asia, the Middle East, and Africa. It caused the deaths of hundreds of thousands of people worldwide.

(f) *Sixth Cholera Pandemic (1899-1923):* This pandemic began in India and then spread to other countries through trade routes. By the end of the 19th century, cholera had become endemic in parts of Africa and Asia.

(g) *Seventh Cholera Pandemic (1961-ongoing):* This pandemic began in Indonesia and spread to other parts of Asia, the Middle East, and Africa. The World Health Organization reported approximately 1.3 million cases of cholera in 2018 alone.

It is important to note that data on cholera are often incomplete and underreporting is common. Several countries do not have reporting systems for cholera (www.who.int). In 2017 and 2019, Yemen accounted for 84 per cent and 93 per cent of all cholera cases respectively (Weekly Epidemiological Report 2018, 2020). In 2021, 23 countries reported cholera outbreaks, mainly in the WHO Regions of Africa and the Eastern Mediterranean. This trend has continued into 2022 with over 29 countries reporting cholera cases or outbreaks, namely Pakistan, Bangladesh, Syria, Cameroon, Somalia etc. All these countries have poor hygienic and sanitation conditions. Deaths were high in Cameroon, Malawi, Nigeria, Syrian Arab Republic and Lebanon etc.

India experienced the first cholera pandemic in 1817, which spread to other countries and continues to be a significant public health concern in India and other parts of the world today. During the 19th century, cholera spread across the world from its original reservoir in the Ganges delta in India. Six subsequent pandemics killed millions of people across all continents. Between 1816 and 1923, the first six cholera pandemics occurred consecutively and continuously over time. Increased commerce, migration, and pilgrimage are credited for its transmission (Tatem *et al.*, 2006). Cholera cases in India have reduced significantly in the past few decades. The case incidence has decreased from more than 1,00,000 per year in the 1980s to less than 1,000 per year in recent years. However, cholera is still a significant public health concern in some regions of India, particularly during the monsoon season when water and sanitation infrastructure are affected.

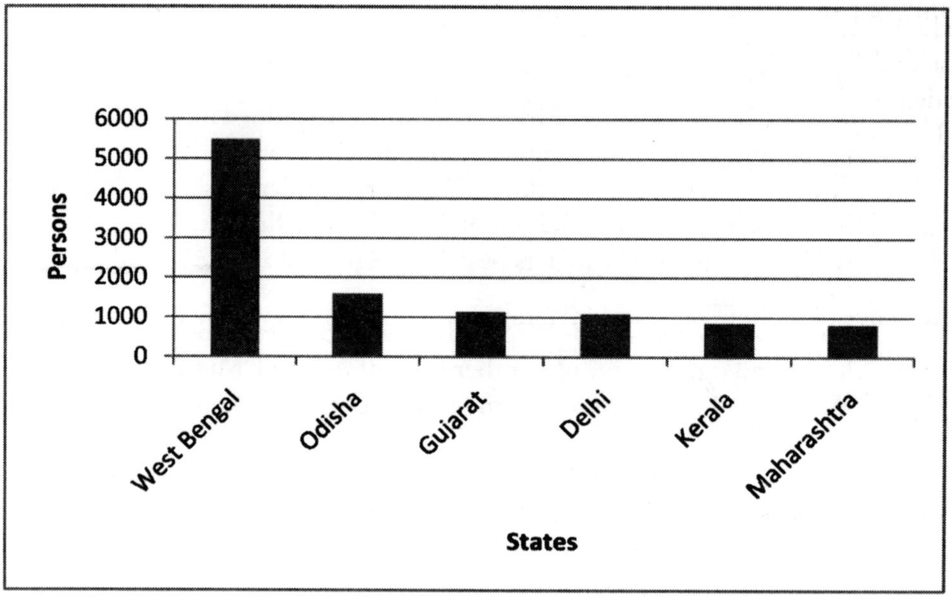

Fig. 4.7: Cholera Cases in India.

Source: National Health Profile, 2020.

Currently, according to National Health Profile 2020, released by Central Bureau of Health Intelligence, West Bengal has the highest cases, i.e., 5489 followed by Odisha 1582, Gujarat 1142, Delhi, Kerala, Maharashtra, Tamil Nadu, Karnataka, Bihar etc.

Despite the availability of vaccines, antibiotics, and better sanitation and hygiene practices, cholera outbreaks still occur today, especially in areas with poor sanitation and inadequate access to clean water. In conclusion, cholera has a history of pandemics that have caused significant global loss of life, but the development of public health initiatives over time has mitigated the effects of the disease in many regions.

4.2.5 *Typhoid*

Typhoid fever is a bacterial infection caused by the bacterium Salmonella typhi. The disease is commonly transmitted through contaminated food and water and is particularly prevalent in regions with poor sanitation and hygiene practices. As of 2019, an estimated 9 million people get sick from typhoid and 1,10,000 people die from it every year. Symptoms include prolonged fever, fatigue, headache, nausea, abdominal pain, and constipation or diarrhoea. Some patients may have a rash. Severe cases may lead to serious complications or even death (who. int). It is still a public health problem in many developing areas of the WHO African, Eastern Mediterranean, South-East Asia and Western Pacific Regions. The number of typhoid cases in developed countries greatly decreased, as a result of changes in sanitation and hygiene. Today, cases of typhoid fever occur throughout the world. Countries with a high endemicity, classified as high-risk regions (incidence >100 cases per 1,00,000 population per year), include South-Central Asia, South-East Asia, and possibly southern Africa (more detailed incidence studies are needed). Medium risk areas (10-100 cases per 1,00,000) are the rest of Asia, Africa, Latin America, and Oceania, except for Australia and New Zealand. In the other parts of the world, the incidence of typhoid fever is low (<10 per 1,00,000) (Colomba *et al.,* 2008).

In India, typhoid fever has been a significant public health concern for many years. Historically, typhoid fever has been a major health problem in India. The disease has caused significant morbidity and mortality, particularly in rural areas where access to health services is limited. The first cases of typhoid fever were recorded in India during the British colonial period, and since then, the disease has continued to be a concern. In recent years, there has been a decline in the incidence of typhoid fever in India, following successful public health interventions such as vaccination and improvements in sanitation and hygiene practices. However, the disease still remains a significant public health problem, particularly in certain states. Fig. 4.8 shows that typhoid cases are highest in Uttar Pradesh followed by Bihar, Madhya Pradesh, Gujarat, Rajasthan, Maharashtra, Assam and Odisha respectively.

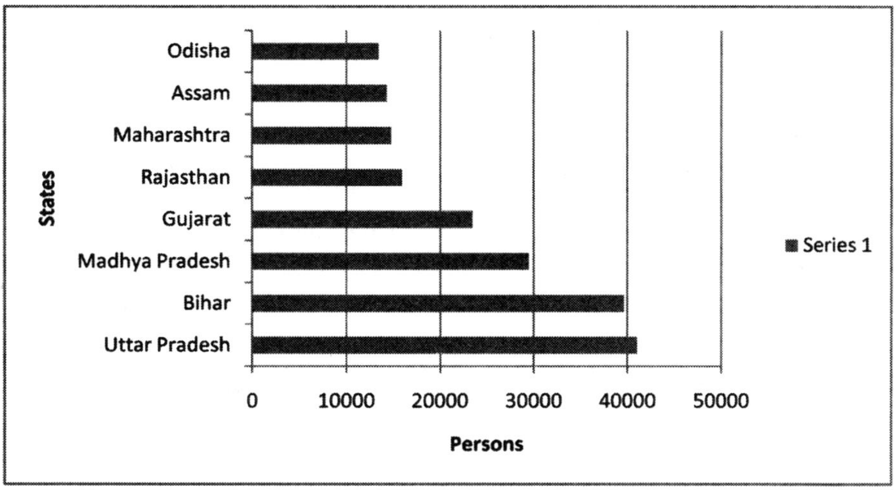

Fig. 4.8: Typhoid cases in India, 2019.

4.2.6 *Hepatitis and Others*

Hepatitis is a group of viral infections that affects the liver. WHO estimated that, in 2019, 296 million people were living with chronic Hepatitis B infection (defined as Hepatitis B surface antigen positive), including about 1.5 million people newly infected with the virus during that year. Hepatitis B prevalence is highest in the WHO African and Western Pacific regions where an estimated 7.5 per cent and 5.9 per cent, respectively, of the adult population have acquired the virus. Prevalence is lower in the South-East Asia (3.0%), Eastern Mediterranean (2.5%) and European regions (1.5%), and in the Region of the Americas (0.5%):

(a) *Hepatitis A (1947—Present):* Hepatitis A is an acute liver infection caused by the Hepatitis-A virus. The first recorded outbreak occurred in 1947 in New Delhi, India. Today, the disease is most prevalent in developing countries, where it is often linked to contaminated food and water.

(b) *Hepatitis B (1965—Present):* Hepatitis B is a viral infection that causes liver inflammation and can lead to serious liver disease. It was first identified in the 1960s. The disease is most prevalent in Asia and Africa, where it is often transmitted from mother to child during birth or early childhood.

(c) *Hepatitis C (1975—Present):* Hepatitis C is a viral infection that can lead to chronic liver disease. It was first identified in the 1970s. Hepatitis C often spreads through infected blood, and people who inject drugs or have unprotected sex are at a higher risk of infection.

(d) *Hepatitis E (1980—Present):* Hepatitis E is a liver infection caused by the Hepatitis E virus. It is often related to contaminated food or water. The disease is most common in developing countries with poor sanitation and hygiene practices.

While much advancement has been made in the prevention and treatment of hepatitis, it remains a significant global health concern. Viral Hepatitis caused an estimated 1.34 million deaths in 2015, with an ongoing prevalence in certain regions. Vaccines have significantly reduced the incidence of Hepatitis A and B, and antiviral treatments are available for hepatitis C. Prevention efforts continue to address the spread of these infections and progress towards global elimination goals.

(e) *Smallpox (1947—1977):* Smallpox is an infectious disease caused by the variola virus that was once prevalent in India. Smallpox was known to be a significant public health threat in India for thousands of years, with evidence of the disease's impact noted in ancient Indian texts. The smallpox vaccine was introduced to India in 1802, and a national vaccination campaign was launched in 1962. With continued efforts to vaccinate, India was declared smallpox-free in 1975. Prior to the eradication of smallpox, India experienced several smallpox epidemics, including the last known outbreak in 1974 in the state of West Bengal.

The distribution of smallpox cases varied across different regions and states in India. In the pre-vaccine era, smallpox was widespread in rural areas where the population had little to no access to healthcare facilities. The disease was often associated with overcrowding, poor sanitation, and low vaccination rates.

According to historical records, the western state of Gujarat was one of the hardest-hit regions by smallpox. Between 1918-19, an estimated 50,000 people in Gujarat died due to smallpox. Other states such as Maharashtra, Uttar Pradesh, and Madhya Pradesh also experienced high smallpox mortality.

During the smallpox vaccination campaign, the Indian government took several measures to ensure a widespread and efficient distribution of the vaccine. Efforts were made to reach remote areas and communities that did not have access to healthcare facilities. Those who were already infected with smallpox were isolated to prevent the spread of the disease. Smallpox was eradicated from India in 1977 after a successful nationwide vaccination campaign.

Respiratory Diseases

Respiratory diseases are any of the diseases and disorders of the airways and the lungs that affect human respiration. Chronic respiratory diseases (CRDs) affect the airways and other structures of the lungs. Some of the most common are chronic obstructive pulmonary disease (COPD), asthma, occupational lung diseases and pulmonary hypertension. In addition to tobacco smoke, other risk factors include air pollution, occupational chemicals and dusts, and frequent lower respiratory infections during childhood (who.int).

4.2.7 *Flu or Influenza*

Influenza is a highly infectious respiratory illness caused by the influenza virus. Seasonal influenza is characterized by a sudden onset of fever, cough (usually dry), headache, muscle and joint pain, severe malaise (feeling unwell), sore throat and a running nose and sometimes the lungs, leading to a range of symptoms from mild to severe. Influenza viruses can undergo genetic changes through two main processes: antigenic drift and antigenic shift. Antigenic drift refers to minor genetic changes that occur over time, leading to gradual changes in the surface proteins of the virus. Antigenic shift, on the other hand, refers to the sudden emergence of a new influenza A virus subtype through significant genetic reassortment. Antigenic shift events have the potential to cause pandemics if the new virus subtype has the ability to efficiently spread in humans.

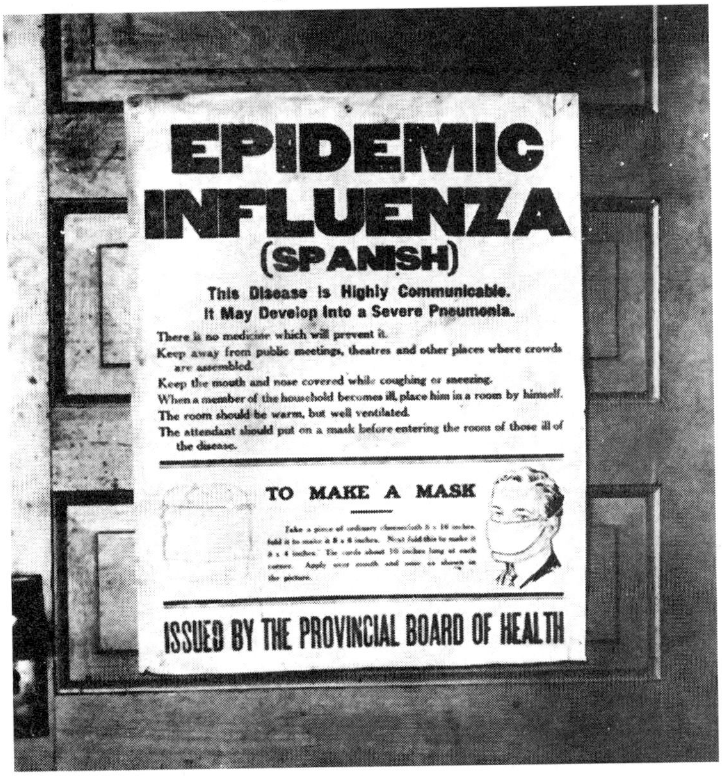

Fig. 4.9: The similarities between instructions issued during the Influenza of 1918 regarding protective protocols and how to make a face mask, and those issued today are startlingly similar...100 years later! Retrieved from/www.gatewayhouse.in/1918-flu-india/

(a) *The Great Influenza Pandemic (1918-19):* The most devastating flu pandemic in history, known as the Spanish flu, killed millions of people worldwide, including an estimated 5,00,000 people in the United States. The pandemic originated in military camps and trenches during World War I and affected more than one-third of the world's population.

(b) *The Asian Flu Pandemic (1957-58):* This pandemic began in China and quickly spread to South-East Asia, Hong Kong, and the United States. The Asian Flu resulted in the deaths of approximately 1.1 million people, including 1,16,000 Americans.

(c) *The Hong Kong Flu Pandemic (1968-69):* The Hong Kong Flu originated in China and quickly spread to Europe and the United States. The pandemic claimed approximately one million lives globally and caused over 1,00,000 deaths in the United States.

(d) *The Swine Flu Pandemic (2009-10):* The H1N1 virus was first detected in Mexico and caused a pandemic that spread to the United States and other countries. It is estimated that the Swine Flu caused approximately 2,84,000 deaths worldwide, including an estimated 12,000 in the United States alone.

(e) *The COVID-19 Pandemic (2019—ongoing):* COVID-19, caused by the SARS-CoV-2 virus, is a respiratory illness that has turned into a global pandemic. The disease was first identified in Wuhan, China in December 2019. It quickly spread across the globe and has since caused millions of deaths worldwide. The COVID-19 pandemic caused by the SARS-CoV-2 virus. According to American Institute for Economic Research, the two primary theories of the origin of SARS-CoV-2 are natural transmission from animals to humans, also called zoonotic transmission, and manipulation in a virus laboratory, most likely the Wuhan Institute of Virology, or WIV. Both theories have merit; neither has been proven or disproven. SARS-CoV-2 is one of seven corona viruses known to infect humans. SARS-CoV-1, MERS-CoV and SARS-CoV-2 are the more dangerous members of the family, while HKU1, NL63, OC43 and 229E are milder (Kristian, 2020). The outbreak of COVID-19 due to the new coronavirus (SARS-CoV-2) began in December 2019 from Wuhan, China, and then spread rapidly throughout China and 202 other countries, including Iran, where it became a tremendous public *health threat*. According to WHO, there have been 8,41,173 cases of COVID-19 virus worldwide, of which 1,80,271 were in USA and 6,60,902 in other countries. Reports also indicate that there was 3,573 deaths in USA and 37,829 deaths in other countries. Countries such as Japan, Thailand, Singapore, Taiwan, and South Korea are among the first countries involved due to their proximity to China. Japan is one of the countries most affected by COVID-19, where officials say was the first to have a cruise ship... Italy is among other European countries where the spread of the disease was extremely worrying. The number of cases in the country has reached 80,589 by March 26, 2020. In addition, European countries such as Spain, Germany, France, Austria, Switzerland, and UK have also reported high cases of COVID-19 conflict (Ahmadi, Dashti and Delgosha, 2020).

India was severely affected during the Spanish flu pandemic that swept across the globe in 1918. The disease claimed an estimated 12.5 million lives in India alone. India has experienced several influenza outbreaks since then, including the H1N1 swine flu pandemic in 2009. Influenza typically spreads through respiratory droplets when an infected person coughs or sneezes. As per Indian government data, the western state of Maharashtra topped the list of states with the highest number of reported cases of influenza in recent years, followed by Gujarat and Karnataka. The northern states of Uttar Pradesh and Delhi are also among the top five states with the highest number of influenza cases. Fig. 4.10 shows that in 2019 Uttar Pradesh reported highest cases of influenza followed by Karnatka, Maharashtra, Tamil Nadu, Rajasthan respvetively.

While influenza occurs year-round in India, the seasonal peak typically occurs during the monsoon season (June-September). To combat the spread of influenza, the Indian government has implemented strategies such as vaccination campaigns, increased surveillance and early detection, and public awareness campaigns. Despite these efforts, the flu remains a significant public health concern in India, particularly among vulnerable populations such as the elderly, young children, and those with compromised immune systems.

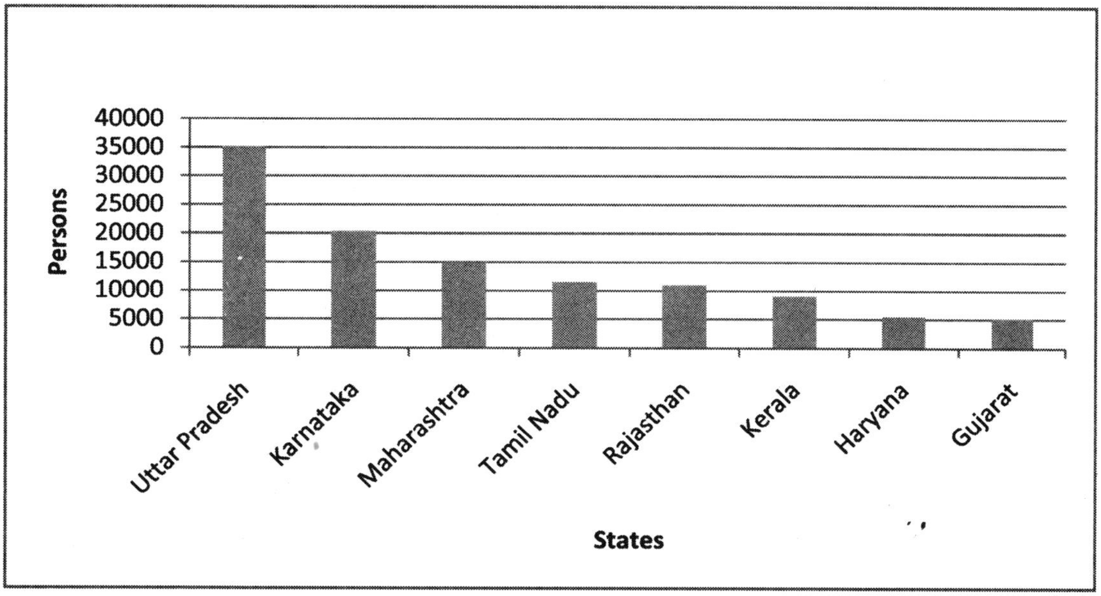

Fig. 4.10: Influenza Cases in India.

Source: National Health Profile 2020 released by the Central Bureau of Health Intelligence.

Influenza outbreaks have the potential to cause severe health concerns, especially among vulnerable groups such as the elderly, young children, and those with weakened immune systems. However, in modern times, preventative vaccines have proven useful in helping to prevent the spread of the flu and minimizing its impact.

4.2.8 *Tuberculosis*

Tuberculosis (TB) is considered to be one of the most infectious diseases in the world. TB is caused by Mycobacterium tuberculosis. It is transmitted through inhalation (droplets of coughing and sneezing), ingestion (unboiled milk and uncooked meat) and surface implantation. Tuberculosis (TB) was called "phthisis" in ancient Greece, "tabes" in ancient Rome, and "schachepheth" in ancient Hebrew. In the 1700s, TB was called "the white plague" due to the paleness of the patients. TB was commonly called "consumption" in the 1800s even after Schonlein named it tuberculosis. During this time, TB was also called the "Captain of all these men of death." Johann Schonlein coined the term "tuberculosis" in the 1834 (www.cdc.gov). It is believed that first trace of TB was found in Atlit Yam, a city now under the Mediterranean Sea, off the coast of Israel.

Tuberculosis is more prevalent in Africa, Asia, and Eastern Europe than in North America and Western Europe. This may be due, in part, to variations in healthcare access, lifestyle, and population density. Reductions in TB case notification were evident in five of the six WHO regions (with large absolute and relative reductions in the South-East Asia (24.0%) and Western Pacific Regions (19.5%). Taken together, these two regions accounted for most (84%) of the

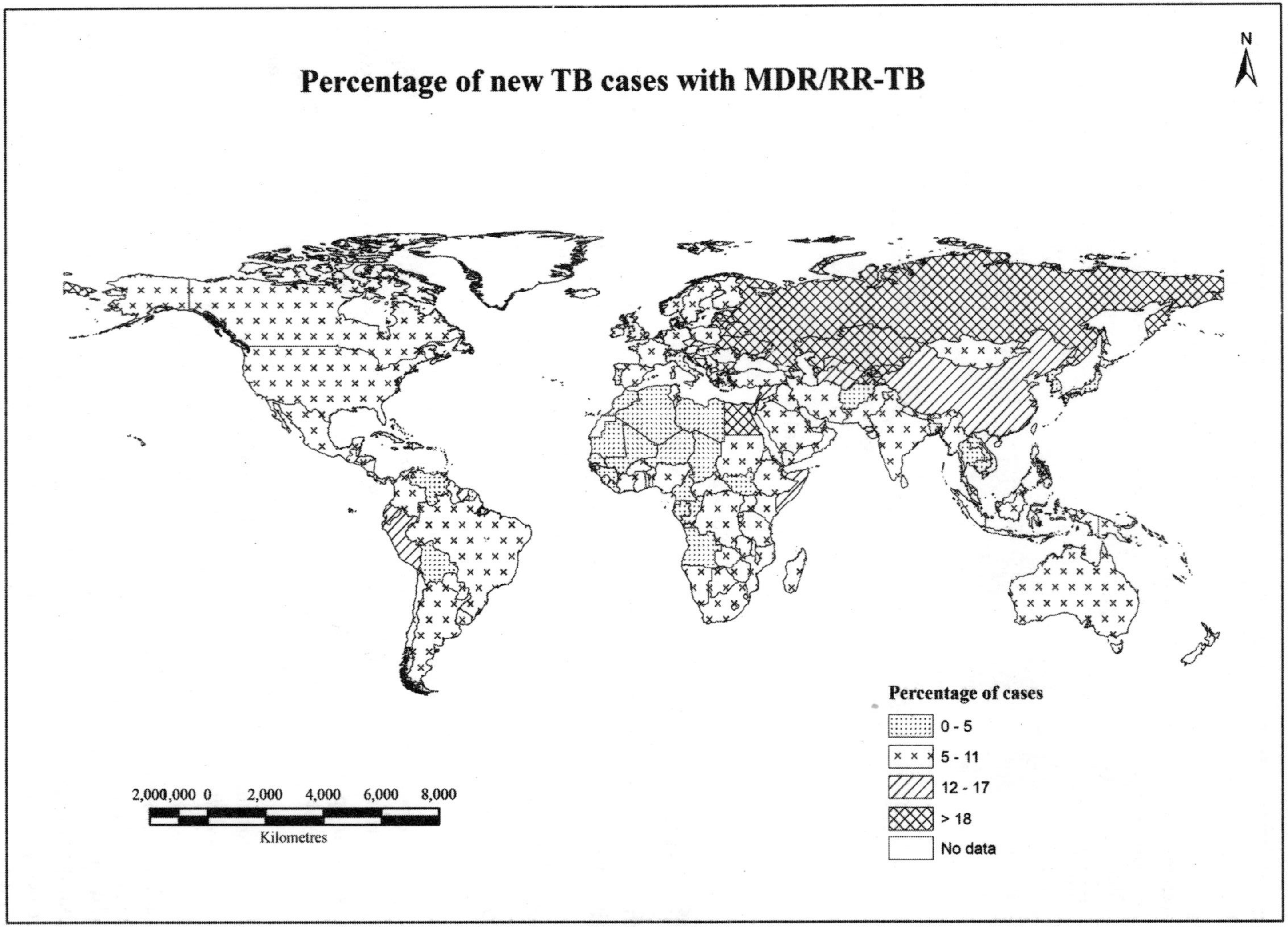

Fig. 4.11: Percentage of New TB Cases.

Source: Adopted from WHO, 2017.

global reduction in notifications of people newly diagnosed with TB between 2019 and 2020. The decline in the WHO African Region was more modest (2.5%). Provisional data up to June 2021 show ongoing shortfalls in diagnoses and reporting. Fewer people received TB preventive treatment in 2020 than in 2019 (3.6 million compared with 2.8 million, a 21% decrease) and fewer people were treated for drug-resistant TB in 2020 than in 2019 (1,50,000 compared with 1,70,000, a 15% decrease) (WHO, 2022). China and El Salvador were certified by WHO as malaria-free in 2021, while the Islamic Republic of Iran attained three consecutive years of zero indigenous cases in 2020 (World Health Report, 2022). According to WHO, a total of 1.6 million people died from TB in 2021 (including 1,87,000 people with HIV). In fact, TB is the thirteenth leading cause of death and the second leading infectious killer after COVID-19 (above HIV and AIDS). In 2021, an estimated 10.6 million people fell ill due to tuberculosis (TB) worldwide. Out of which six million were men, 3.4 million women and 1.2 million children. TB is present in all countries and age groups (who.int).

In India, according to National Tuberculosis Institute, TB is responsible for 53 deaths per lakh population per year. The mortality is higher in older age people. India accounts for 27 per cent of the global estimated 10 million cases and 25 per cent of the estimated 1.6 million deaths. The global burden of disease analysis estimated the number of incident cases to be 3 million people in the year 2016 (Arinaminpathy *et al.,* 2016). A study based on data from the National Family Health Survey (NFHS-4) estimates that the self-reported incidence of TB in India is 304/1,00,000 (Mazumdar *et al.,* 2019).

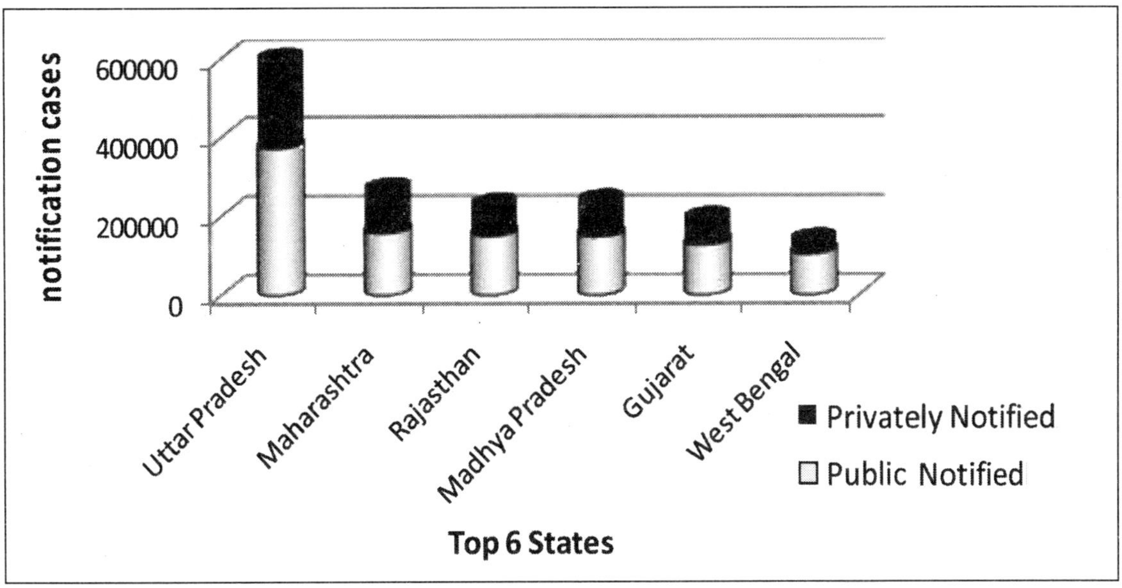

Fig. 4.12: TB notification in India, 2021.

Source: www.statista.com

In 2021, the state of Uttar Pradesh notified highest number of TB cases followed by Maharashtra, Rajasthan, Madhya Pradesh, Gujarat and West Bengal respectively. Very less cases were being reported in North-Eastern states and states of Jammu & Kashmir, Himachal Pradesh, Uttarakhand etc. Reported TB death totals decreased across 28 states, with the largest per cent decrease being seen in Lakshadweep (100% decrease with zero deaths in 2020), Andaman and Nicobar Islands (36.0% decrease), Andhra Pradesh (30.5% decrease), and Manipur (25.7% decrease). Notably, there was a decrease of 3,496 total TB deaths in Uttar Pradesh over this time period (19.0% decrease). Total TB deaths increased in seven states, with the largest per cent increase occurring in Goa (23.6% increase), Arunachal Pradesh (21.9% increase), and Jharkhand (19.3% increase) (Varshney *et al.*, 2015).

4.2.9 *COVID-19*

COVID-19 has spread globally and has rapidly become a pandemic. Coronavirus disease (COVID-19) is an infectious disease caused by the SARS-CoV-2 virus. Most people infected with the virus will experience mild to moderate respiratory illness. The virus can spread from an infected person's mouth or nose in small liquid particles when they cough, sneeze, speak, sing or breathe. These particles range from larger respiratory droplets to smaller aerosols (who.int). The spread and severity of the disease have varied greatly in different regions depending on factors such as population density, access to healthcare, and public health interventions.

The first case of COVID-19 was reported on December 1, 2019 in Wuhan. It is believed that virus originating in bats and mutated to become dangerous to humans. The prevalence of this disease is very high in the western hemisphere, the prevalence of the disease is not very high in the eastern hemisphere irrespective of the economic levels of the countries. A majority of countries with a prevalence of more than 10,000 cases per million are located in the Americas, while a small number of countries in the eastern hemisphere have such a high prevalence. The variation in the COVID-19 mortality rate is much wider than the disease, prevalence in the western and eastern hemispheres. The vast of the countries with death rates of more than 200 death per million are located in the western hemisphere including the Americas and Western European countries while such a high mortality rate has rarely occurred in the countries of the eastern hemisphere (Poorolajal, 2020).

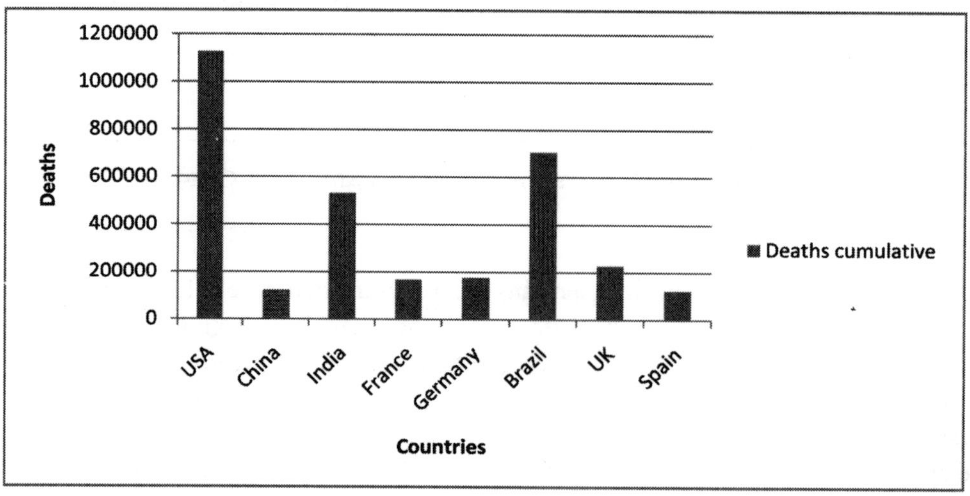

Fig. 4.13: Deaths cumulative due to Coronavirus.

Source: https://covid19.who.int/

Deaths cumulative were high in countries of USA and Europe. China also experienced high mortality during COVID-19. India also registered high mortality due to COVID in 2020-21.

The WHO-defined diseases and disease groups mostly affect impoverished populations in tropical areas. In 2020, approximately 1.73 billion people worldwide required treatment and care for NTDs (Neglected Tropical Diseases). This was considerably fewer than the 2.19 billion people in 2010 and a slight decline (9.5 million) compared with 2019, despite the COVID-19 pandemic, which caused significant disruptions to NTD services (21). In the least developed countries, 502 million people required treatment and care for NTDs in 2020 (representing 48% of those countries' populations, down from 79% in 2010). However, more than 1.2 billion people still required treatment and care for NTDs outside these countries (World Health Report, 2022).

India has experienced a significant outbreak of COVID-19 since 2020, with a high number of cases and deaths and significant strain on the country's healthcare system. The spatial distribution of COVID-19 in India has been uneven, with some regions and states being more affected than others. The pandemic started in India in early 2020 and has spread rapidly, with the entire country reporting cases of the disease.

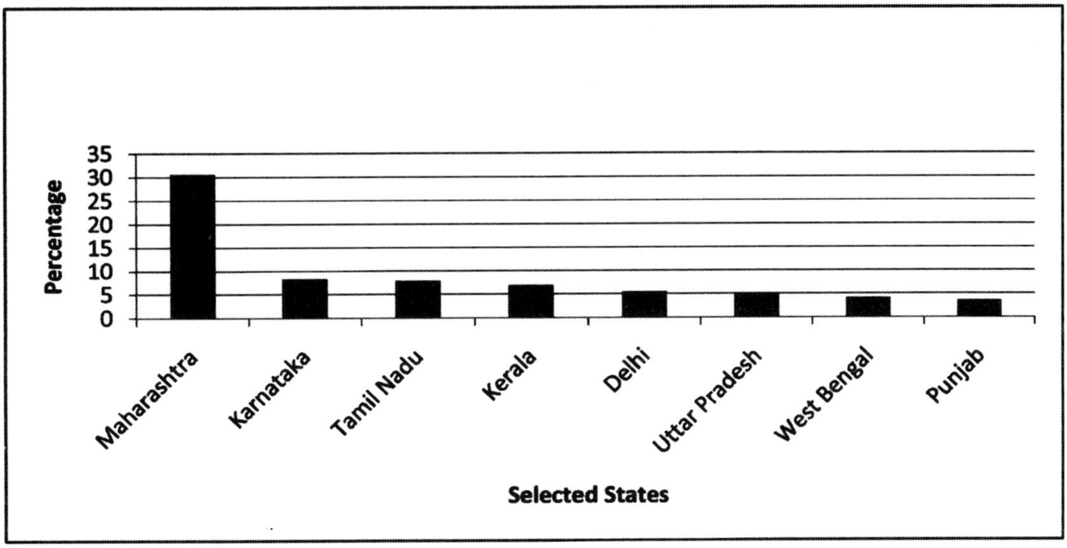

Fig. 4.14: COVID-19 (Percentage of Deceased to Total Cases).

Source: https://www.covid19india.org/

As of November 2021, Maharashtra remains the worst-affected state in India with the highest number of confirmed cases and deaths. Other states that have been significantly impacted by the virus include Kerala, Tamil Nadu, Karnataka, and Delhi. The reasons for the high number of cases in these states are likely due to factors such as population density, urbanization, and inadequate healthcare resources (Fig. 4.14).

The spread of COVID-19 in India has also been influenced by factors such as travel, socio-economic status, and adherence to preventive measures such as wearing masks and social distancing. The disease has affected both urban and rural areas, with the latter being more vulnerable due to lower levels of healthcare facilities and a larger proportion of vulnerable communities such as migrant workers.

Several states in India have implemented measures such as lockdowns, travel restrictions, and curfews to control the spread of the virus. The government has also launched several initiatives such as vaccination drives and community-based surveillance measures to reduce the impact of the pandemic. COVID-19 in India continues to evolve, with new outbreaks and clusters emerging in different parts of the country. The situation remains a significant public health concern, and it is essential to continue to monitor the spread of the virus and implement targeted interventions to control the pandemic.

Contact Diseases: Contact diseases are caused due to surface infection. It can be caused due to coming in direct or indirect contact with the infected person. Contact diseases are also called contagious diseases as they are caused by direct contact. Some are even caused by touching, kissing, sexual intercourse etc.

4.2.10 *Sexually Transmitted Diseases (STDs)*

Sexually transmitted diseases (STDs) have been prevalent throughout history. Sexually transmitted diseases (STDs) are caused by microorganisms that reside on the human skin or in body fluids like blood, semen, and vaginal fluids. When these microorganisms are transmitted from an infected individual to a healthy person, they can result in illness. According to WHO, more than 1 million sexually transmitted infections (STIs) are acquired everyday worldwide, the majority of which are asymptomatic. According to WHO, each year there are an estimated 374 million new infections with 1 of 4 curable STIs: chlamydia, gonorrhea, syphilis and trichomoniasis. When used correctly and consistently, condoms offer one of the most effective methods of protection against STIs, including HIV. Although highly effective, condoms do not offer protection for STIs that cause extra-genital ulcers (i.e. syphilis or genital herpes). When possible, condoms should be used in all vaginal and anal sex. Safe and highly effective vaccines are available for 2 viral STIs: Hepatitis B and HPV. These vaccines have represented major advances in STI prevention (www.who.int).

- **(a)** *Syphilis (1495-ongoing):* Syphilis is a bacterial infection that has been present throughout history and was first documented during the 1495 French invasion of Italy. The disease spreads sexually and can cause severe health problems if left untreated.
- **(b)** *Gonorrhea (1882-ongoing):* Gonorrhea is a bacterial infection that has been recorded throughout history and was first identified in 1882. It is one of the most prevalent sexually transmitted diseases worldwide and can cause infertility and other health complications.
- **(c)** *Chlamydia (1960-ongoing):* Chlamydia is a bacterial infection that mainly affects the genital region and can cause infertility and other complications if left untreated. It was first identified in the early 1960s.
- **(d)** *HIV/AIDS (1980s-ongoing):* HIV/AIDS is a viral infection that damages the immune system and can be transmitted sexually. In Kinshasa in Belgian Congo first case of HIV-1 infection was found in 1959. The disease was reported in the United States in the early 1980s and has since become a global pandemic, affecting millions of people worldwide.
- **(e)** *Human Papilloma Virus (HPV) (1990s-ongoing):* HPV is a viral infection that spreads through sexual contact and is the most common sexually transmitted disease. The

infection often clears up on its own, but certain strains can cause cancer and other health complications.

Sexually transmitted infections have been a global public health issue, and the transmission and prevalence of these infections have been significantly reduced through public education, improved access to healthcare, and innovative treatments. However, the stigma surrounding these diseases remains a significant barrier to encouraging people to seek testing and treatment.

4.2.11 *HIV/AIDS*

The Immunodeficiency Virus (HIV) is classified within the Lenti (slow) viruses of Retroviruses. The virus can generate complimentary DNA upon entry into the host cell. According to WHO, there are two types of viruses in this category, i.e., HIV 1 and HIV 2. Out of these two, HIV-1 is lethal and is widespread in Asia, Europe, Africa and American Continent. HIV 2 is mainly found in West Africa as it is similar to the virus found in monkeys. Studies show that HIV infection in humans came from a type of chimpanzee in Central Africa as far back as the late 1800s. The chimpanzee version of the virus is called simian immunodeficiency virus. It was probably passed to humans when humans hunted these chimpanzees for meat and came in contact with their infected blood. Over decades, HIV slowly spread across Africa and later into other parts of the world. The virus has existed in the United States since at least the mid to late 1970s (www.cdc.gov).

There are different stages of this disease: Stage 1 is called acute HIV infection where a person experiences flu like symptoms. Stage 2 is called chronic HIV infection virus is active in body and can reproduce. It can infect other healthy person too. In stage 3, there is high viral load and severe infection. Person is considered to have AIDS and can live up to three to four years.

The prevalence of HIV/AIDS varies significantly around the world. Sub-Saharan Africa has the highest number of HIV/AIDS cases, but the disease is also prevalent in certain areas of Asia, Eastern Europe, and North America. This is due to a variety of factors, including access to healthcare, education, prevention methods, and rates of high-risk behaviours. According to Global HIV statistics, 38.4 million (33.9 million-43.8 million) people globally were living with HIV in 2021. AIDS-related deaths have been reduced by 68 per cent since the peak in 2004 and by 52 per cent since 2010. In 2021, around 6,50,000 (5,10,000-8,60,000) people died from AIDS-related illnesses worldwide, compared to 2.0 million (1.6 million-2.7 million) people in 2004 and 1.4 million (1.1 million-1.8 million) people in 2010. Certain sub-populations continued to be at heightened risk of HIV infection. In the WHO African Region, adolescent girls and young women (aged 15-24 years) accounted for approximately 25 per cent of all HIV infections in 2020, although they represented only 10 per cent of the total population (UNAIDS, 2021). In all regions, people belonging to key populations are considerably more likely to acquire HIV compared with the overall adult population. According to the Joint United Nations Programme on HIV/AIDS, almost two-thirds of new HIV infections in 2020 were among persons belonging to key populations and their sex partners (UNAIDS, 2021).

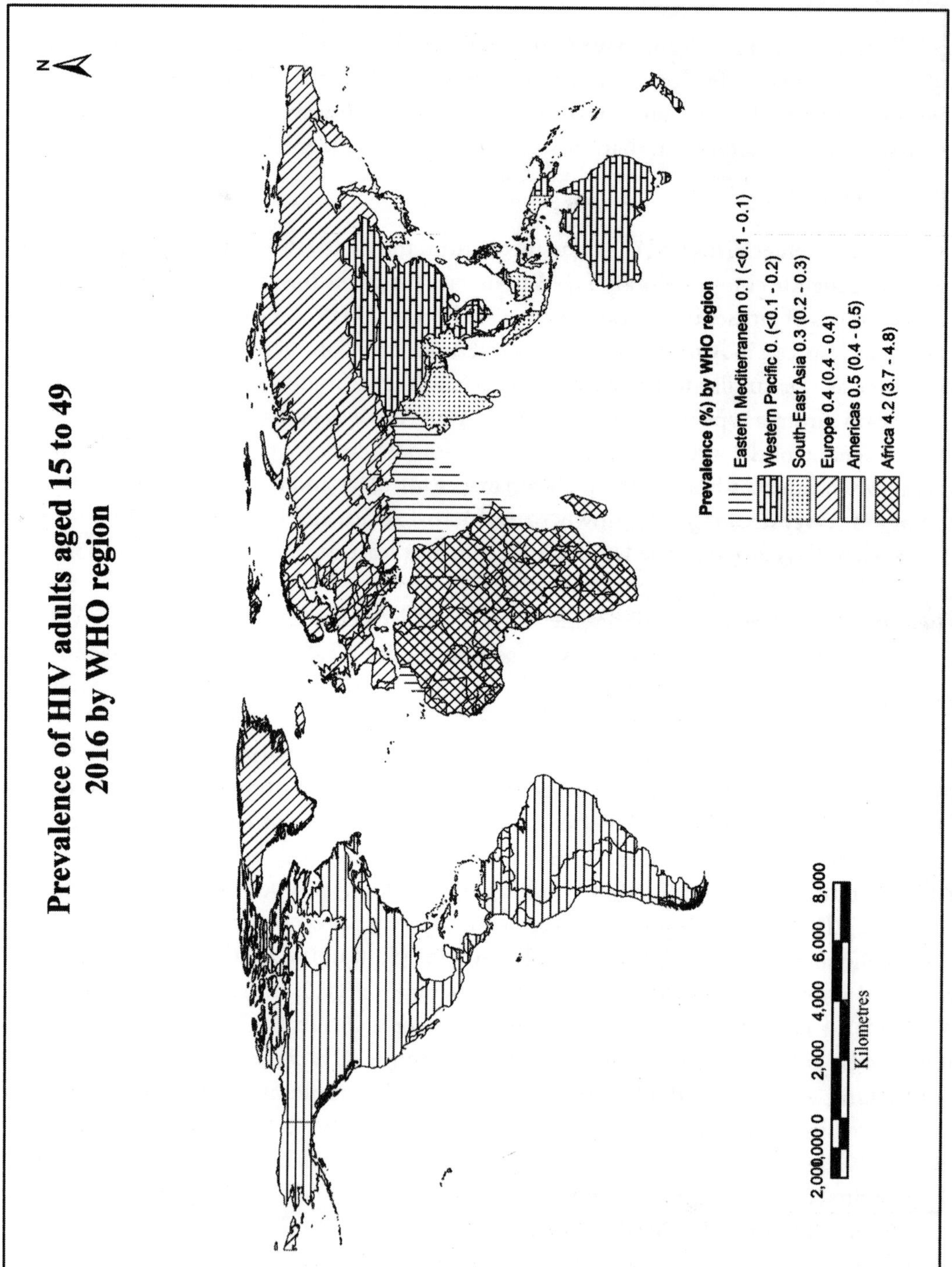

Fig. 4.15: Prevalence of HIV/AIDS age 15-49.

Source: Adopted from WHO, 2017.

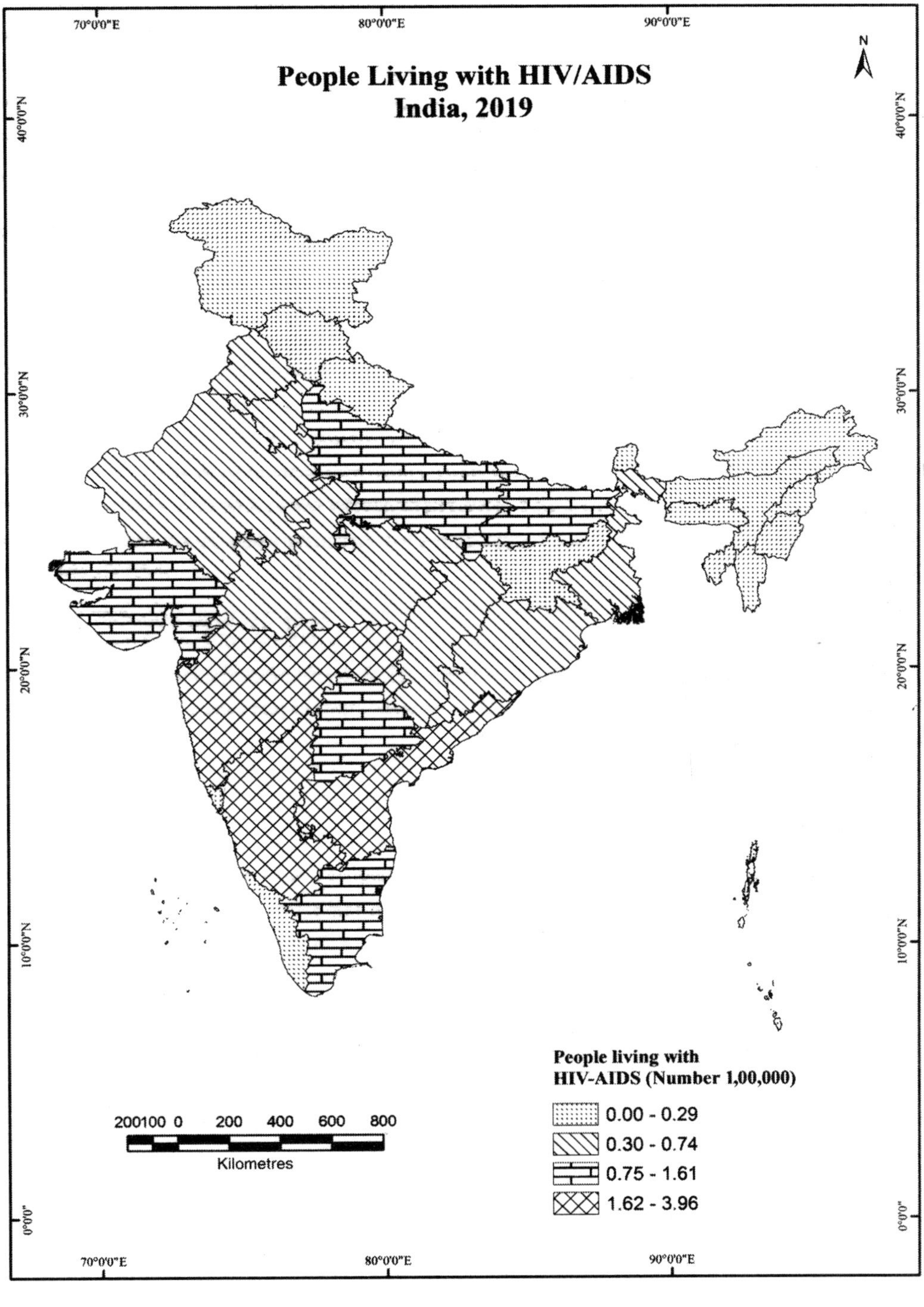

Fig. 4.16: Number of People living with HIV/AIDS, India.

Source: www.unaids.org

According to WHO, HIV remains a major global public health issue, having claimed 40.4 million (32.9-51.3 million) lives so far with ongoing transmission in all countries globally; with some countries reporting increasing trends in new infections when previously on the decline. There were an estimated 39.0 million (33.1-45.7 million) people living with HIV at the end of 2022, two-thirds of whom (25.6 million) are in the WHO African Region. In 2022, 6,30,000 (4,80,000-8,80,000) people died from HIV-related causes and 1.3 million (1.0-1.7 million) people acquired HIV (who.int).

India's first HIV/AIDS case was diagnosed among sex workers in Chennai in 1986. According to 2021 statistics, India has 2.4 million people with HIV and 42,000 AIDS related deaths happened in 2021. As per the recently released, India HIV Estimation 2019 report, Overall, the estimated adult (15-49 years) HIV prevalence trend has been declining in India since the epidemic's peak in the year 2000 and has been stabilizing in recent years. The estimate for this indicator was 0.22 per cent (0.17-0.29%) in 2019. In the same year, HIV prevalence among adult males (15-49 years) was estimated at 0.24% (0.18-0.32%) and among adult females at 0.20 per cent (0.15-0.26%) (naco.gov.in). At the sub-national level, three states with the highest adult HIV prevalence were from the north-eastern part of the country, namely Mizoram (2.32%), Nagaland (1.45%), and Manipur (1.18%). Other states/UTs estimated to have adult HIV prevalence higher than the national average were Andhra Pradesh (0.69%), Meghalaya (0.54%), Telangana (0.49%), Karnataka, Delhi, Maharashtra respectively (naco.gov.in). Since 2007, when the number of AIDS Related Deaths (ARD) started to show a declining trend, the annual number of AIDS related deaths has declined by 54 per cent. In 2015, an estimated 67.6 (46.4-106.0%) thousand people died of AIDS related causes nationally. The reason for decline is government targettted intervention and programmes to make people aware, HIV testing to identify and Vaccine initiatives.

4.2.12 *Leprosy*

Leprosy is a long-term infection caused by the bacteria *Mycobacterium leprae* or *Mycobacterium lepromatosis*. It is believed to spread through cough and cold of an infected person. Genetic and immunity factors are also found to play significant role in how easily a person catches it. It is a highly contagious tropical disease that occurs in around more than 120 countries and is still prevalent with more than 2,00,000 cases every year. In the 1980s, there were 5.2 million cases globally but they went down to fewer than 200 thousand by 2020 (Global leprosy situation, 2019). As per WHO data of 2019, Brazil, India and Indonesia reported more than 10,000 new cases, while 13 other countries (Bangladesh, Democratic Republic of the Congo, Ethiopia, Madagascar, Mozambique, Myanmar, Nepal, Nigeria, Philippines, Somalia, South Sudan, Sri Lanka and the United Republic of Tanzania) each reported 1,000-10,000 new cases. Forty-five countries reported 0 cases and 99 reported fewer than 1,000 new cases. Due to multidrug therapy (MDT) in 1982, the leprosy reduced drastically in world from over 5 million cases in the mid-1980s to less than 2,00,000 at the end of 2016. India declared itself as leprosy free nation when the cases decreased from the rate of 57.8/10,000 in 1983 to less than 1/10,000 by the end of 2005.

The prevalence rate of leprosy has come down from 0.69 per 10,000 population in 2014-15 to 0.45 in 2021-22. Further, annual new case detection rate per 1,00,000 population has come down from 9.73 in 2014-15 to 5.52 in 2021-22. After achieving elimination status at national level, National Leprosy Eradication Programme (NLEP) has taken a number of initiatives to encourage early case detection of leprosy patients to prevent Grade 2 Disabilities, and to ensure free of cost treatment of leprosy patients. There are few districts within States/UTs, where leprosy is endemic. With various interventions introduced under NLEP in the last few years, number of new leprosy cases detected have come down to 75,394 in 2021-22 from 1,25,785 in 2014-15, accounting for 53.6 per cent of global new leprosy cases (pib.gov.in).

Zoonotic Diseases: A zoonotic disease is a disease or infection that can be transmitted naturally from vertebrate animals to humans or from humans to vertebrate animals. More than 60 per cent of human pathogens are zoonotic in origin. This includes a wide variety of bacteria, viruses, fungi, protozoa, parasites, and other pathogens. Factors such as climate change, urbanization, animal migration and trade, travel and tourism, vector biology, anthropogenic factors, and natural factors have greatly influenced the emergence, re-emergence, distribution, and patterns of zoonoses (Rahman *et al.,* 2020). The diseases are more common in rural areas where people come in direct contact with the animals like cattle, horses, pigs, goats etc. The zoonotic diseases get transmitted either through direct contact or through animal origin food. Some zoonotic diseases that can be transmitted to humans from domestic animals include anthrax, rabies, tuberculosis, brucellosis, bovine pustular stomatitis, rotavirus infection etc. Animal deaths caused by zoonotic diseases can impose massive economic losses on the livestock sector of any country. Even if animals do not die, animal health and productivity can still be negatively impacted. This can lead to a significant loss of animal products such as meat, milk, and eggs, which can be more than 70 per cent. Human health and nutrition are also affected due to the reduced supply of high-protein food of animal origin such as milk, meat, and eggs (Arámbulo III and Thakur, 1992).

4.2.13 *Rabies*

Rabies is caused by a virus that spreads by an infected animal biting to another animal or person. It is a disease that affects the nervous system of mammals. Rabies has clinically two forms: Furious rabies—characterized by hyperactivity and hallucinations, and Paralytic rabies—characterized by paralysis and coma. According to WHO, rabies is estimated to cause 59,000 human deaths annually in over 150 countries, with 95 per cent of cases occurring in Africa and Asia. Due to underreporting and uncertain estimates, this number is likely a gross underestimate. The burden of disease is disproportionally borne by rural poor populations, with approximately half of cases attributable to children under 15 years of age (who.int). Interestingly, rabies is present in all the countries leaving aside Antartica. Around 95 per cent of deaths due to rabies occur in Asia and Africa. It basically impacts vulnerable and poor sections of the society.

When the ecological system gets disturbed many zoonotic diseases start impacting human health. For example, we all know that scavengers play role in disease regulation by reducing host and vector densities, through local competitive exclusion, minimising the pathogen numbers or feeding on the hosts directly. For example, leopards in Mumbai (India) have played an important role in controlling of dog population and thus, reduction in the cases of dog bites and transmission of rabies to humans (O'Bryan *et al.,* 2018). On the basis of existing evidences, many studies reinforce the fact that absence of vultures will increase the transmission of infectious diseases to humans as well as their livestock (Markandya *et al.,* 2008; Ogada *et al.,* 2011, 2012; Moleón *et al.*, 2014). A study by Ogada shows that due to the decrease in the vulture population in Kenya, the number of animal carcasses (dead body of animals) increased three times, so did the amount of time to clear them out. Correlating this with the probability of disease spread, he added that the risk posed on human health (Ogada *et al.*, 2012) and the economic burden surged threefold. Vultures are known to dispose more than 22 per cent of the organic waste in urban areas. Decaying carcasses are undoubtedly a huge lingering threat to human health (Shearer *et al.*, 2018). They act as breeding grounds for a large number of pathogens that can lead to transmission of infections. Water-borne diseases easily spread through the fouling of watercourses by rotting carcasses, however, this link is not that easy to establish (Markandya *et al.*, 2008). The reduction in the number of vultures leaves quite a few carcasses un-scavenged, invariably increasing other organisms and abiotic resources exposed to a large number of diseases. The absence of vultures can cause the "piling up of corpses in the land of the living" (Van Dooren, 2010).

4.2.14 *Swine Flu/Influenza (2009-10)*

Swine-origin influenza virus (S-OIV) also H1N1, H1N2, H2N1, H3N1, H3N2, and H2N3, refers to any strain of the influenza family of viruses that is endemic in pigs. Swine flu was first identified in Mexico in 2009 and quickly spread to other parts of the world, resulting in a global pandemic. H1N1 epidemic spread in US from June 2009 to August 2010. In June 2009, the WHO declared the swine flu outbreak as a global pandemic. This designation reflected the widespread nature of the virus rather than its severity. During the swine flu pandemic, numerous countries implemented public health measures to prevent the spread of the virus. This included school closures, travel restrictions, and vaccination campaigns. Pharmaceutical companies also developed H1N1 vaccines. The Centres for Disease Control and Prevention (CDC) estimated that globally, there were approximately 1.4 billion cases of swine flu from April 2009 to April 2010, leading to around 2,84,500 deaths. Since the initial pandemic, the swine flu has continued to circulate as a seasonal influenza virus. It has been included in the annual flu vaccine to provide protection against H1N1 strains.

In India, the first case of swine flu was reported in May 2009 in Hyderabad, and since then, the disease has a significant impact on public health in the country leading to a significant number of cases and deaths. The distribution of swine flu in India has been uneven, with some regions and states being more affected than others. The disease has been reported in almost all states of India, with the highest number of cases being reported in Maharashtra, Gujarat, and Rajasthan, among others. The reason for the high incidence of swine flu infection in some states is likely due to factors such as population density, low levels of hygiene, and inadequate healthcare resources. Swine flu has a significant impact on public health in India over the years, with several outbreaks and epidemics being reported. In 2015, there was a major outbreak of swine flu in different parts of the country, with over 31,000 cases being reported and more than 2,000 deaths recorded. Similarly, in 2017, there was another outbreak of swine flu in India, with over 38,000 cases and more than 2,000 deaths.

To combat the spread of swine flu in India, the government has implemented various measures, including effective surveillance and monitoring systems, rapid diagnostics, public health education, and promotion of good hygiene practices. Vaccination is also an important strategy in preventing the disease. The Government of India has recommended the vaccination of high-risk groups such as healthcare workers and people with underlying health conditions. In recent years, the incidence of swine flu in India has been relatively lower, with fewer cases and deaths being reported. However, the disease remains a significant public health concern in the country, and continuous efforts are required to control and prevent its spread.

Communicable diseases are a great matter of concern due to their ability to spread rapidly from person to person, potentially causing widespread illness, death, and socio-economic impact. Communicable diseases can easily cross borders and affect populations worldwide. With increasing international travel and interconnectedness, the risk of global outbreaks rises, as seen with diseases like COVID-19, Ebola, and Zika. They can also lead to severe illness, long-term disabilities, and even death. They often disproportionately affect vulnerable populations with limited access to healthcare, exacerbating existing health inequalities.

Outbreaks of communicable diseases can place a significant burden on healthcare systems, disrupt economies, and lead to productivity losses. The cost of prevention, treatment, control measures, and containment efforts can be substantial.

As the leading global health agency, the WHO provides technical guidance, coordinates responses, and supports countries in preventing, detecting, and responding to communicable diseases. They establish surveillance systems, conduct research, and facilitate the development of vaccines and treatment options. Vaccine development and distribution: Organizations such as the Coalition for Epidemic Preparedness Innovations (CEPI) and Gavi, the Vaccine Alliance, work to accelerate the development and equitable distribution of vaccines against communicable diseases. They support research, development, and global vaccination campaigns. Communicable diseases have been a significant public health concern in world for centuries. While many efforts have been made to control and eradicate these diseases, outbreaks continue to occur.

4.3 Managing Communicable Diseases

Managing communicable diseases is critical for public health and requires a multi-disciplinary approach. It is very challenging to manage infectious diseases. Countries can take various steps to manage communicable diseases, such as the following examples worldwide.

4.3.1 *Disease Surveillance*

Most countries have established disease surveillance systems to track communicable diseases. These systems use various data sources, such as reports from healthcare providers, laboratories, and hospitals, to monitor incidence rates and identify outbreaks. According to Health Protection Surveillance Centre, disease surveillance is an information-based activity involving the collection, analysis and interpretation of large volumes of data originating from a variety of sources. The goals of infectious disease surveillance are threefold: (1) to describe the current burden and epidemiology of disease, (2) to monitor trends, and (3) to identify outbreaks and new pathogens (Murray and Cohen, 2017).

The information collated is then used in a number of ways to:

- Evaluate the effectiveness of control and preventative health measures.
- Monitor changes in infectious agents, e.g., trends in development of antimicrobial resistance.

- Support health planning and the allocation of appropriate resources within the healthcare system.
- Identify high risk populations or areas to target interventions.
- Provide a valuable archive of disease activity for future reference.

To be effective, the collection of surveillance data must be standardized on a national basis and be made available at local, regional and national level (www.hpsc.ie).

For example, in 1998, the IDSR (Integrated Disease Surveillance and Response) strategy was first drafted by the WHO Regional Office for Africa in order to harmonize existing surveillance networks (including AFP and neonatal tetanus) in the African region (WHO, 2010). The Global Outbreak and Response Network (GOARN) is a WHO-coordinated network comprised over 600 partners worldwide, including government, technical, and academic institutions involved in epidemic surveillance. GeoSentinel is a global network of clinics assessing travellers' and migrants' health for illnesses acquired while abroad (Leder *et al.*, 2013).

4.3.2 *Vaccination*

Vaccination is a highly effective approach to prevent the spread of communicable diseases. Vaccination is a simple, safe, and effective way of protecting you against harmful diseases, before you come into contact with them. It uses your body's natural defences to build resistance to specific infections and makes your immune system stronger (www.who.int). Vaccination not only prevents occurrence of disease to the one who is vaccinated rather it also helps others not to get infected. There are small children who cannot be given vaccination. Vaccination is also not administered to patients who are seriously ill. But in both the cases, the probability to catch a virus is high, so by vaccinating most of the population helps to halt the spread of the disease. Many countries have comprehensive immunization programmes that offer routine vaccinations to their population. For instance, the United States and Canada have well-established vaccination programmes that have helped control and prevent diseases such as measles, rubella and mumps. According to Ministry of Health and Family Welfare, Government of India, India's immunization programme, launched in 1985, is one of the largest health programmes of its kind in the world, catering to a birth cohort of 2.7 crore (27 million) children annually. The programme provides vaccination against eight life threatening diseases (diphtheria, whooping cough, Haemophilus influenzae type B (Hib) causing pneumonia and meningitis, tetanus, polio, tuberculosis, measles and Hepatitis B) in the entire country. In addition, vaccination against Japanese Encephalitis (JE) is provided in the selected endemic districts/states of the country. Recently, rotavirus vaccine (RVV) has been introduced in the four selected states (Andhra Pradesh, Haryana, Himachal Pradesh and Odisha) (main.mohfw.gov.in). The Indian mission of immunization, i.e., Mission Indradhanush (rainbow), launched in December 2014, is to identify, enlist, mobilize, vaccinate and track to achieve full immunization.

4.3.3 *Contact Tracing*

Contact tracing involves identifying individuals who have come into contact with an infected person and ensuring that they are evaluated, tested, or treated accordingly. This approach can be critical in controlling the spread of communicable diseases, especially when it comes to highly infectious diseases such as tuberculosis or sexually transmitted infections (STIs). According to WHO, the monitoring process or contact tracing can be broken down into 3 basic steps:

- *Contact identification:* Once someone is confirmed as infected with a virus, contacts are identified by asking about the person's activities and the activities and roles of the people around them since onset of illness. Contacts can be anyone who has been in contact with an infected person: family members, work colleagues, friends, or healthcare providers.
- *Contact listing:* All persons considered to have contact with the infected person should be listed as contacts. Efforts should be made to identify every listed contact and to inform them of their contact status, what it means, the actions that will follow, and the importance of receiving early care if they develop symptoms. Contacts should also be provided with information about prevention of the disease. In some cases, quarantine or isolation is required for high risk contacts, either at home, or in hospital.
- *Contact follow-up:* Regular follow-up should be conducted with all contacts to monitor for symptoms and test for signs of infection (www.who.int).

Contact tracing is a primary means of disease control for infectious diseases with low prevalence. In the USA, contact tracing is required for TB, recommended for human immunodeficiency virus (HIV) and not uncommon for other sexually transmitted diseases (STDs). Contact tracing has also been used (and modelled) for severe acute respiratory syndrome (SARS), foot-and-mouth-disease, smallpox and avian influenza (Armbruster and Brandeau, 2007). Recently digital contact tracing uses technology to track and trace contacts. Individuals download an app onto their smartphones and record location and symptom information, or their devices might use location-finding technology, like Bluetooth or GPS (global positioning system). If the user is infected, the technology identifies close contacts and/or secondary infections (people to whom they passed the disease), and informs people whom they have been near. The technology identifies where the infection was passed on and its duration (NIHR, 2023).

4.3.4 *Health Education Campaigns*

Education campaigns can help inform the public about how to prevent the spread of communicable diseases. These campaigns can cover areas such as how to properly wash hands, prevent mosquito bites, and practice safe sex. Australia, for example, has run a highly effective nationwide awareness campaign targeting various communicable diseases such as HIV/AIDs, Hepatitis, STIs, and other infectious diseases. For example, CDC's Let's Stop HIV Together (Together) campaign is the national campaign of the Ending the HIV Epidemic in the U.S. (EHE) initiative and the National HIV/AIDS Strategy. Together is an evidence-based campaign created in English and Spanish. It aims to empower communities, partners, and healthcare providers to reduce HIV stigma and promote HIV testing, prevention, and treatment (www.cdc.gov).

Table 4.2: Health Days/Campaigns

Health Day or Campaigns	Detail
World Health Day	*April 7:* This day, established by the World Health Organization (WHO), aims to raise awareness on a specific health topic each year. It also commemorates the founding of WHO.
World AIDS Day	*December 1:* This day is dedicated to spreading awareness about HIV/AIDS, remembering those who have lost their lives to AIDS, and showing support for people living with the virus.

(*Contd.*)

Health Day or Campaigns	Detail
World Cancer Day	*February 4:* It aims to raise awareness, promote prevention, and support individuals affected by cancer globally. The day focuses on the importance of early detection, treatment, and research.
World Mental Health Day	*October 10:* This day raises awareness about mental health issues and aims to reduce stigma while advocating for mental health support, treatment, and care.
World Diabetes Day	*November 14:* It is observed to raise global awareness about diabetes, its prevention, treatment, and possible complications. The day emphasizes the importance of lifestyle changes and effective diabetes management.

Source: Compiled by Author.

4.3.5 *Quarantine and Isolation*

Quarantine and isolation are measures taken to separate individuals who may be infected with a communicable disease to prevent the spread of the disease to others. Isolation and quarantine help protect the public by preventing exposure to people who have or may have a contagious disease.

- Isolation separates sick people with a contagious disease from people who are not sick.
- Quarantine separates and restricts the movement of people who were exposed to a contagious disease to see if they become sick (www.cdc.gov).

Many countries, including China, India, South Korea and Taiwan, have used quarantine and isolation effectively to control the spread of communicable diseases such as COVID-19.

4.3.6 *Build-up Herd Immunity*

'Herd immunity' also known as 'population immunity', is the indirect protection from an infectious disease that happens when a population is immune either through vaccination or immunity developed through previous infection. WHO supports achieving 'herd immunity' through vaccination, not by allowing a disease to spread through any segment of the population, as this would result in unnecessary cases and deaths (www.who.int). The percentage of people who need to be immune in order to achieve herd immunity varies with each disease. For example, herd immunity against measles requires about 95 per cent of a population to be vaccinated. The remaining 5 per cent will be protected by the fact that measles will not spread among those who are vaccinated. For polio, the threshold is about 80 per cent. The proportion of the population that must be vaccinated against COVID-19 to begin inducing herd immunity is not known. This is an important area of research and will likely vary according to the community, the vaccine, the populations prioritized for vaccination, and other factors (www.who.int).

A comprehensive approach is needed to manage Communicable diseases. It needs to involve multiple interventions. Efforts should focus on surveillance, vaccination, contact tracing, health education, and quarantine and isolation measures. Countries should have strong public health systems to respond to the outbreaks of communicable diseases as they arise.

4.4 Epidemiological Transition in India

As discussed earlier, epidemiology is the study and analysis of the distribution, patterns and determinants of health and disease conditions in a defined population. The epidemiological transition theory outlines the changes in patterns of diseases and health conditions that occur as a population undergoes socio-economic and demographic shifts. Abdel. R. Omran, the pioneer of Epidemiological Transition theory, highlights following propositions of the theory:

1. The theory of epidemiological transition begins with the major premise that mortality is a fundamental factor in population dynamics.
2. During the transition, a long term shift occurs in mortality and disease patterns whereby pandemics of infection are gradually displaced by degenerative and man-made diseases as the chief form of morbidity and primary cause of death.
3. During the epidemiologic transition, profound inequities or differentials in health and disease changes occur according to age, gender, race or ethnic origin, social class and indigenous status.
4. During the transition, systematic variations in the pattern, pace, determinants and consequences of health, survival and population changes distinguish several models of the epidemiologic transition (Omran, 1971).

Omran originally identified three stages of 'epidemiologic transition'—(i) the 'age of pestilence and famine', (ii) the 'age of receding pandemics', and (iii) the 'age of degenerative and man-made diseases'. In the 'age of pestilence and famine', mortality remained at very high levels for thousands of years. He initially identified three models of transition: the 'western model' based on the experience of England and other Western countries, an 'accelerated model' for Japan and other countries that experienced a more rapid transition during industrialisation and a 'delayed model' for developing countries where the decline in infectious disease mortality was more recent (Omran, 1971). He later added a fourth 'transitional variant' of the delayed model in which rapidly declining mortality was followed relatively quickly by fertility decline, which occurred in developing countries with well-organised family planning services (Omran, 1983). Later he added, Fourth stage: Age of declining cardiovascular mortality, ageing, lifestyles modification, emerging and resurgent diseases and Fifth stage (Futuristic stage): Age of aspired quality of life, with paradoxical longevity and (futuristic stage) persistent inequities (Omran, 1971).

After that numerous modifications happened in Omran's theory. Currently considering larger part of the world, four commonly referred stages of epidemiological transition can be considered:

Stage 1: *Age of Pestilence and Famine:* This stage is characterized by high mortality rates, societies are predominantly agrarian and experience widespread infectious diseases, malnutrition, and high infant and child mortality. Countries that largely fit this stage historically include pre-industrial societies, particularly those in Sub-Saharan Africa.

Stage 2: *Age of Receding Pandemics:* During this stage, infections and malnutrition gradually decline due to improving living conditions, sanitation, and nutrition. Many countries in Europe and North America went through this stage during the 19th and early 20th centuries.

Stage 3: *Age of Degenerative and Man-Made Diseases:* As societies continue to develop, chronic diseases like heart disease, stroke, diabetes, and cancer become more prevalent. Countries in parts of Latin America, Asia, and the Middle East have transitioned or are transitioning through this stage.

Stage 4: *Age of Delayed Degenerative Diseases:* In this stage, chronic diseases remain the primary health concern, but a decline in mortality rates is observed due to advancements in medical technology, healthcare access, and disease management. Many developed countries, such as the United States, Canada, Japan, and those in Western Europe, have reached this stage.

Non-communicable diseases are rapidly increasing in many developing countries, largely due to demographic and lifestyle changes. It is estimated that nearly half of the disease burden in low- and middle-income countries is from non-communicable diseases, and more than 21 per cent of deaths in such countries are due to cardiovascular diseases (Quigley, 2006). Overall, India has been experiencing rapid structural changes in disease pattern within the short span of the last three decades. Advances in mortality and morbidity transition to later stages point towards an upheaval in epidemiological transition (Yadav *et al.*, 2014). The share of communicable diseases has not been entirely replaced by chronic NCDs. In addition to Visaria's study (2004), John *et al.* (2011) have recently demonstrated the heavier burden of communicable diseases, which is as high as 30 per cent of the total. Therefore, India's current stage of epidemiological transition can be characterized by low mortality, high morbidity, and by the double burden of communicable diseases and NCDs. The burden of communicable diseases had been dominant around the world until the mid-twentieth century. In Africa and Asia (including India), the trilogy of smallpox, plague, and malaria remained the 'top killer' diseases until the 1960s. However, by the late 1970s, smallpox was eradicated in India through sustained vaccination programmes; better sanitation and housing reduced the overall burden of communicable diseases (Banthia and Dyson, 1999). Nevertheless, by the mid-1990s, other communicable diseases, such as tuberculosis of lungs (5.3%), gastroenteritis/dysentery (3%), and pneumonia (4.7%) were responsible for a considerable number of deaths, signifying the burden of communicable diseases. Overall, the manifold rise in morbidity rates in recent decades concomitant with a decline in mortality rates is a manifestation of the progression of 'health transition' (Johansson, 1991); this is a phenomenon where the survival rate of the population led to an increase in the level of morbidity and a decline in mortality. The data also point to significant variation between the states with the greatest morbidity rates (such as Kerala's rate of 255/1000 people) and the lowest rate (in poorer states like Jharkhand, where the rate is 33/1000 people). Additional information from India's National Sample Survey Organisation (NSSO) shows a significant rise in morbidity during the previous two decades (16-18). Non-communicable disease (NCD) risk factors include inadequate physical activity, tobacco use, a low intake of fruits and vegetables, a high body mass index (BMI), and more have all been linked to an increase in NCDs.

India lies primarily in the transitional stage between Stage 3 and Stage 4 of the epidemiological transition. India has experienced a decline in infectious diseases over the years, but they still remain a significant health issue, particularly in rural areas. However, the burden of non-communicable diseases (NCDs) such as cardiovascular diseases, diabetes, chronic respiratory diseases, and cancer is rapidly rising. For example, India has contributed to the largest drop in cases region-wide, from approximately 20 million to about 6 million. The percentage drop in the malaria cases was 71.8 per cent and deaths were 73.9 per cent between 2000 and 2019. India achieved a reduction of 83.34 per cent in malaria morbidity and 92 per cent in malaria mortality between the year 2000 (20,31,790 cases, 932 deaths) and 2019 (3,38,494 cases, 77 deaths) (HFW/World Malaria Report/2nd December 2020/21). In India in 2016, Cardio Vascular Disease (CVDs) contributed to 28·1 per cent of total deaths and 14·1 per cent of total Disability-Adjusted Life Years (DALYs) compared with 15·2 per cent and 6·9 per cent, respectively in 1990. Within India, the rates of CVD vary markedly with highest in states of

Kerala, Punjab and Tamil Nadu (Kumar and Sinha, 2020). Life expectancy in India has been steadily increasing. According to the UN-World population prospects, the life expectancy at birth in India has risen from 57.66 years in 1990 to 70 years in 2020, indicating improved healthcare and disease management (Fig. 4.17).

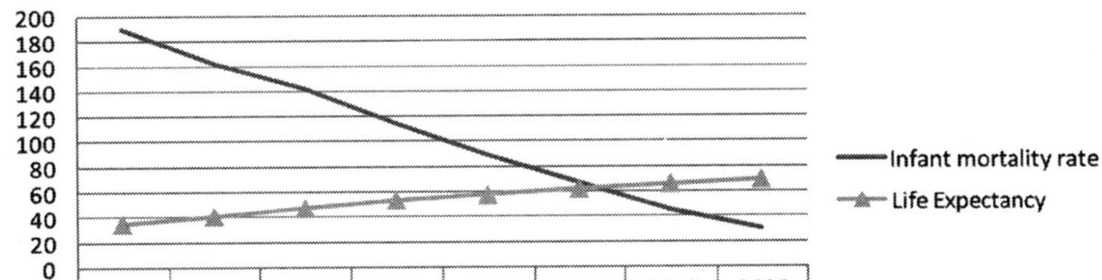

	1950	1960	1970	1980	1990	2000	2010	2020
Infant mortality rate	189.62	161.74	141.822	114.743	88.79	66.72	45.3	29.84
Life Expectancy	35.21	41.13	47.4	53.47	57.66	62.28	66.42	69.73

Fig. 4.17: Infant Mortailty Rate and Life Expectancy (India).

Source: UN—World Population Prospects: Macro trends.

According to the Global Burden of Disease Study, the leading causes of death in India are Ischemic heart disease, Chronic obstructive pulmonary disease (COPD), and Diabetes. These diseases are typically associated with Stage 3 and Stage 4 of the epidemiological transition. India is also experiencing a demographic shift with a rapidly growing aging population. The proportion of the population aged 60 and above is projected to reach 13 per cent by 2025, which is characteristic of countries in Stage 4. India can be examined under various stages of epidemiological transition as under:

Stage 1: Age of Pestilence and Famine

In this stage, India faced high mortality rates due to infectious diseases, epidemics, and famines. Historically, India experienced numerous outbreaks of diseases like cholera, smallpox, and malaria, leading to high level of morbidity and mortality. Limited healthcare infrastructure and inadequate public health measures contributed to the prevalence of infectious diseases.

During 1970s and 1980s, the mortality was very high due to infectious diseases. For example, rural population was more susceptible to diarrhoea, cough and fever. These infections were responsible for 45 per cent of deaths in 1972. In urban areas, the deaths were mainly due to parasitic diseases, respiratory diseases or digestive disorders. This amounts for nearly 42 per cent of total deaths in urban areas.

Stage 2: Age of Receding Pandemics

During this stage, India began to experience a decline in infectious disease-related mortality rates. The advancements in healthcare, improved sanitation, and access to clean water reduced the impact of diseases. Immunization programmes, widespread use of antibiotics, and better disease surveillance systems further contributed to this decline. From 1982 to 1997, the deaths due to infectious diseases like diarrhoea, cough and fever reduced to 36-38 per cent. The deaths were more attributable to tuberculosis, gastroenteritis, dysentery and pneumonia. The deaths in urban areas due to parasitic diseases, respiratory diseases or digestive disorders declined to 28 per cent in 1995.

Stage 3: Age of Degenerative and Man-made Diseases

With the improving healthcare system and changing lifestyle patterns, India started witnessing a rise in chronic diseases such as cardiovascular diseases, diabetes, respiratory diseases, and cancers. Factors like urbanization, sedentary lifestyles, tobacco use, unhealthy diets, and environmental pollution have been significant contributors to the increasing burden of non-communicable diseases (NCDs) in India. The stage began from 1997 with the rise of non-communicable diseases in India. In 1997, around 28 per cent of deaths in rural areas can be attributed to NCD. In urban areas, the deaths due to NCD contributed to around 36 per cent. After 2004, non-communicable diseases (NCDs) became the major cause of deaths in India.

Stage 4: Age of Delayed Degenerative Diseases

India is currently in the earlier phases of this stage. This stage represents a further transition where the focus shifts to healthcare advancements, early detection, treatment, and management of chronic diseases. Additionally, there is an increasing emphasis on preventive measures, lifestyle modifications, and public health interventions to reduce the burden of chronic diseases. Currently India has made significant progress in reducing the burden of communicable diseases such as malaria, tuberculosis, and HIV/AIDS. The National Health Mission, initiated by the Indian Government, has implemented several programmes targeting communicable diseases. For example, the Revised National Tuberculosis Control Programme (RNTCP) aims to detect and treat tuberculosis, significantly reducing morbidity and mortality rates. Similarly, National Malaria Control Programmes have been initiated to combat malaria in high-risk areas. However, the burden of communicable diseases remains a challenge, particularly in densely populated areas and among vulnerable population. The recent COVID-19 pandemic has further highlighted this issue, straining healthcare systems and leading to a higher number of infections and deaths.

In addition to communicable diseases, India is experiencing a rising burden of non-communicable diseases (NCDs) such as cardiovascular diseases, diabetes, respiratory diseases, and cancer. The changing lifestyle patterns, urbanization, sedentary behaviour, and adoption of unhealthy diets contribute to the increasing prevalence of NCDs. To address this challenge, the Indian Government has launched various initiatives like the National Programme for Prevention and Control of Cancer, Diabetes, Cardiovascular Diseases, and Stroke (NPCDCS). These programmes focus on creating awareness, early detection, and treatment of NCDs. The government has also emphasized the importance of promoting healthy lifestyles, including regular physical activity and balanced diets, to prevent NCDs.

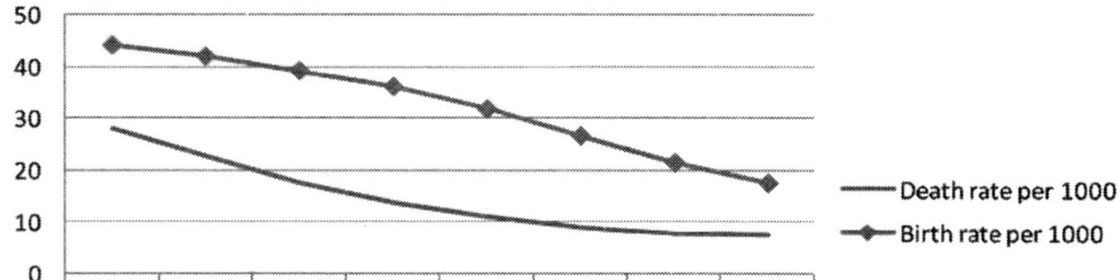

	1950	1960	1970	1980	1990	2000	2010	2020
Death rate per 1000	28	22.48	17.45	13.49	11	8.8	7.58	7.3
Birth rate per 1000	44.17	42.06	39.23	36.21	31.81	26.63	21.5	17.59

Fig. 4.18: Birth Rate and Death Rate (per thousand), India.

Source: UN—World Population Prospects: Macro trends.

The country is also undergoing a demographic transition, with potential prospects for a demographic dividend complemented by a large and growing share of working-age population being set against an increasing elderly population. Predictably, a growing burden of non-communicable conditions alongside its traditional concerns of communicable diseases and reproductive health outcomes adds to its worries. India's progress on reducing the infant mortality rate (IMR) is remarkable, from a high IMR of 88 per 1000 live births in 1990 to about 32 in 2020. Similarly, the maternal mortality ratio (MMR) declined from 556 in 1990 to 113 per 1,00,000 live births during 2016-18, but the progress has been uneven with economically weaker states continuing to report higher rates. The mixed performance on communicable diseases shows that although polio has been eliminated and the human immunodeficiency virus infection and acquired immune deficiency syndrome (HIV/AIDS) epidemic contained, significant disease burden from tuberculosis remains, with rising numbers of multidrug-resistant variants. Dengue and Chikungunya have posed a regular threat to urban health planners. Non-communicable diseases (NCDs) are increasingly emerging as a challenge, with NCDs and injuries together accounting for over half the disease burden (Mahal, 2022).

Despite these efforts, access to quality healthcare, especially in rural areas, hilly areas or other vulnerable areas remain a significant challenge. When examining the spatial epidemiology of diseases in India region-wise, it is important to consider the country's vast size and diverse population. Northern regions of India face various health challenges. Uttar Pradesh and Bihar have a high burden of communicable diseases like tuberculosis, malaria, and diarrhoeal illnesses. Additionally, water-borne diseases like typhoid and Hepatitis A are prevalent due to inadequate water and sanitation infrastructure. States in South India generally have better healthcare infrastructure and display lower morbidity and mortality rates for many diseases. However, non-communicable diseases like diabetes, cardiovascular diseases, and cancer are on the rise in this region, potentially due to changing lifestyles and economic development. Parts of Western India, such as Maharashtra and Gujarat, have shown higher incidence rates of lifestyle-related diseases like obesity, diabetes, and hypertension. Occupational hazards, such as those encountered by labourers in industries and mining, also contribute to disease patterns in some areas. Certain states in Eastern India, like West Bengal and Odisha, have a significant burden of infectious diseases. Malaria, dengue fever, and Japanese encephalitis are prevalent in some regions. These states also have a higher prevalence of water-borne diseases due to inadequate sanitation facilities and limited access to safe drinking water. North-east India presents unique challenges in terms of disease patterns due to its geographical isolation and diverse ethnic communities. Diseases like malaria, tuberculosis, and vector-borne diseases such as dengue and chikungunya are prevalent in this region. Additionally, endemic diseases like leprosy and filariasis are of concern in specific areas. On the whole, there is a significantly visible shift of India from high birth rate to low birth rate, high death rate to low death rate, low life expectancy to higher life expectancy and from high mortality from communicable diseases to non-communicable diseases.

REFERENCES

Ahmadi, K., Dashti, M.F., Delgosha, M.S. (2020, Aug. 25). Geographical distribution of COVID-19 in the World and Iran; Investigation of possible transmission roots. *J Family Med Prim Care*, 9(8): 4473-4475. doi: 10.4103/jfmpc.jfmpc_733_20. PMID: 33110890; PMCID: PMC7586559

Arámbulo III, P.V., Thakur, A.S. (1992). Impact of zoonoses in tropical America. *Ann. N.Y. Acad. Sci*, 653: 6-18. doi: 10.1111/j.1749-6632.1992.tb19624.x

Arinaminpathy, N., Batra, D., Khaparde, S., Vualnam, T., Maheshwari, N., Sharma, L., Dewan, P. (2016). The number of privately treated tuberculosis cases in India: an estimation from drug sales data. *Lancet Infect Dis.*, 16(11): 1255-60.

Armbruster, B., Brandeau, M.L. (2007 Dec.). Contact tracing to control infectious disease: when enough is enough. *Health Care Manag Sci.*, 10(4): 341-55. doi: 10.1007/s10729-007-9027-6. PMID: 18074967; PMCID: PMC3428220.z

Beale, L., Abellan, J.J., Hodgson, S., Jarup, L. (2008 Aug.). Methodologic issues and approaches to spatial epidemiology. *Environ Health Perspect*, 116(8): 1105-10. doi: 10.1289/ehp.10816. PMID: 18709139; PMCID: PMC2516558

Centers for Disease Control Prevention (CDC) (21 October, 1994). "International Notes Update: Human Plague—India, 1994". *MMWR Morb. Mortal. Wkly. Rep.* 43 (41): 761-762. PMID 7935308. Retrieved 26 December 2015.

C. Colomba, L. Saporito, L. Titone (2008). *Typhoid Fever, Editor(s): Harald Kristian (Kris) Heggenhougen, International Encyclopedia of Public Health*, Academic Press, pp. 414-420, ISBN 9780123739605, https: //doi.org/10.1016/B978-012373960-5.00619-5

Confronting inequalities: Lessons for pandemic responses from 40 years of AIDS Global AIDS Update Geneva: UNAIDS; 2021 (https: //www.unaids.org/sites/default/files/media_asset/2021-global-aids-update_en.pdf, accessed 3 May 2022).

Doll, R. (1980). The epidemiology of cancer. *Cancer*. 1980 May 15; 45(10): 2475-85. doi: 10.1002/1097-0142(19800515)45: 10<2475: : aid-cncr2820451004>3.0.co;2-6. PMID: 7378985

Edemekong, P.F., Huang, B. (2023 Jan.). Epidemiology of Prevention of Communicable Diseases. [Updated 2022, Oct. 24]. In: *StatPearls* [Internet]. Treasure Island (FL): StatPearls Publishing; available from: https: //www.ncbi.nlm.nih.gov/books/NBK470303/

Elliott, P., Wartenberg, D. (2004 June). Spatial epidemiology: current approaches and future challenges. *Environ Health Perspect*, 112(9): 998-1006. doi: 10.1289/ehp.6735. PMID: 15198920; PMCID: PMC1247193.

Global leprosy situation (2012). *Weekly Epidemiological Record.* 87(34): 317-328. August 2012. PMID 22919737

Global tuberculosis report, Geneva: World Health Organization; (https: //apps.who.int/iris/rest/ bitstreams/1379788/retrieve, accessed 3 May, 2022).

Gupta, N., Srivastava, S., Jain, A., Chaturvedi, U.C. (2012 Sep.). Dengue in India. *Indian J Med Res.*, 136(3): 373-90. PMID: 23041731; PMCID: PMC3510884 https: //arc-w.nihr.ac.uk/research/projects/are-digital-contact-tracing-technologies-effective-during-infectious-disease-outbreaks/

Keys, A. (1980). *Seven Countries—A Multivariate Analysis of Death and Coronary Heart Disease.* Boston: Harvard University Press.

Kristian, G. Andersen *et al.* (2020). "The proximal origin of SARS-CoV-2", *Nature Medicine*, April.

Leder, K., Torresi, J., Libman, M.D., Cramer, J.P., Castelli, F., Schlagenhauf, P., Wilder-Smith, A., Wilson, M.E., Keystone, J.S., Schwartz, E., Barnett, E.D., von Sonnenburg, F., Brownstein, J.S., Cheng, A.C., Sotir, M.J., Esposito, D.H., Freedman, D.O. (2013). for the GeoSentinel Surveillance Network GeoSentinel surveillance of illness in returned travellers, 2007-2011. *Ann. Intern. Med.,* 158(6): 456-468.

Mahal, A., Selvaraj., S., *et al.,* (ed.) (2022). India Health System Review in *Health System in Transition,* Vol. 11, No. 1, 202, WHO Pub.

Markandya, A., Taylor, T., Longo, A., Murty, M.N., Murty, S., Dhavala, K. (2008). Counting the cost of vulture decline—an appraisal of the human health and other benefits of vultures in India. *Ecol Econ,* 67(2): 194-204.

Mazumdar, S., Satyanarayana, S., Pai, M. (2019). Self-reported tuberculosis in India: evidence from NFHS-4. *BMJ Glob Health.,* 4(3): e001371

Moleón, M., Sánchez-Zapata, J.A., Margalida, A., Carrete, M., Owen-Smith, N., Donázar, J.A. (2014). Humans and scavengers: the evolution of interactions and ecosystem services. *Bioscience.,* 64(5): 394-403. doi: 10.1093/biosci/biu034

Murray, J., Cohen, A.L. (2017). *Infectious Disease Surveillance. International Encyclopedia of Public Health,* 222-9. doi: 10.1016/B978-0-12-803678-5.00517-8. Epub 2016 Oct. 24. PMCID: PMC7149515

O'Bryan, C.J., Braczkowski, A.R., Beyer. H.L., Carter, N.H., Watson, J.E., McDonald-Madden, E. (2018). The contribution of predators and scavengers to human well-being. *Nat Ecol Evoln.,* 2(2): 229-236. doi: 10.1038/s41559-017-0421-2

Ogada, D.L., Keesing, F., Virani, M.Z. (2011). Dropping dead: causes and consequences of vulture population declines worldwide. *Ann N Y Acad Sci.,* doi: 10.1111/j.1749-6632.2011.06293.x

Omran, O.R. (1971). The epidemiologic transition. *Milbank Memorial Fund Quarterly,* 49, 509-538.

Omran, O.R. (1983). The epidemiologic transition theory. A preliminary update. *Journal of Tropical Paediatrics,* 29, 305-316.

Poorolajal, J. (2020, Sep. 30). Geographical Distribution of COVID-19 Cases and Deaths Worldwide. *J Res Health Sci.,* 20(3): e00483. doi: 10.34172/jrhs.2020.24. PMID: 33169715; PMCID: PMC7585770

Rahman, M.T., Sobur, M.A., Islam, M.S., Ievy, S., Hossain, M.J., El Zowalaty, M.E., Rahman, A.T., Ashour, H.M. (2020, Sep. 12). Zoonotic Diseases: Etiology, Impact, and Control. *Microorganisms.* 8(9): 1405. doi: 10.3390/microorganisms8091405. PMID: 32932606; PMCID: PMC7563794

Roy, R.N. and Saha, I. (revised) (2013). *Mahajan and Gupta Text Book of Preventive and Social Medicine,* Jaypee Pub., India.

Sakai, T., Morimoto, Y. (2022, Oct. 4). The History of Infectious Diseases and Medicine. *Pathogens,* 11(10): 1147. doi: 10.3390/pathogens11101147. PMID: 36297204; PMCID: PMC9609744

Shearer, J.K., Griffin, D., Cotton, S.E. (2018). Humane Euthanasia and Carcass Disposal. *Vet Clin Food Anim Pract.,* 34(2): 355-374. doi: 10.1016/j.cvfa.2018.03.004

Tatem, A.J.; Rogers, D.J.; Hay, S.I. (2006). "Global Transport Networks and Infectious Disease Spread". *Adv Parasitol. Advances in Parasitology.* National Institute of Health, 62: 293-343. doi: 10.1016/S0065-308X(05)62009-X

Van Dooren, T. (2010). Vultures and their people in India: equity and entanglement in a time of extinctions. *Austral Hum Rev.* 22(2): 130-145. http: //australianhumanitiesreview.org/2011/05/01/vultures-and-their-people-in-india-equity-and-entanglement-in-a-time-of-extinctions/. Accessed 9 August, 2020.

Varshney, K., Patel, H., Kamal, S. (2023 April 29). Trends in Tuberculosis Mortality Across India: Improvements Despite the COVID-19 Pandemic, *Cureus,* 15(4): e38313. doi: 10.7759/cureus.38313. PMID: 37261163; PMCID: PMC10226868.

WHO second ed. WHO Document Production Services; Geneva (2010). *Technical Guidelines for Integrated Disease Surveillance and Response in the African Region*; pp. 5-17 http: //www.afro.who.int/en/clusters-a-programmes/dpc/integrated-disease-surveillance/integrated-disease-surveillance-and-response.html [online] Available at: (accessed 22.07.16.)

www.who.int

Chapter

5

Non-Communicable and Lifestyle Diseases

Trends and Pattern

Lifestyle refers to the way a person lives his life. Human lifestyle is ever changing and evolving. The pattern and need of food consumption, usage of resources, pursuing various activities etc. have been constantly changing. Many diseases in the world are linked to the way we live. Diseases caused due to eating, sleeping, working disorders and are not transmissible are called non-communicable diseases (NCDs) or lifestyle diseases. Early humans were constantly on move. They were hunters and gatherers. Later, humans got confined to a particular region or place when they started following agriculture, fishery, mining or any other primary activity. The secondary or tertiary activity made them live an inert life. Better means of transport and communication further effected the physical movement of human body.

According to WHO, 60 per cent of related factors to individual health and quality of life are correlated to lifestyle (Ziglio, E., Currie, C., Rasmussen, V.B., 2004). Today, many changes have occurred in life of all people. Malnutrition, unhealthy diet, smoking, alcohol consumption, drug abuse, stress and so on, are the presentations of unhealthy lifestyle that they are used as dominant form of lifestyle. Varied lifestyles have varied challenges of sustenance. For instance, emerging new technologies within IT such as the internet and virtual communication networks, lead our world to a major challenge that threatens the physical and mental health of individuals. The challenge is the overuse and misuse of the technology (Farhud, 2015). Unhealthy lifestyle can lead to problems like metabolic diseases, joint and skeletal problems, cardio-vascular diseases, hypertension, overweight, hormonal imbalance etc.

According to WHO, the causes of NCDs can be divided into three broad categories, i.e., modifiable behavioural risk factors, non-modifiable risk factors and metabolic risk factors.

1. **Modifiable Behavioural Risk Factors:** Behavioural risk factors such as excessive use of alcohol, bad food habits, eating and smoking tobacco, physical inactivity, wrong body

posture and disturbed biological clock increase the likelihood of NCDs. The modern occupational setting (desk jobs) and the stress related to work is also being seen as a potent risk factor for NCDs. According to the WHO, more than 7million people die each year due to the use of tobacco and the fatality rate is projected to increase markedly in the years to come. Excessive use of sodium in the diet causes 4.1million deaths per year while alcohol intake leads to around 1.65 million deaths due to NCDs. A simple lack of physical activity has been claiming 1.6 million lives annually.

2. **Non-modifiable Risk Factors:** Risk factors that cannot be controlled or modified by the application of an intervention can be called non-modifiable risk factors and include: (a) Age, (b) Race, (c) Gender, and (d) Genetics.
3. **Metabolic Risk Factors:** Metabolic risk factors lead to four major changes in the metabolic systems that increase the possibility of NCDs: (i) Increased blood pressure, (ii) Obesity, (iii) Increased blood glucose levels or hyperglycemia, and (iv) Increased levels of fat in the blood or hyperlipidemia (Tabish, 2017).

According to WHO, NCDs claim 41 million lives annually, which is over 70 per cent of all deaths across the globe. Of these over 15 million deaths occur among people in the age band of 30-69 years. In India, NCDs claim 6 million lives. Cardiovascular diseases account for most NCD deaths of the world followed by cancer, chronic respiratory diseases and diabetes respectively.

Figure 5.1 shows that deaths due to non-communicable diseases are high in Turkey, Ghana, Liberia, Afghanistan, Mangolia, Angola etc. also experience high deaths due to non-communicable diseases. The poor healthcare services, political unrest and poverty are the major causes of high mortality in these areas. The deaths in such cases are evidently low in case of North and South America, Australia and Europe. This is because of the improved healthcare system in these countries.

5.1 Factors Influencing Lifestyle Diseases

Lifestyle diseases are result of various behavioural patterns followed over the period of time. Chronic diseases, often referred to as non-communicable diseases (NCDs), usually emerge in middle age after long exposure to an unhealthy lifestyle involving tobacco use, a lack of regular physical activity, and consumption of diets rich in highly saturated fats, sugars, and salt, typified by "fast foods". This lifestyle results in higher levels of risk factors, such as hypertension, dyslipidemia, diabetes, and obesity that act independently and synergistically. The risk factors are frequently undiagnosed or inadequately managed in health services designed to treat acute conditions (Steyn and Damasceno, 2006).

5.1.1 *Food Consumption*

Poor food choices and eating habits lead to various lifestyle diseases. Nutritional imbalance in body is caused by both overconsumption and underconsumption of food. Overeating or consumption of 'junk food' has risen in almost all-over the world. Developed nations and urban population both consume diets high in calorie, sugar, salt and saturated oil. The excessive consumption of such foods is leading to obesity. Almost all of the world's population now has

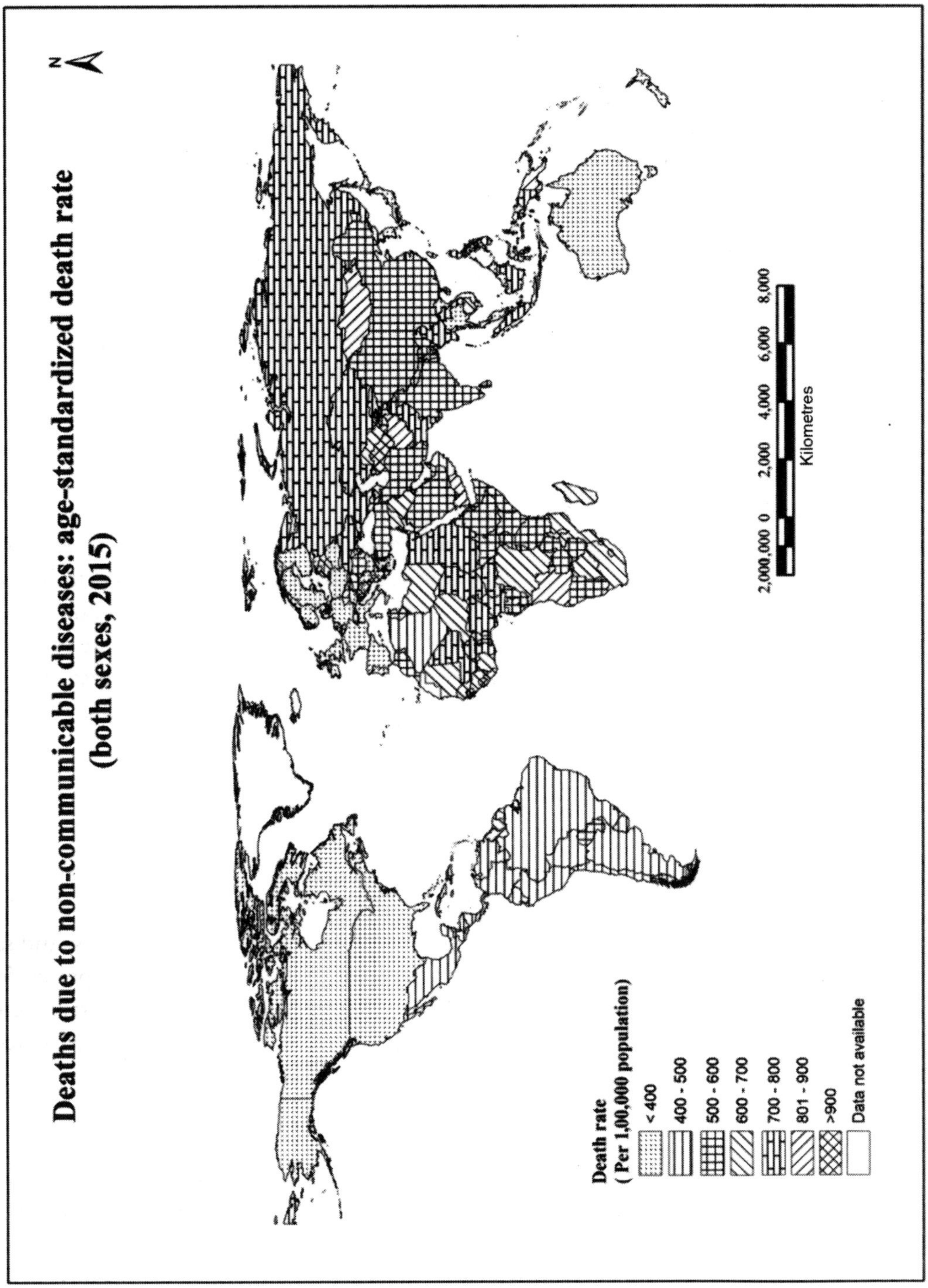

Fig. 5.1: Deaths due to non-communicable diseases.

Source: Adopted from WHO, 2018.

ubiquitous access to low-cost, but highly-processed, energy-dense, nutrient-poor food products. These changes in the food supply, rather than decreases in physical activity, are most likely the primary driver of population weight gain and obesity (Crino *et al.,* 2015). Supermarkets and a growing fast-food industry have transformed our dietary pattern. Ultra-processed food rich on sugars and saturated fat is now the major source of energy in most countries. The shift in food supply is considered a major driver of the obesity epidemic and the increasing prevalence of accompanying complications, such as type 2 diabetes, cardiovascular disease and cancer (Zobel *et al.,* 2016). To obtain good health and longevity of healthy life one must consume a balanced diet especially cooked at home. A balanced diet contains an adequate amount of all the nutrients required by the body to grow, remain healthy and be disease-free. In addition, a healthy, balanced diet provides the necessary energy requirement, protects against vitamin, mineral, and other nutritional deficiencies, and builds up immunity. Excessive consumption of junk food can cause diseases like atherosclerosis, hypertension, type 2 diabetes, cancer etc. On contrary, consuming healthy and balanced diet can help to live healthy life and build immunity in our body to fight against diseases. According to WHO, these diseases are driven by common dietary risk factors, including:

- *High salt intake*—a leading dietary risk factor for death and illness worldwide. High salt consumption increases blood pressure, which increases the risk of cardiovascular disease and stroke, chronic kidney disease and some cancers.
- *High sugar intake*—excess sugars can contribute to tooth decay and weight gain, leading to overweight and obesity, as well as higher blood pressure, cardiovascular disease and stroke, and some cancers.
- *High trans fats intake*—linked to cardiovascular disease and stroke.
- *Low fruit and vegetables intake*—linked to several cancers, cardiovascular disease and stroke.
- *Low intake of fibres, grains, nuts, seeds, micronutrients*—linked to diabetes, cardiovascular disease and stroke, and some cancers (www.who.int).

According to a study published in *Lancet* journal, 2019, a small number of dietary risks had a large impact on health outcomes. In 2017, more than half of diet-related deaths and two-thirds of diet-related DALYs (Disability-adjusted life years) were attributable to high intake of sodium (3 million deaths and 70 million DALYs), low intake of whole grains (3 million deaths and 82 million DALYs), and low intake of fruits (2 million deaths and 65 million DALYs (Afshin *et al.,* and GBD, 2017).

5.1.2 *Physical Activity or Exercise*

Physical activity is defined as any bodily movement produced by skeletal muscles that require energy expenditure. Physical activity includes exercise, as well as other activities which involve bodily movement and are done as part of playing, working, active transportation, household chores and recreational activities (WHO, 2015). Sedentary lifestyle coupled with unhealthy food habits can turn to be disastrous. It can lead to development of chronic disease like cancer, diabetes etc. According to Brannon and Feist most deaths in the 20th and 21st century result from diseases that are associated with individual lifestyle/behaviour (Brannon and Feist, 2007). A relationship between Sedentary Lifestyles and ill health was revealed as early as the 17th century by Bernadino Ramazzini, an occupational physician who discovered that sedentary lifestyle with its associated physical inactivity has an adverse effect on human metabolism, cardiac output, physical function and well-being. Technological advancement and increase in knowledge have provided man with so many facilities that reduce physical and muscular activities such as cars, airplane, accelerators and a corresponding increase in the amount of time spent sitting down at workplace, school, home and public places. According to WHO, current global estimates show one in four adults and 81 per cent of adolescents do not do enough physical activity. Furthermore, as countries develop economically, levels of inactivity increase and can be as high as 70 per cent, due to changing transport patterns, increased use of technology for work and recreation, cultural values and increasing sedentary behaviours (www.who.int). In 2010, the Region had the highest prevalence of insufficient physical activity globally, which reached 31 per cent. Women were less active than men, with differences of 10 per cent and greater of prevalence between men and women (Insufficient is defined as attaining less than 150 minutes of moderate-intensity physical activity per week, or less than 75 minutes of vigorous-intensity physical activity per week, or equivalent) (Global Status Report on Non-communicable Diseases, 2014).

Among children and adolescents, the numbers were striking. Globally, 81 per cent of adolescents aged 11-17 were insufficiently physically active in 2010 (insufficient is defined as attaining less than 60 minutes of moderate-intensity daily physical activity). Adolescent girls were less active than adolescent boys (WHO, 2014).

5.1.3 *Sleep Disorders*

Researches have found that sleep/meditation and relaxation are equally important for body and its fitness. Quality sleep and meditation is required for happy and healthy life. It gives better physical and mental growth. The American Sleep Association says that 50-70 million adults in the US have a sleep disorder. Insomnia is the most common in the short term (30% of Americans), but it also affects 10 per cent in the long-term (www.happiness.com). Sleep is regulated by neuro-chemicals in the brain. Sufficient and sound sleep relaxes your mind and helps in better concentration and active functioning of the brain and body. So, when poor sleep is ongoing, just about everything you think, feel and do can be negatively affected.

5.1.4 *Smoking/Alcohol/Drug Consumption*

Cigarette smoking increases the risk of all histological types of lung cancer and is also associated with cancer at other locations and with cardiovascular diseases (Lopez, 2003). Each cigarette contains a mixture of carcinogens, tumour promoters, and co-carcinogens. Most tobacco carcinogens require metabolic activation to exert their carcinogenic effects and competing detoxification pathways also exist (Padrão *et al.*, 2007). People who drink and smoke are at higher risk for certain types of cancer, particularly those of the mouth and throat (Franceschi, 1990; Zeng, 1990; Negri, 2004). Alcohol and tobacco cause approximately 80 per cent of cases of cancer of the mouth and throat in men and about 65 per cent in women. For people who both smoke and drink, the danger of mouth and throat cancer increases dramatically—in fact, the combined risk is greater than or equal to the risk associated with alcohol multiplied by the risk associated with tobacco (Negri, 1993). Alcohol and tobacco co-use appears to substantially increase the risk of at least one type of cancer of the esophagus (Hove, 2001). Drug consumption may damage or destroy nerve cells, either in the brain or the peripheral nervous system. Drug use can also increase the risk of contracting infections. HIV and Hepatitis C (a serious liver disease) can occur from sharing injection equipment or from unsafe practices such as condomless sex (WSIPP, 2017; Bassel *et al.*, 2014). Infection of the heart and its valves (endocarditis) and skin infection (cellulitis) can occur after exposure to bacteria by injection drug use (Klevens, 2012).

5.1.5 *Environmental Factors (Pollution)*

The urban people are prone to various health risks. Harmful pollutants like PM 2.5, nano particles, carbon dioxide, ozone etc. are prevalent in urban environment. These pollutants attack the lung system (upper and lower respiratory track), skin, eyes etc. This leads to respiratory disorders. Epidemiological evidence shows that PM10 particles are easily inhalable and cannot be filtered because of their smaller size directly reach to the upper part of the lungs. The PM2.5 can easily penetrate to lower part of the lungs and mix up with the blood stream that allows all harmful chemicals enter into different organs of the body and cause adverse health effects such as cancer, brain damage, cardiovascular and respiratory disease and finally, leads to premature mortality. In addition, that the PM2.5 surface was rich in iron, copper, zinc, manganese, and other transition elements, as well as polycyclic aromatic hydrocarbons and lipopolysaccharide etc. These components can increase free radical production in the lung, consume antioxidant ingredients and cause oxidative stress (Donaldson and Beswick, 1996).

It is very difficult to identify any one factor that is responsible for a particular health issue. Lifestyle diseases are thus outcome of multiple factors.

5.2 Characteristics of NCDs

1. **Complex etiology (causes):** Non-communicable diseases are driven by seemingly unrelated multiple causes such as unhealthy food consumption, sedentary lifestyle, rapid unplanned urbanization, globalization of unhealthy lifestyles and population ageing. Apparent causes such as raised blood pressure, increased blood glucose, elevated blood lipids and obesity may be representations of deep lying lifestyle habits.
2. **Multiple risk factors:** There are a number of risk factors that lead to the onset and development of NCDs. The various types of risks can be divided into three primary risk sets: modifiable behavioural risk factor, non-modifiable risk factor and metabolic risk factor, many of which are common for a number of diseases.
3. **Long latency period:** The latency period of NCDs is generally long, often stretching from many years to several decades.
4. **Non-contagious origin (non-communicable):** NCDs are not communicated from one person to another, so it is given that these diseases develop in a person from non-contagious origins.
5. **Prolonged course of illness:** NCDs are chronic in nature and thus the course of illness if often prolonged and takes years before a patient may be forced to opt for medical care or intervention.
6. **Functional impairment or disability:** NCDs usually give rise to circumstances that make it difficult for the patients to lead a normal life. Patients with chronic NCDs may not be able to take part in regular physical activity, go to the office or eat normally (Tabish, 2017).

5.3 Spatial Epidemiology of major Non-Communicable Diseases

According to World Heart Organization over 17 million deaths in the world are due to Coronary Vascular Disease (CVDs). This is followed by Cancer that is 8.2 million, respiratory disease, i.e., 4 million and Diabetes, i.e., 1.5 million in the world. In India, Coronary Heart disease, stroke and hypertension attribute to 45 per cent of the deaths; chronic respiratory disorder amounts to 23 per cent, cancer 12 per cent and diabetes 3 per cent of the total deaths in 2019.

5.3.1 *Obesity*

According to World Health Organization, overweight and obesity are defined as abnormal or excessive fat accumulation that may impair health. Body mass index (BMI) is a simple index of weight-for-height that is commonly used to classify overweight and obesity in adults. It is defined as a person's weight in kilograms divided by the square of his height in meters (kg/m^2).

It has become a severe epidemic health problem. It is continuing to be increasing among students (Bray, 1996; Tayem *et al.*, 2012). Obesity leads to so many disorders such as diabetes, hypertension, cardiovascular problems and many more (Warren *et al.*, 2010; Baig *et al.*, 2015). WHO data shows that obesity has tripled by 1975. In 2016, around 650 million people were obese. It is also remarkably prevalent in the children between 5-19 years of age with figure as high as 340 million. Approximately, 2.8 million deaths are reported as a result of being overweight or obese (WHO, 1998).

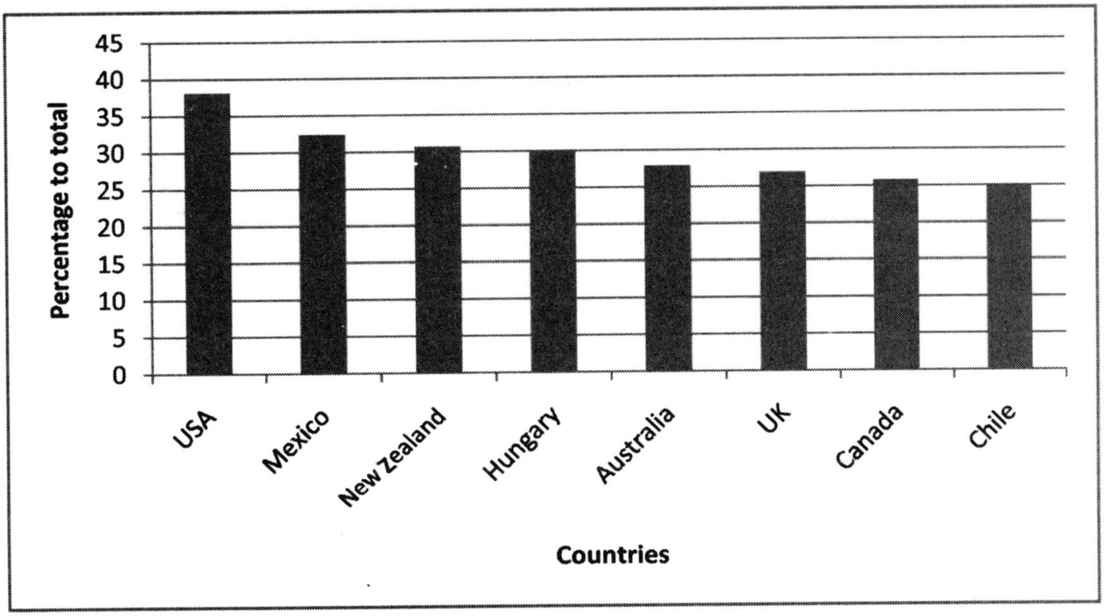

Fig. 5.2: Obese Population with countries more than 25 per cent of Population.

Source: OECD (2017), OECD Health Statistics, 2017. www.oecd.org/health/health-data.htm

In 2015, across the OECD, 19.5 per cent of the adult population was obese. This rate ranges from less than 6 per cent in Korea and Japan to more than 30 per cent in Hungary, New Zealand, Mexico and the United States. More than one in four adults is obese in Australia, Canada, Chile, South Africa and the United Kingdom. Overweight and obesity rates have grown rapidly in England. Obesity levels are expected to be particularly high in the United States, Mexico and England, where 47 per cent, 39 per cent and 35 per cent of the population respectively are projected to be obese in 2030. On the contrary, the increase is expected to be weaker in Italy and Korea, with obesity rates projected to be 13 per cent and 9 per cent in 2030, respectively. The level of obesity in France is projected to nearly match that of Spain, at 21 per cent in 2030. Obesity rates are projected to increase at a faster pace in Korea and Switzerland where rates have been historically low (OECD, 2017).

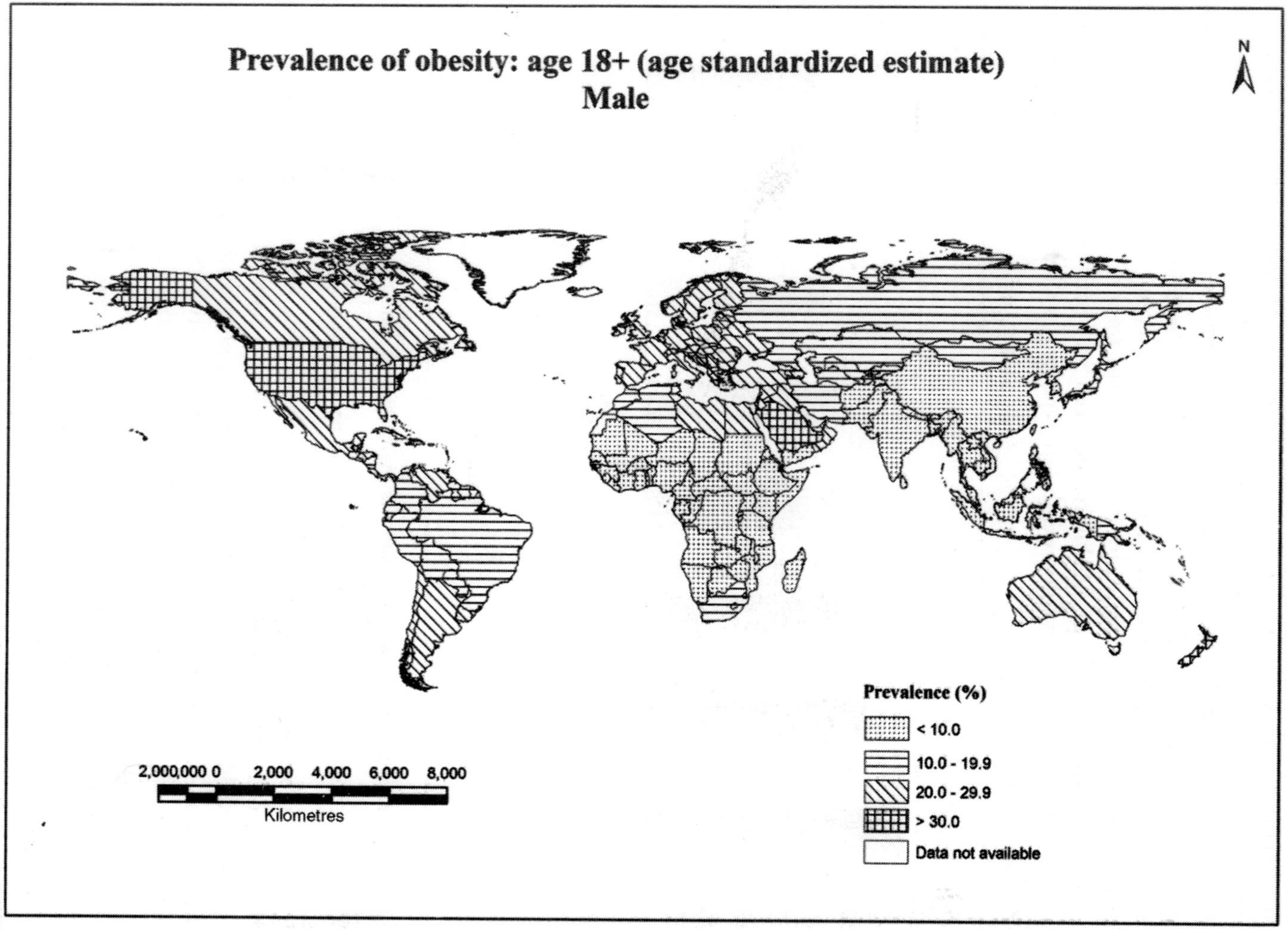

Fig. 5.3: Prevalence of Obesity : Age 18+ (Male).

Source: Adopted from WHO, 2017.

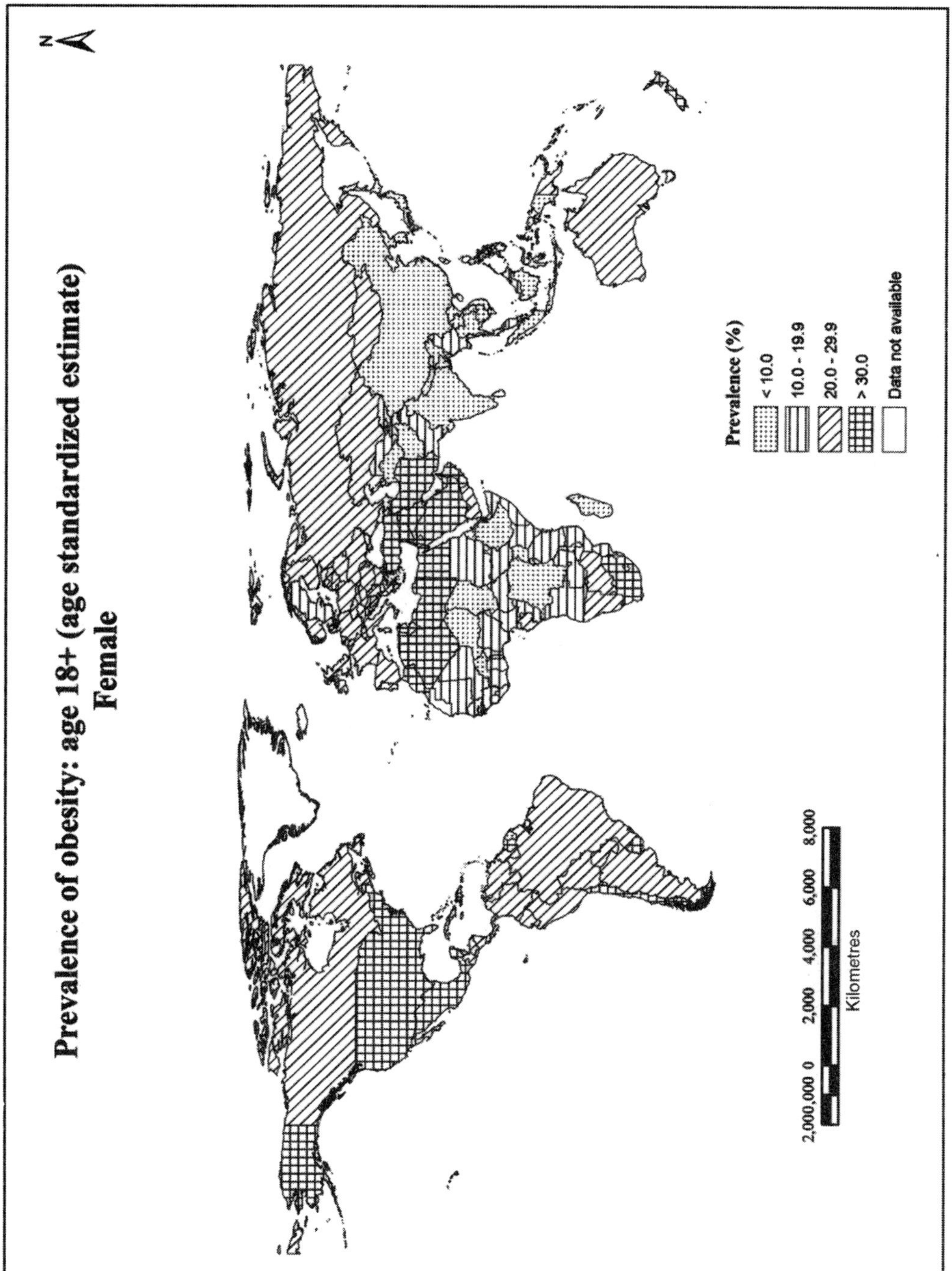

Fig. 5.4: Prevalence of Obesity : Age 18+ (Female).

Source: Adopted from WHO, 2017.

Major factors that contribute to increase in obese population are linked to changing lifestyle. Urbanization is on record high. People are migrating from rural and suburban to urban areas. People adopt complex urban lifestyle and indulge in faulty eating disorders. Higher consumption of packaged food and sedentary form of jobs lead to obesity. Together with these changes it has been reported that groups moving from rural to urban areas experience an increased intake of energy, sugar, refined grains and fat (Monteiro *et al.*, 1992). This dietary profile, referred to as a "western" diet, has been reported to be associated with diabetes, heart disease and excessive caloric intake and obesity (Popkin *et al.*, 1995; Drewnowski and Popkin, 1997; WHO, 1998).

Fig. 5.3 shows that obesity in males is highly prevalent in United States of America and Saudi Arabia. The WHO data show that more than 30 per cent of the population above the age of 18 is obese. In Canada, Euproe and Australia, the data varies between 20-29 per cent. Obesity in males is lowest, i.e., less than 10 per cent in Asia and African countries.

Fig. 5.4 shows that Obesity is high in females in United States of America, South Africa, Algeria, Libya, Egypt, Iran, Iraq etc. The obesity in females is low in parts of Central Africa and South Asia. This can be attributed to low physical activity and energy dense food consumption.

Due to the consumption of energy dense food (i.e. unhealthy food habits), sedentary lifestyle, lack of healthcare services and financial support, the developing countries are facing high risk of obesity and their adverse consequences (i.e. diabetes, ischemic heart disease etc.). In Africa, the number of overweight children under 5 has increased by nearly 24 per cent since 2000. Almost half of the children under 5 who were overweight or obese in 2019 lived in Asia. In India, more than 135 million individuals were affected by obesity (Ahirwar and Mondal, 2019).

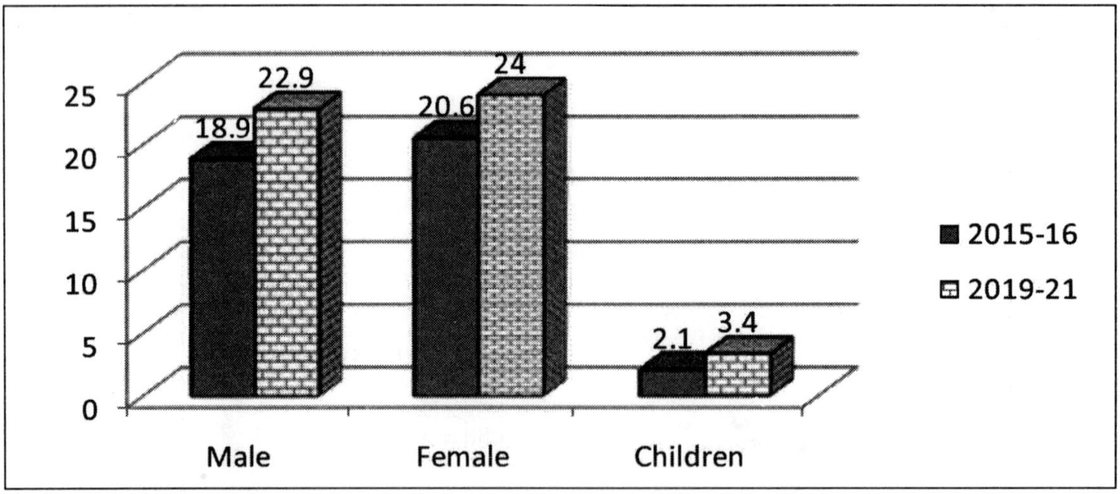

Fig. 5.5: Obesity among Males and Females in India (2005-19).

Source: NFHS, 2021.

According to the fifth round of the NFHS conducted between 2019 and 2021, about 6.4 per cent of women and 4.0 per cent of men aged 15-49 in India are obese. Around 17.6 per cent women and 18.9 per cent men in the same age group are overweight, but not obese. Studies showed that obesity also causes problems in thyroid function (Menon and Thenmozhi, 2016). Obesity also affects you psychologically by being bullied by the society which leads to a state of depression. As shown in Fig. 5.5, obesity among males have risen from 18.9 per cent to 22.9 per cent and in females from 20.6 per cent to 24 per cent from 2015-16 to 2019-21 NFHS rounds.

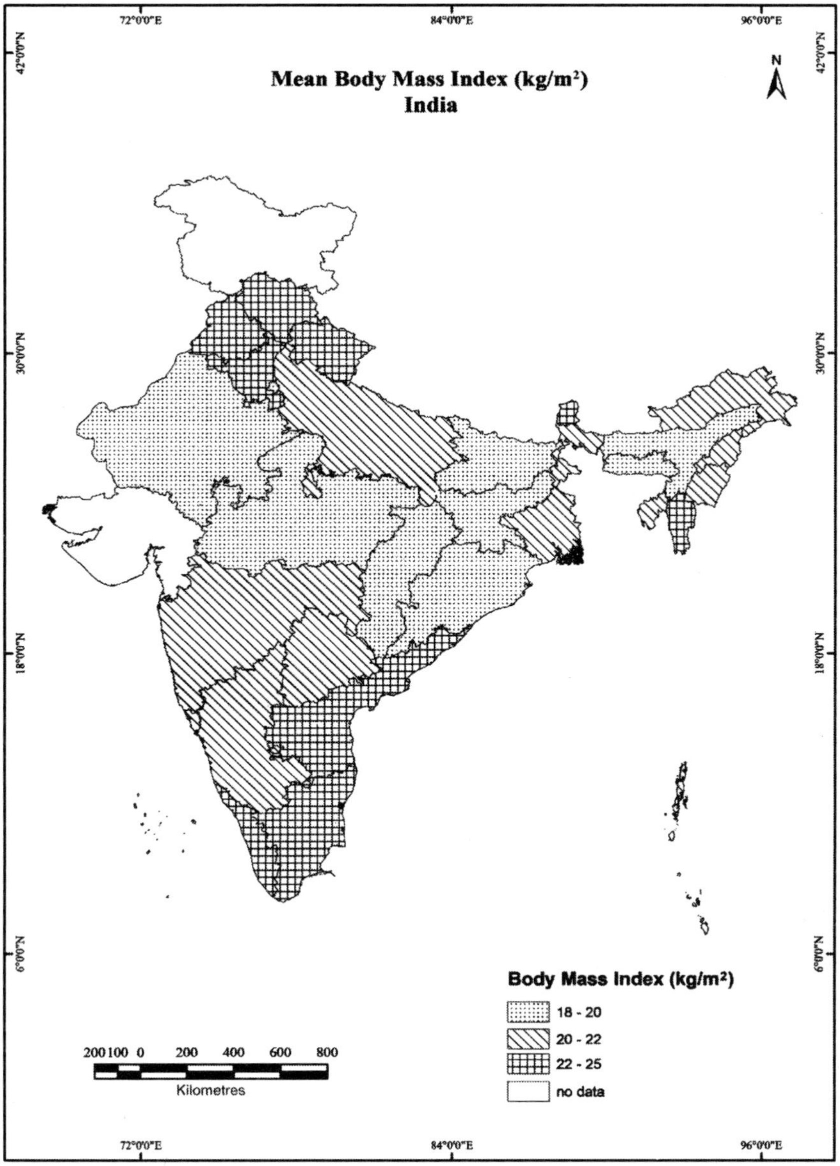

Fig. 5.6: Body Mass Index, India.

Source: Adopted from Geldsetzer *et al.,* 2018.

As per a study by Geldsetzer (Fig. 5.6), Mean BMI was high in both northern (Haryana, Himachal Pradesh, Punjab, and Uttarakhand) and southern states (Andhra Pradesh, Goa,

Karnataka, Kerala, Tamil Nadu), ranging from 22.8 kg/m^2 among males in Uttarakhand to 25.1 kg/m^2 among females in Punjab. Body Mass Index is less than 20 kg/m^2 in Rajasthan, Madhya Pradesh, Bihar, Jharkhand, Odisha, Assam etc. This can be linked to the type of economic activity and food consumption in this region. Regions where food is available in abundance and accessible easily, the BMI seems to be high. But there can be other reasons too.

5.3.2 *Malnutrition and Deficiency Diseases*

Where on one hand world is struggling from health challenges linked to obesity, overeating and consumption of high energy foods, on the other hand it is also struggling from health challenges linked to low consumption of required calaries and lesser consumption of nutrients. Malnutrition is associated not only with reduced body mass index but also with obesity. In fact, Obesity is defined as a paradoxical state of malnutrition, which despite excessive energy consumption is associated with a shortage of individual microelements (Kobylinska *et al.,* 2022). Malnutrition is a condition in which a deficiency of one or many nutrients has an adverse effect on cells, tissues, organs, and the body understood as a whole, which is manifested in the deterioration of its functioning and a negative change in the overall clinical picture. The European Society for Clinical Nutrition and Metabolism (ESPEN) defines malnutrition as a state of the body in which due to insufficient supply or incorrect absorption of essential nutrients, body composition changes, physical and mental impairment of the body and adverse effects on the outcome of the underlying disease (Burgos, 2018). According to UNICEF, 1 in 5 deaths among children below 5 years of age are attributed to severe wasting (Low weight for height) or stunting (low weight for age). It is caused by a lack of nutritious food and repeated bouts of diseases such as diarrhoea, measles and malaria, which in turn compromise a child's immunity (www.unicef.org). According to WHO, Malnutrition, in all its forms, includes undernutrition (wasting, stunting, and underweight), inadequate vitamins or minerals, overweight, obesity, and resulting diet-related non-communicable diseases. It is estimated that around 9 billion adults are overweight or obese, while 462 million are underweight. Globally in 2020, 149 million children under 5 were estimated to be stunted (too short for age), 45 million were estimated to be wasted (too thin for height), and 38.9 million were overweight or obese. Around 45 per cent of deaths among children below 5 years of age are linked to undernutrition. These mostly occur in low- and middle-income countries. At the same time, in these same countries, rates of childhood overweight and obesity are rising (who.int). Fig. 5.7 shows people who are undernourished mainly concentrated in areas of Central and Southern Africa, South Asia and Central America. This is because of high population density, poverty and high food insecurity.

Iron deficiency is prominent in Sub-Saharan Africa and South Asia, where more than 40 per cent of pregnant women suffer from Anaemia. Anaemia is a condition that is marked by low level of haemoglobin in the blood basically caused by iron deficiency. North America, Europe and Central Asia has less than 25 per cent of pregnant women with anaemia.

According to WHO, vitamin A deficiency's prevalence rates are typically highest across Africa and Asia. Across North Africa, the Middle East and Central/East Asia, between 20 and 25 per cent of pregnant women was vitamin-A deficient. Most countries across Sub-Saharan Africa and South Asia had slightly lower rates between 15 and 20 per cent. In children, prevalence rates

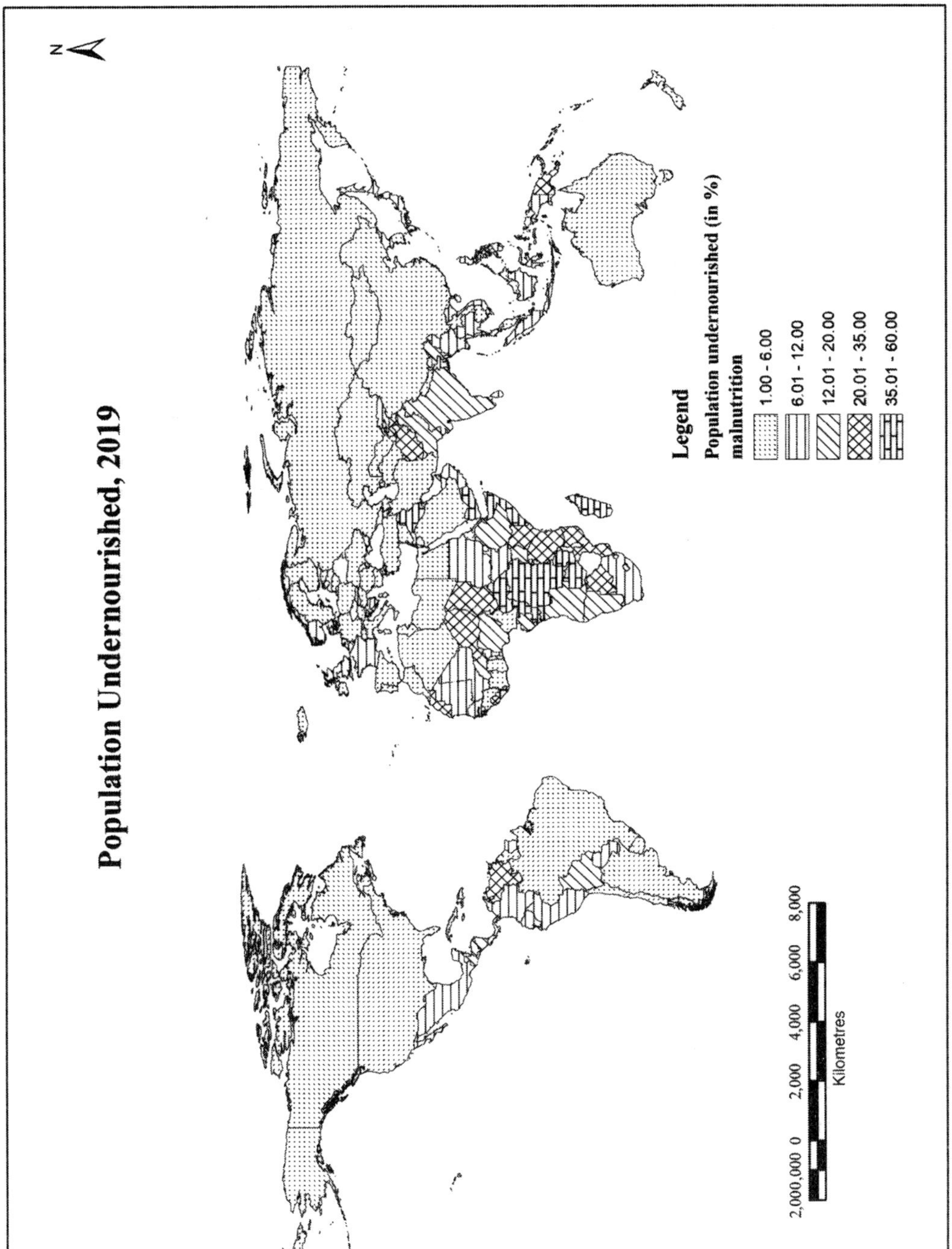

Fig. 5.7: Population Undernourished, 2019.

Source: Adopted from WHO, 2020.

are typically highest across Sub-Saharan Africa and South Asia, often reaching up to 60-70 per cent. The highest prevalence rate occurs in Kenya, where almost 85 per cent of children suffer from vitamin-A deficiency.Three main regions in the world where deficiency diseases can be prominently identified are: Sub Saharan Africa, South Asia and Central America.

1. **Sub-Saharan Africa:** Sub-Saharan Africa has a high prevalence of Vitamin A deficiency (VAD), which can lead to blindness and weakened immune systems, especially among children. According to the World Health Organization (WHO), around 48.1 per cent of preschool-aged children in the region are affected by VAD. Anaemia is another major health challenge here. It is a common deficiency disease in Sub-Saharan Africa, primarily affecting women and children. WHO reports that 52 per cent of pregnant women and 76 per cent of children under five in the region suffer from anaemia. Limited access to nutritious food due to poverty, inadequate food distribution, and limited health infrastructure are predominant reasons for deficiency diseases in Sub-Saharan Africa. Additionally, agricultural challenges, such as poor soil quality and climate conditions, can affect food production, leading to nutrient deficiencies.
2. **South Asia:** Iodine Deficiency Disorders (IDD) is prevalent in countries like Nepal, Bangladesh, and India. Lack of iodine in the diet can lead to goiter, mental retardation, and impaired cognitive development in children. According to UNICEF, around 94 million children in India have iodine deficiency. Inadequate dietary intake of iodine and a lack of awareness about the importance of iodized salt contribute to IDD in South Asia. In some regions, the availability and affordability of iodized salt may also be limited, exacerbating the problem.
3. **Central America:** Protein-Energy Malnutrition (PEM) is commonly prevalent in Guatemala and Honduras, especially among children. PEM can result in stunted growth and impaired cognitive development. According to the Food and Agriculture Organization (FAO), approximately 30 per cent of children under five in Guatemala suffer from chronic malnutrition. Poverty, limited access to diverse and nutritious foods, and inadequate nutrition education are key factors contributing to PEM in Central America. Inadequate healthcare infrastructure and lack of clean water and sanitation can also worsen the situation.

Even developed regions of the world are also facing one or the other vitamin and nutrient deficiency. Despite being a developed region, North America experiences a high prevalence of vitamin D deficiency due to various factors, including lifestyle choices and limited sun exposure. According to a study published in Nutrition Research Reviews, about 42 per cent of adults in the United States have inadequate vitamin D levels. Iron deficiency is also observed in North America, particularly among certain population groups like infants, women of childbearing age, and athletes. The Centres for Disease Control and Prevention (CDC) estimates that approximately 5 per cent to 12 per cent of women in the United States have iron deficiency.

Some European countries face challenges related to calcium deficiency, which can increase the risk of osteoporosis and fractures. For instance, a study published in the journal *Osteoporosis International* found that the prevalence of osteoporosis in men and women over 50 years old varied between 8 per cent and 37 per cent in different European countries. In Europe, vitamin

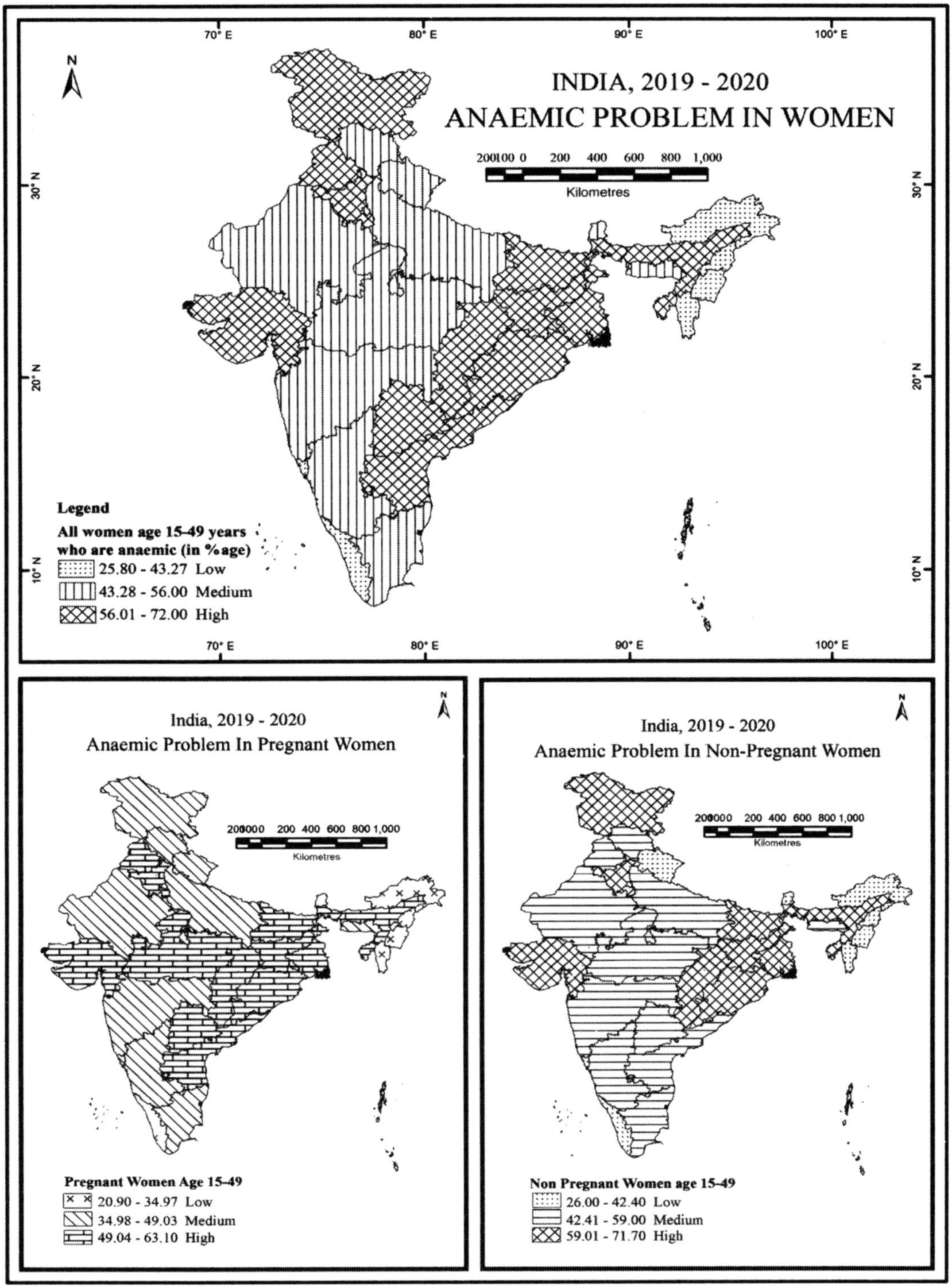

Fig. 5.8: Anaemic Problem in Women (India 2019-20).

Source: NFHS, 2020.

B12 deficiency can be an issue, particularly among older adults and vegetarians. According to a study published in *Clinical Biochemistry*, the prevalence of vitamin B12 deficiency among people aged 65 and above in various European countries ranged from 4 per cent to 6 per cent. Certain areas of Oceania, such as parts of Australia and New Zealand, experience iodine deficiency due to limited iodine in the soil and a decline in seafood consumption. The Australian Health Survey reported that around 45 per cent of Australians aged 2 years and above have insufficient iodine intake. A study published in the Australian and New Zealand *Journal of Public Health* found that 13.7 per cent of Australians in low socio-economic areas had inadequate vitamin C level.

According to *Worldometer*, India is the largest contributor of undernourished people in the world. This means roughly 194.4 million people, or 14.37 per cent of its population not receiving enough nutrition. Child malnutrition scenario is one of the worst in the world, with one-third of malnourished children of the world being Indian. As per the Government of India's National Family Health Survey 5 (NFHS-5), "Thirty-six per cent of children under age five years are stunted; 19 per cent are wasted; 32 per cent are underweight; and 3 per cent are overweight. Children born to illiterate mothers or children in the lowest wealth quintile are most likely to be undernourished" (www.thehindu.com). Geographically, Maharashtra followed by Bihar and Gujarat have the worst levels of malnourishment in children in the country. Madhya Pradesh, Andhra Pradesh, and Jharkhand have very high rates of undernutrition. Incidentally, these regions also have the highest population of children, and the highest poverty rates. Even states with the lowest percentage of undernutrition, such as Mizoram, Sikkim and Manipur have much higher malnutrition rates than developed nations. India's anaemia burden has grown alarmingly with NFHS-5 (2019-21) finding that 57 per cent of women in the age group 15-49 and 67 per cent children between six months and 59 months are anaemic (from the corresponding 53% and 58.6% respectively) in NFHS-4 (2015-16). Anaemia is like epidemic in India. (Fig. 5.8). Anaemia prevalence is high in women and children. It is high in Ladhak, Daman and Diu, West Bengal, Tripura and Chandigarh, where it is close to 70 per cent of women in age group 15-49 years. Mostly, the eastern coast of India is more affected by iron deficiency. In Gujarat, Ladhak, Chandigarh, Haryana and Jharkhand it is nearly 70 per cent among the children of less than 6 years of age.

1. **Northern India (Bihar, Uttar Pradesh, Rajasthan):** Iron deficiency anaemia is prevalent in northern India, particularly among women and children. According to the National Family Health Survey (NFHS) 4, the prevalence of anaemia among women aged 15-49 in Bihar is around 53.1 per cent. Vitamin A Deficiency (VAD) is also a matter of concern in northern India. NFHS-4 data shows that in Uttar Pradesh, around 54.9 per cent of children aged 6-59 months have vitamin A deficiency. Limited access to nutrient-rich foods, poor sanitation practices, and inadequate healthcare facilities contribute to these deficiency diseases in northern India. Socio-economic factors, cultural practices, and lack of awareness about proper nutrition can also play a role.
2. **Eastern India (West Bengal, Odisha, Jharkhand):** Iodine deficiency is a major concern in eastern India. According to a study published in the *Indian Journal of Public Health*, the prevalence of goiter (a consequence of IDD) in school-age children in West Bengal is as high as 32.6 per cent. Vitamin D deficiency is also observed in this region. A study conducted in Odisha reported that 51.6 per cent of adolescent girls had deficient or

insufficient levels of vitamin D. Protein Energy Malnutrition is also prevalent in Odisha and Jharkhand. This is mainly due to extreme poverty and hunger. Limited availability and consumption of iodized salt, lack of awareness about the importance of iodine, and limited exposure to sunlight contribute to IDD and vitamin D deficiency in eastern India. Poverty, inadequate healthcare infrastructure, and cultural factors may also contribute to these deficiencies.

3. **Southern India (Kerala, Tamil Nadu, Karnataka):** Calcium deficiency is a prominent issue in Southern India. According to a study published in the *Indian Journal of Clinical Biochemistry*, the prevalence of calcium deficiency among pregnant women in Karnataka is approximately 50 per cent. Vitamin B12 deficiency is also observed in Southern India, particularly among vegetarians. A study published in the *Indian Journal of Community Medicine* reported that in Tamil Nadu, around 16 per cent of participants had vitamin B12 deficiency. Dietary factors, such as low intake of milk and dairy products, contribute to calcium deficiency in southern India. Vegetarian diets and inadequate consumption of vitamin B12-rich foods, such as meat, fish, and eggs, contribute to vitamin B12 deficiency. Poor awareness and access to fortified foods may also play a role.

5.3.3 *Cardiovascular Diseases* (*Stroke and Heart Diseases*)

Cardiovascular diseases (CVDs) are a group of disorders of the heart and blood vessels. They include:

- *Coronary heart disease*—a disease of the blood vessels supplying the heart muscle;
- *Cerebrovascular disease*—a disease of the blood vessels supplying the brain;
- *Peripheral arterial disease*—a disease of blood vessels supplying the arms and legs;
- *Rheumatic heart disease*—damage to the heart muscle and heart valves from rheumatic fever, caused by streptococcal bacteria;
- *Congenital heart disease*—birth defects that affect the normal development and functioning of the heart caused by malformations of the heart structure from birth; and
- *Deep vein thrombosis and pulmonary embolism*—blood clots in the leg veins, which can dislodge and move to the heart and lungs (WHO, 2021).

CVD burden attributable to modifiable risk factors continues to increase globally. Prevalent cases of total CVD nearly doubled from 271 million in 1990 to 523 million in 2019, and the number of CVD deaths steadily increased from 12.1 million in 1990, reaching 18.6 million in 2019. Out of the 17 million premature deaths (under the age of 70) due to non-communicable diseases in 2019, 38 per cent were caused by CVDs. According to a paper in the *Journal of the American College of Cardiology* , the number of people dying from cardiovascular disease (CVD) is steadily rising, including one-third of all deaths globally in 2019. Further, it analyses the highest number of CVD deaths occurred in China, followed by India, Russia, the US and Indonesia. At the country level, age-standardized mortality rates for total CVD were lowest in France, Peru and Japan where rates were six-fold lower in 2019 than in 1990 (ACC, 2020).

The most common reason for this is a build-up of fatty deposits on the inner walls of the blood vessels that supply the heart or brain. Strokes can be caused by bleeding from a blood vessel

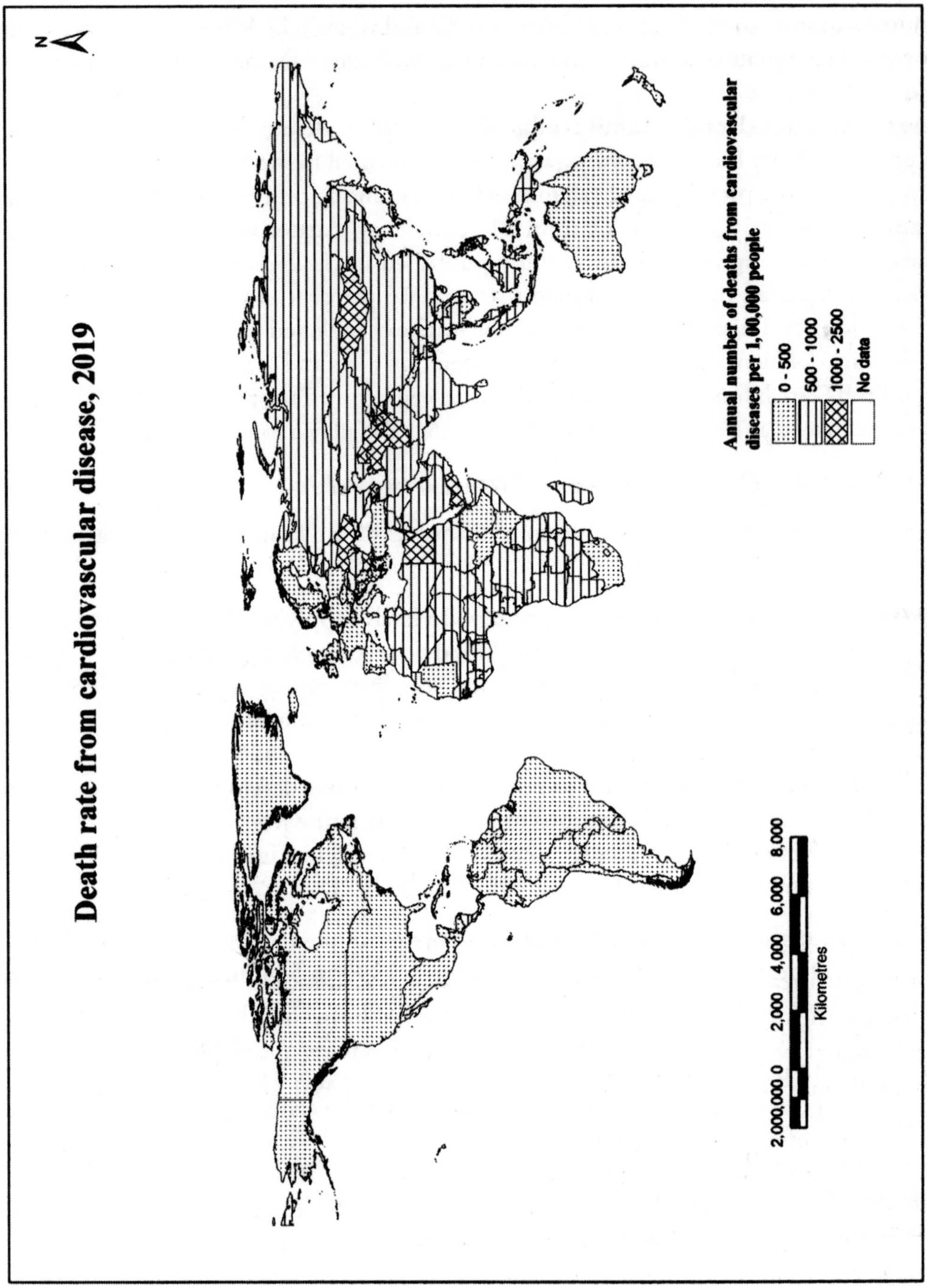

Fig. 5.9: Death Rate from Cardiovascular disease, 2019.

Source: Adopted from WHO, 2020.

in the brain or from blood clots. It can be caused genetically as well as due to lifestyle disorders. Unhealthy diet, physical inactivity, tobacco use and harmful use of alcohol are prominent factors responsible for Heart diseases.

Fig. 5.9 shows that death rate due to cardiovascular diseases is high in parts of Europe, Middle East and Central Asia. Almost entire Asia and Africa has 500-1000 annual number of deaths from cardiovascular diseases. The deaths due to CVD are remarkably high in between 500-1000 per one lakh, in almost entire Asia, Africa and Russia. This is because of less impactful health systems and huge population base in these countries.

In India in 2016, CVDs contributed to 28·1 per cent of total deaths and 14·1 per cent of total disability-adjusted life years (DALYs) compared with 15·2 per cent and 6·9 per cent, respectively in 1990. Within India, the rates of CVD vary markedly with highest in states of Kerala, Punjab and Tamil Nadu (Kumar and Sinha, 2020).

The age-standardized state-level mean 10-year CVD risk (across all age groups) varied from 10.2 per cent among females in Assam to 24.2 per cent among males in Nagaland and Himachal Pradesh. Similarly, the age-standardized prevalence of a high CVD risk varied from 5.0 per cent among females in Assam to 30.4 per cent among males in Kerala. Among both males and females, CVD risk tended to be highest in South India (including Goa), the 3 most northern states (Himachal Pradesh, Punjab, and Uttarakhand), the north-eastern states (except Assam), and West Bengal, particularly among males (Geldsetzer *et al.,* 2018).

5.3.4 *Cancer*

According to estimates from the International Agency for Research on Cancer (IARC), in 2018 there were 17.0 million new cancer cases and 9.5 million cancer deaths worldwide.

By 2040, the global burden is expected to grow to 27.5 million new cancer cases and 16.3 million cancer deaths simply due to the growth and aging of the population. However, the future cancer burden will probably be considerably larger due to increasing prevalence of factors that increase risk, such as smoking, unhealthy diet, physical inactivity, and fewer pregnancies. Cancers related to these factors, such as lung, breast, and colorectal cancers, are already on the rise in economically transitioning countries, a trend that will continue if preventive measures are not widely applied (American Cancer Society, 2018).

According to a reaserch, only 5-10 per cent of all cancer cases can be attributed to genetic defects, whereas the remaining 90-95 per cent has their roots in the environment and lifestyle. The lifestyle factors include cigarette smoking, diet (fried foods, red meat), alcohol, sun exposure, environmental pollutants, infections, stress, obesity, and physical inactivity. The evidence indicates that of all cancer-related deaths, almost 25-30 per cent are due to tobacco, as many as 30-35 per cent are linked to diet, about 15-20 per cent are due to infections, and the remaining percentage are due to other factors like radiation, stress, physical activity, environmental pollutants etc. (Anand *et al.,* 2008).

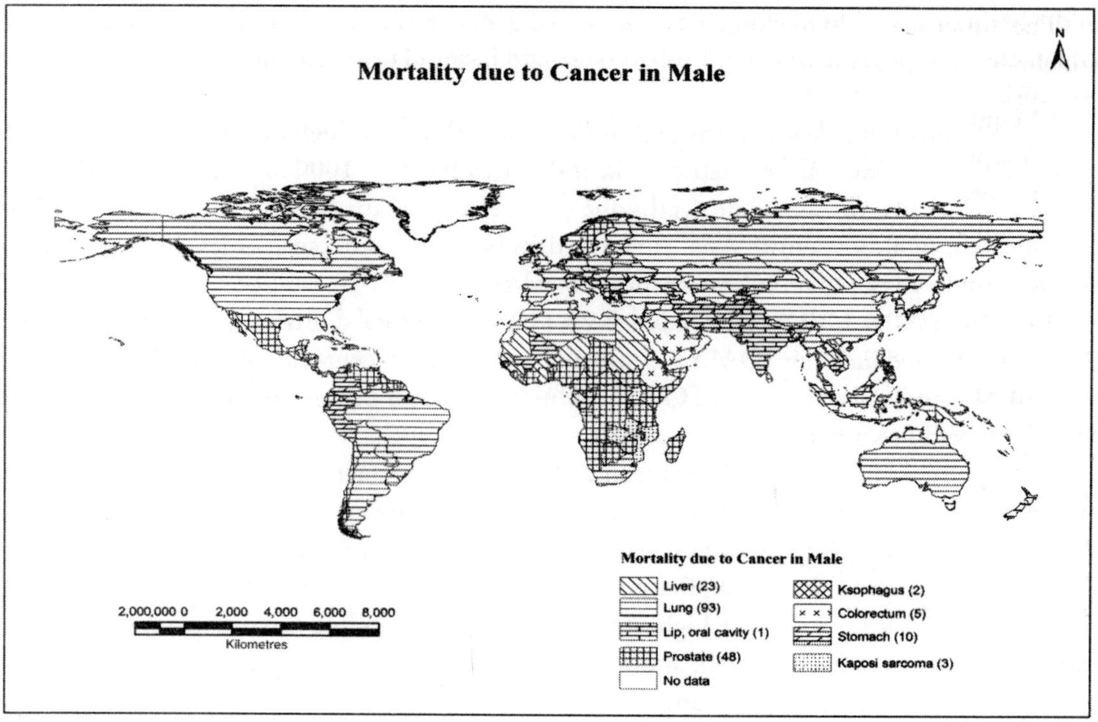

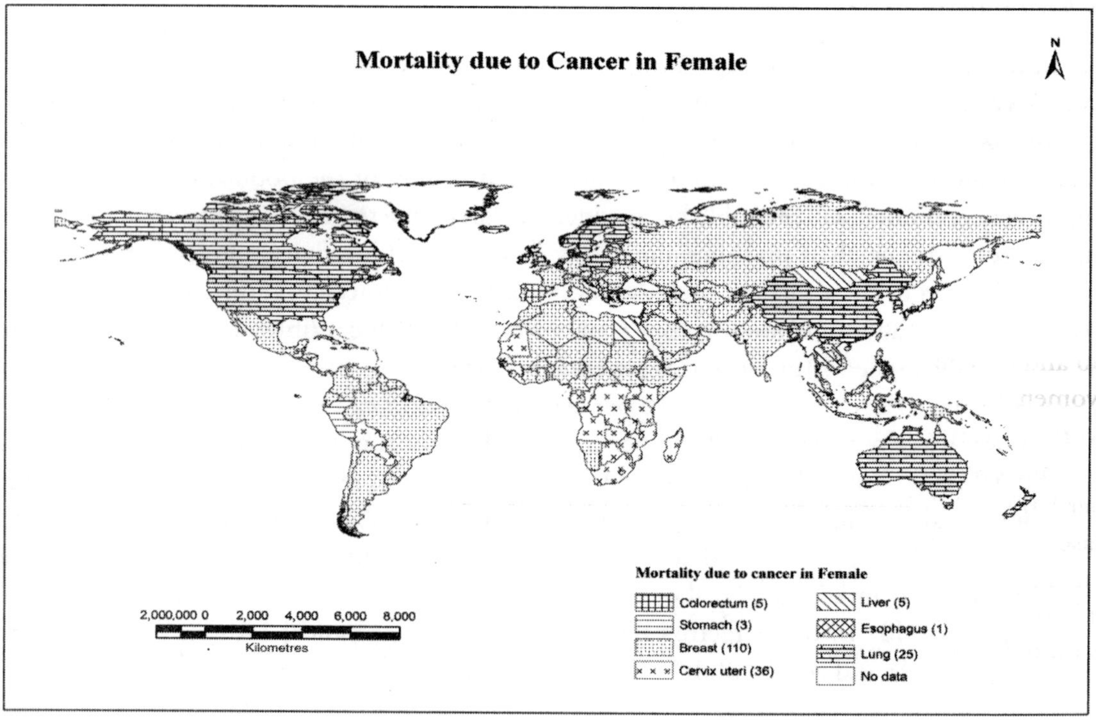

Fig. 5.10: Mortality due to type of Cancer Prevalent in different parts of the World among Males and Females.
Source: Adopted from WHO, 2020.

The American Cancer Society recently released updated dietary and physical activity guidelines for cancer prevention. The current guidelines support the following:

- Maintaining a healthy body weight throughout life;
- Adopting a physically active lifestyle;
- Consuming a healthy diet with an emphasis on plant food sources; and
- Limit alcoholic beverage consumption.

According to the National Centre for Health Statistics, 65 per cent of US adults over the age of 20 are overweight, with 30 per cent of those considered to be obese: (1) Obesity, particularly increased abdominal obesity, is associated with increased risk for the development of reduced insulin sensitivity; (2) predisposing to the development of metabolic syndrome, cardiovascular disease, diabetes, and some cancers. Most epidemiological studies support a role for obesity as a risk factor for endometrial (39%), esophageal (12%), kidney, and colon cancers (25%); and (3) For colorectal cancers, the effect of obesity as measured by body mass index (BMI) seems limited to the colon with no effect in the rectum, stronger in the proximal colon, and stronger in men than in women. In the case of hormonal cancer, a BMI above 30 kg/m^2 at age of 30 years has been associated with a significant increase in risk for developing hormone-related cancers including breast, ovarian, and uterine cancers (Carmichael, 2006).

According to the World Bank data, deaths due to liver and lung cancer are more prominent in middle income countries while kidney cancer is more in high income countries. Lip and oral cancer deaths are high in low income countries.

Fig. 5.10 shows mortality in males due to lung cancer is high in North America, South America, Australia, Europe, Central Asia etc. mortality is also high due to prostrate cancer among 48 per cent men, especially in Central Africa and Central America. Mortality in females is high due to breast cancer. It is prominent in South America, North and Central Africa, Indian Subcontinent, Russia, Mediterranean region. Cervical cancer, i.e., cancer of uterine cervix is the commonest cancer among women in the world. In developed countries, cervical cancer is a public health problem in developing countries like India, so much so that India alone accounts for one-quarter of the worldwide burden of cervical cancers. It is the one of the leading causes of cancer mortality, accounting for 17 per cent of all cancer deaths among women aged between 30 and 69 years. It is estimated that cervical cancer will occur in approximately 1 in 53 Indian women during their lifetime compared with 1 in 100 women in more developed regions of the world (Institute of Health Matrix and Evaluation, 2011).

According to World Bank data, cancer incidences are very high, i.e., more than 257 cases per 1,00,000 in North America, Australia, and European countries. Countries with low cancer cases, i.e., less than 111 per 1,00,000 are in parts of Central Africa and South Asia. In all high, medium and low income regions of the world tracheal, bronchus and lung cancer are the highest. It is followed by liver cancer, kidney cancer and lip and oral cancer respectively. Number of deaths is more in middle income regions than in high or low income regions (Fig. 5.11).

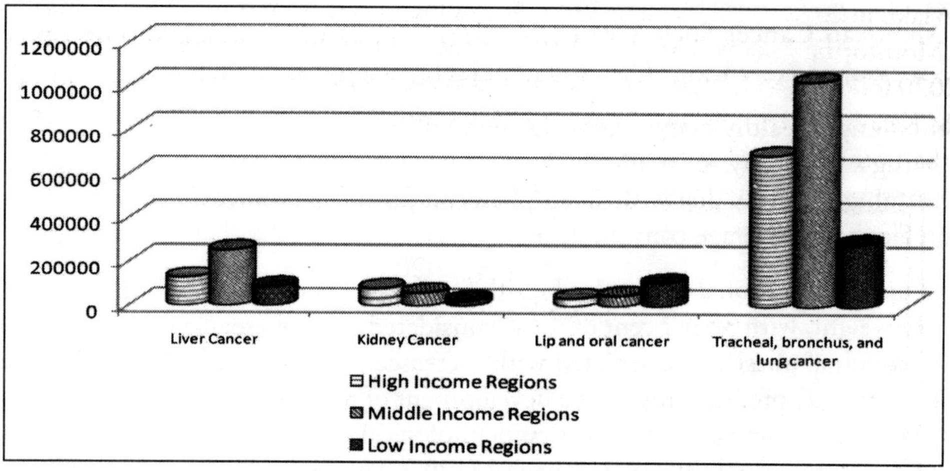

Fig. 5.11: Deaths due to Cancer.

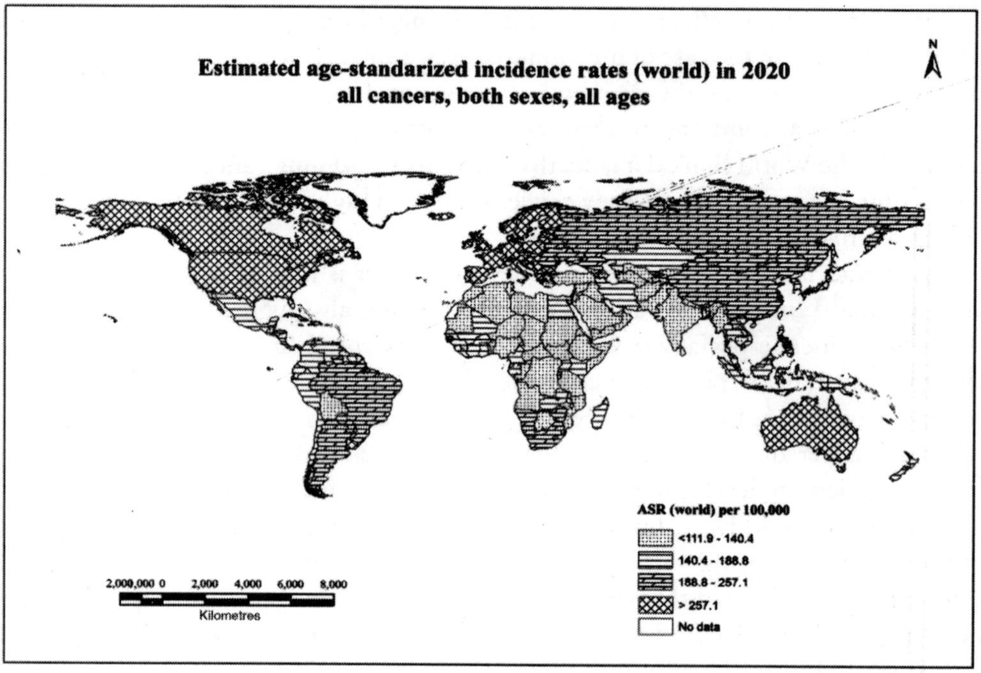

Fig. 5.12: Estimated Age standardised incidence rates in world 2020, all cancers, both sexes, all ages. *Source*: Adopted from WHO, 2017.

In India, some prominent causes for cancer include tobacco and alcohol consumption, unhealthy eating habits, use of chemicals in the form of cosmetics and toiletries. According to Ministry of Health and Family Welfare, tobacco consumption either as chewing tobacco or smoking tobacco will account for 50 per cent of all cancers in men. Dietary practices, reproductive and sexual practices etc. will account for 20-30 per cent of cancers.

According to a report published in one of the leading newspapers of India, *The Hindu*, on 14 March, 2023, according to the Indian Council of Medical Research-National Cancer Registry Programme (ICMR-NCRP), the number of cancer cases in the country is projected to go up from 14.6 lakh in 2022 to 15.7 lakh in 2025. According to data of National Non-Communicable Diseases Monitoring Survey, Uttar Pradesh recorded the highest number of 2.01 lakh cancer cases in 2020 followed by Maharashtra, Bihar and West Bengal. Himachal Pradesh, Uttrakhand, Jammu & Kashmir, Haryana and North Eastern states are also witnessing low level of cancer patients than other states (Fig. 5.13).

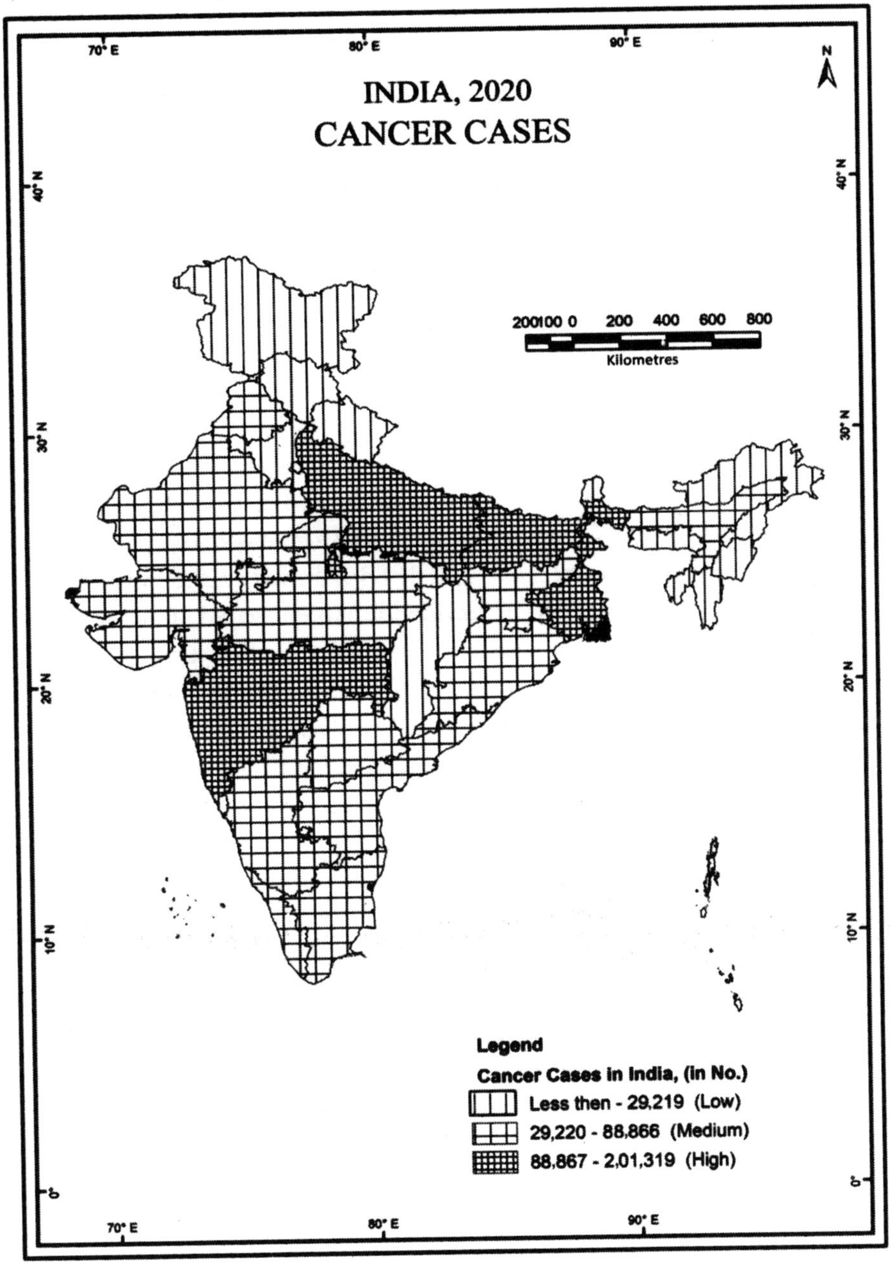

Fig. 5.13: India, Cancer Cases 2020.

Source: National Cancer Registry Programme, 2020.

5.3.5 *Hormonal Imbalance*

Hormones are chemicals that coordinate different functions in your body by carrying messages through your blood to your organs, skin, muscles and other tissues. These signals tell your body what to do and when to do it. Hormones are essential for life and your health. Hormones regulate metabolism, blood pressure, insulin levels, growth and development, sexual function, sleep, moods etc. Too high or too low hormones in a human body can lead to minor to chronic concerns. For example Hyperthyroidism happens when your thyroid gland makes more thyroid hormone than necessary. This can be caused by a range of things, including autoimmune conditions. On the contrary, Hypothyroidism occurs when your thyroid does not produce enough thyroid hormone. Imbalance of thyroid hormone can cause change in energy levels and functioning of various organs. Let's examine some common health challenges due to hormonal imbalance.

5.3.5.1 *Thyroid*

Thyroid is caused due to imbalance in thyroid hormone in thyroid glands. Two types of health disorders associated with it are hypothyroidism (less hormone) and Hyperthyroidism (more hormone). The first description of thyroid diseases as they are known today was that of Graves disease by Caleb Parry in 1786, but the pathogenesis of thyroid disease was not discovered until 1882-1886. Thomas Curling first described hypothyroidism (myxoedema) in 1850 and the cause and suitable treatment were established after 1883 (Ahmed and Ahmed, 2005). Thyroid diseases affect an estimated 200 million people worldwide. An estimated 40 per cent of the world's population—some 2·8 thousand million people—are at risk of iodine deficiency, a nutrient that is essential for the production of thyroid hormones. Iodine deficiency remains a major cause of morbidity worldwide: it contributed to an estimated 4 million disability-adjusted life years lost in 2010. Although substantial improvements have been made in developing countries, mainly through the provision of iodinised salt, iodine deficiency is still increasing in some developed countries—including Australia and the UK (*The Lancet*, 2013). According to the American Thyroid Association (ATA) 12 per cent of US population will develop thyroid conditioned in their lifetime and approximately 20 million Americans have some form of thyroid disease. Thyroid is linked to iodine deficiency. Many studies show poor diet, unhealthy lifestyle and mental stress can lead to thyroid. More sugar, salt and oil consumption with lack of exercise can lead to thyroid issues. Nearly 42 million Indians suffer from thyroid and many remain undiagnosed. Thyroid put many Indians to risk for cardiovascular disease, infertility issues, osteoporosis etc. Kerala is a state in the southern part of India. It is geographically divided in two parts, the coastal region and hilly region. The hilly region, due to deficiency of iodine, is known to report cases of thyroid disorders. But studies have depicted that even the coastal regions are known to report higher cases of goiter. The inland and hilly states report higher cases of thyroid. The capital city of India, Delhi lies in the sub-Himalayan plains of India. This region is known to have iodine deficiency in the soil and in the cultivated vegetables. The universal iodization programme introduced the Iodised salt in 1983, which was almost 4 decades back. Still the population is deficient in iodine and develop goitre, and other thyroid disease (redcliffelabs.com). Telangana is not known for widespread iodine deficiency in its population, the main cause for thyroid disorders, but the state ranks fourth in India when it comes to this endocrine disease, triggered largely by high consumption of junk food. According to the Union Health and Family Welfare Ministry's latest data, Telangana has 5763 women per lakh suffering from thyroid. Dietary changes with healthy lifestyle can bring changes in the metabolism and functioning of various body organs which can perhaps help to mitigate the thyroid issues in body (refer Fig. 5.14).

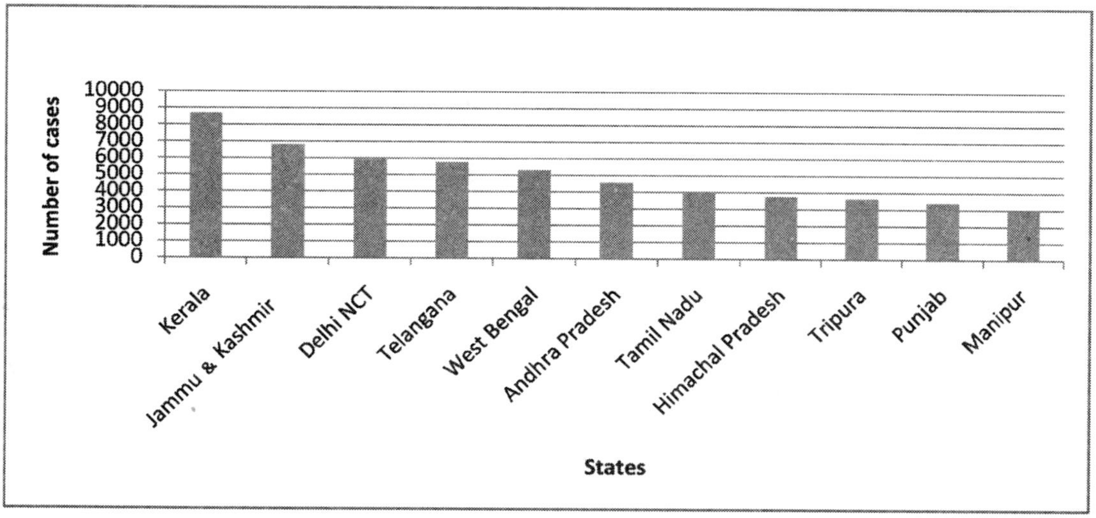

Fig. 5.14: Thyroid cases in Indian States (per lakh).

5.3.5.2 *Diabetes*

Diabetes is a chronic (long-lasting) health condition that affects how human body turns food into energy. Human body breaks down most of the food into sugar (glucose) and releases it into bloodstream. When the blood sugar goes up, it signals your pancreas to release insulin. Insulin acts like a key to let the blood sugar into your body's cells for use as energy. With diabetes, the body does not make enough insulin or cannot use it as well as it should. When there is not enough insulin or cells stop responding to insulin, too much blood sugar stays in your bloodstream. Over time, that can cause serious health problems, such as heart disease, vision loss, and kidney disease (CPCD). Diabetes, especially Type 2 diabetes is an outcome of poor food habits and sedentary lifestyle. The term "diabetes" was first coined by Araetus of Cappodocia (81-133 AD). Later, the word mellitus (honey sweet) was added by Thomas Willis (Britain) in 1675 after rediscovering the sweetness of urine and blood of patients (first noticed by the ancient Indians). It was only in 1776 that Dobson (Britain) firstly confirmed the presence of excess sugar in urine and blood as a cause of their sweetness. In modern time, the history of diabetes coincided with the emergence of experimental medicine. An important milestone in the history of diabetes is the establishment of the role of the liver in glycogenesis, and the concept that diabetes is due to excess glucose production by Claude Bernard (France) in 1857. The role of the pancreas in pathogenesis of diabetes was discovered by Mering and Minkowski (Austria) 1889. Later, this discovery constituted the basis of insulin isolation and clinical use by Banting and Best (Canada) in 1921 (Ahmed, 2002). According to WHO, in the past 3 decades, the prevalence of type 2 diabetes has risen dramatically in countries of all income levels. About 422 million people worldwide have diabetes, the majority living in low- and middle-income countries, and 1.5 million deaths are directly attributed to diabetes each year.

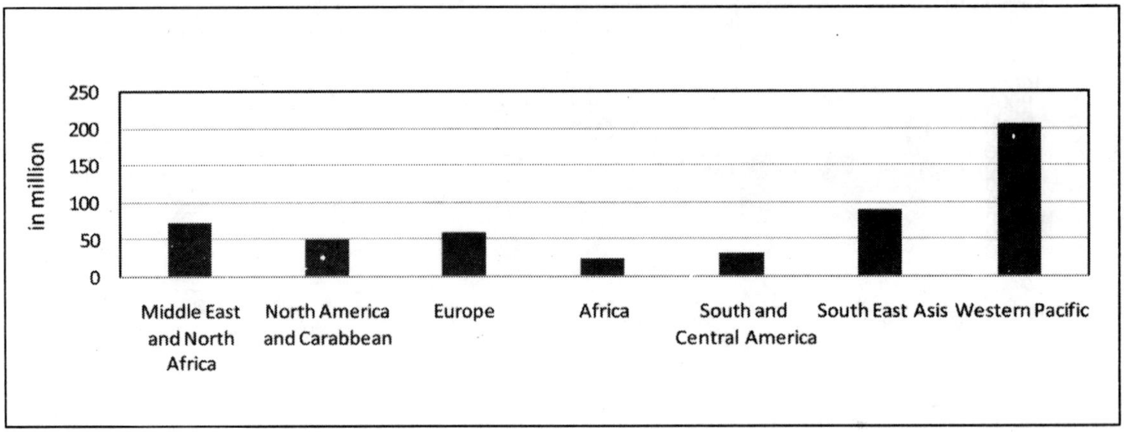

Fig. 5.15: People Living with Diabetes (in millions).

Source: IDF, Diabetes Atlas 2022.

It could be seen from Fig. 5.15, Middle East and North Africa have highest number of people having diabetes followed by South East Asia, Western Pacific, Europe, North America and Caribbean. IDF data further analyses that over 3 in 4 adults with diabetes live in low- and middle-income countries. Diabetes is responsible for 6.7 million deaths in 2021—1 every 5 seconds. By the year 2035, nearly 592 million people are predicted to die of diabetes (Tao *et al.*, 2015). Type 2 diabetes, which constitutes 90 per cent of all cases of diabetes, earlier considered to be a disease of the affluent "Western" countries, has now spread globally, and has become a major cause of disability and death affecting even younger age group (IDF, 2019). Diabetes has reached epidemic proportions in many developing economies, such as China and India (Pradeepa and Mohan, 2021).

Fig. 5.16 shows that prevalence of raised fasting blood glucose levels are high in Middle East and Mediterranean region. Parts of Central Asia and North Africa also experience 10-12 per cent of population experiencing high fasting blood sugar levels. This is low in North America, Canada, Euorpe and Oceania. This in a way reflects, diabetic conditions or insulin resistance conditions in the regions with high blood sugar levels.

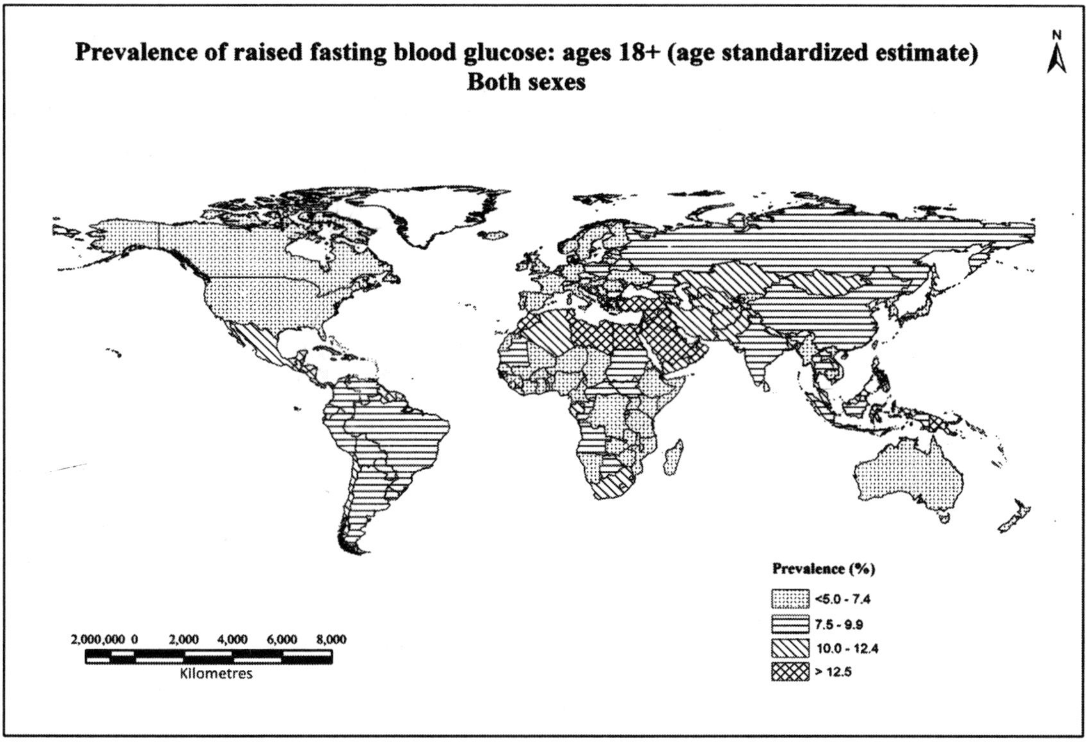

Fig. 5.16: Prevalence of raised fasting blood glucose: Ages 18+ (age standardized estimate), Both sexes.

Source: Adopted from WHO, 2017.

According to WHO in India, there are estimated 77 million people above the age of 18 years are suffering from diabetes (type 2) and nearly 25 million are prediabetics (at a higher risk of developing diabetes in near future). More than 50 per cent of people are unaware of their diabetic status which leads to health complications if not detected and treated early. Adults with diabetes have a two- to three-fold increased risk of heart attacks and strokes. Combined with reduced blood flow, neuropathy (nerve damage) in the feet increases the chance of foot ulcers, infection, and the eventual need for limb amputation. Diabetic retinopathy is an important cause of blindness and occurs as a result of long-term accumulated damage to the small blood vessels in the retina. Diabetes is among the leading causes of kidney failure. According to WHO, healthy diet, regular physical activity, maintaining a normal body weight and avoiding tobacco use are ways to prevent or delay the onset of type 2 diabetes.

Geldsetzer further in his study reported high blood glucose prevalence, however, was relatively low in the northern states (ranging from 4.4% among males in Himachal Pradesh to 10.9% among females in Punjab). Mean systolic BP was highest in the northern states (ranging from 123.7 mm Hg among females in Haryana to 136.2 mm Hg among males in Punjab) as well as in Nagaland and Sikkim (130.7 mm Hg and 132.8 mm Hg among females and 133.6 mm Hg and 133.1 mm Hg among males, respectively). Smoking was most prevalent among males in the north-eastern states of Arunachal Pradesh (46.4%), Manipur (60.3%), Meghalaya (59.7%), and Mizoram (71.7%) and the eastern state of West Bengal (49.5%).

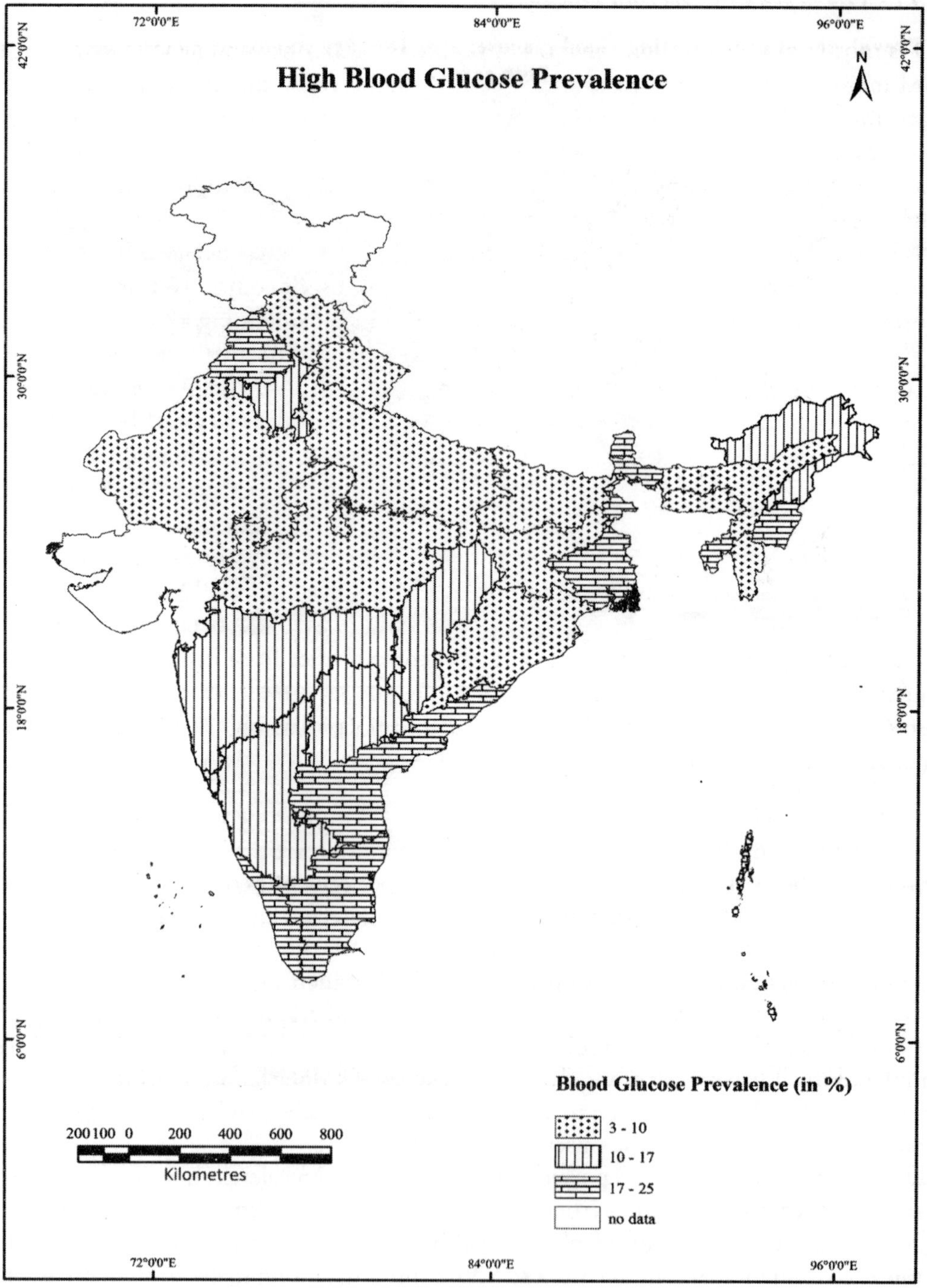

Fig. 5.17: High Blood Glucose, Prevalence in India.

Source: Modified and adopted from Geldsetzer *et al.,* 2018.

5.3.5.3 *PCOD (Polycystic Ovarian Disease)*

PCOD is mostly caused by a combination of hormonal imbalance and genetic tendencies. In a standard menstrual cycle, the two ovaries will alternately release mature, ready-to-be-fertilized eggs each month. This also leads to the ovaries swelling and becoming enlarged. Generally, the ovaries release a limited amount of androgens (male hormones) during the cycle—but in this case, the ovaries will start producing androgens in excess, which leads to symptoms like male pattern hair loss, abdominal weight gain, irregular periods, and in some extreme cases, even infertility. There is no set 'cure' as such for PCOD, but one of the best ways to manage it is by introducing changes in your lifestyle (after having consulted professionals, of course: your gynaecologist, an endocrinologist and a dietician, preferably). Exercising and maintaining a healthy diet (low on sugars and carbohydrates, high on protein and fiber) are the most effective ways to get your PCOD under control. This also cuts out some of the weight gain, which is very helpful, as even a 5 per cent reduction in weight eases treatment considerably (www.unicef.org). Polycystic Ovarian Syndrome is similar to Polycystic ovarian syndrome (PCOS) is a common endocrine/hormonal disorder that affects women, especially after puberty. Alternatively, PCOS may be expanded as polycystic ovary syndrome. Around 5-15 per cent of women in the reproductive age group suffer from hormonal imbalances that lead to menstrual irregularities, cysts in ovaries, infertility, and other health problems that include cardiovascular complications, type 2 diabetes mellitus (T2DM), and endometrial cancer. PCOS is recognized as an important reproductive as well as a metabolic disorder since it affects the ovaries, and 40 per cent of the affected women suffer from insulin resistance and are subsequently predisposed to developing T2DM. The global prevalence of PCOS is estimated between 4 per cent and 20 per cent. The World Health Organization (WHO) data suggest that approximately 116 million women (3.4%) are affected by PCOS globally.

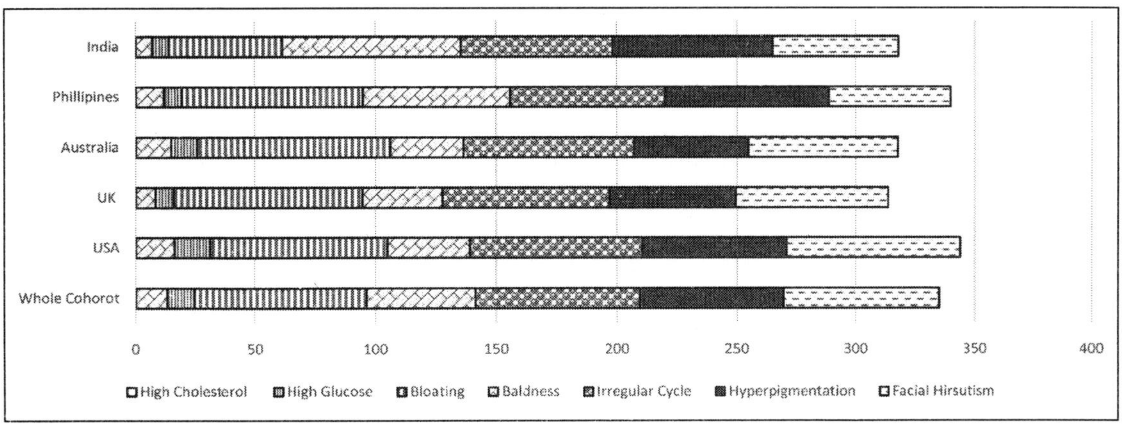

Fig. 5.18: Symptoms of PCOS in women.

Source: Jain *et al.,* 2021.

In the US, UK, and Australia, the most common symptoms of PCOS positive women were bloating, facial hirsutism, and irregular cycles (see Fig. 5.18). In the Philippines, women with PCOS were most likely to have bloating (75.4%), hyperpigmentation (68.5%), irregular cycle (64.4%), and baldness (61.0%). Women with PCOS in India most often reported baldness

(74.4%), hyperpigmentation (66.5%), and irregular cycles (62.2%). In four of the top five countries, the most frequently reported symptom was bloating, seen in 73.8 per cent of US women, 78.6 per cent of UK women, 80.4 per cent of women in Australia, and 75.4 per cent of women in the Philippines with PCOS (Jain *et al.*, 2021).

The data on the prevalence of PCOS in India are scarce. According to the National Health Portal of India, the prevalence rate of PCOS in Maharashtra was noted to be 22.5 per cent. Another previous report from South India, which included adolescents, showed an incidence of 9.13 per cent. However, the diagnostic criteria for PCOS were different in those studies (Jabeen *et al.*, 2022). It is difficult to gather data regarding PCOS/D as females do not discuss about it in open and families too consider it as a taboo to discuss or share information. According to a survey conducted by OZiva, key findings of the Nationwide PCOS Survey were:

1. 35 per cent of women have never spoken about their condition (PCOS) to anyone;
2. Almost 15 per cent of women never want to talk about PCOS to anyone and more than 4.5 per cent consider talking about PCOS a taboo;
3. Almost 48 per cent of women find it uncomfortable speaking about PCOS with their spouses and have never done so. Most women prefer discussing this with their mothers;
4. Around 65 per cent of women have been shamed or know someone who has been shamed for having PCOS or related symptoms (like facial hair, difficulty losing weight, difficulty conceiving etc.); and
5. More than 60 per cent of men do not know what PCOS is (*The Print*, 2021).

5.3.6 *Hypertension*

Hypertension or high blood pressure is a common health challenge faced by people of different age groups. It is when the pressure in your blood vessels is too high (140/90 mmHg or higher). According to WHO, things that increase the risk of having high blood pressure include: older age, genetics, being overweight or obese, not being physically active, high-salt diet, drinking too much alcohol. Lifestyle changes like eating a healthier diet, quitting tobacco and being more active can help lower blood pressure. Some people may still need to take medicines. Prominent symptoms are severe headache, vomiting, dizziness, chest pain etc. Hypertension is leading cause of cardiovascular diseases.

According to WHO, an estimated 1.28 billion adults aged 30-79 years worldwide have hypertension, most (two-thirds) living in low- and middle-income countries. An estimated 46 per cent of adults with hypertension are unaware that they have the condition. Less than half of adults (42%) with hypertension are diagnosed and treated. Approximately, 1 in 5 adults (21%) with hypertension have it under control. Hypertension is a major cause of premature death worldwide. One of the global targets for non-communicable diseases is to reduce the prevalence of hypertension by 33 per cent between 2010 and 2030 (www.who.int).

It can be seen from Fig. 5.19 epidemiology due to hypertension is less prevalent in North America, Australia and Europe, in case of women. In case of men North Africa and Mediterranean region is having less cases of hypertension. Developing countries of Africa and parts of Central Asia and Europe have more than 34 per cent of cases of hypertension.

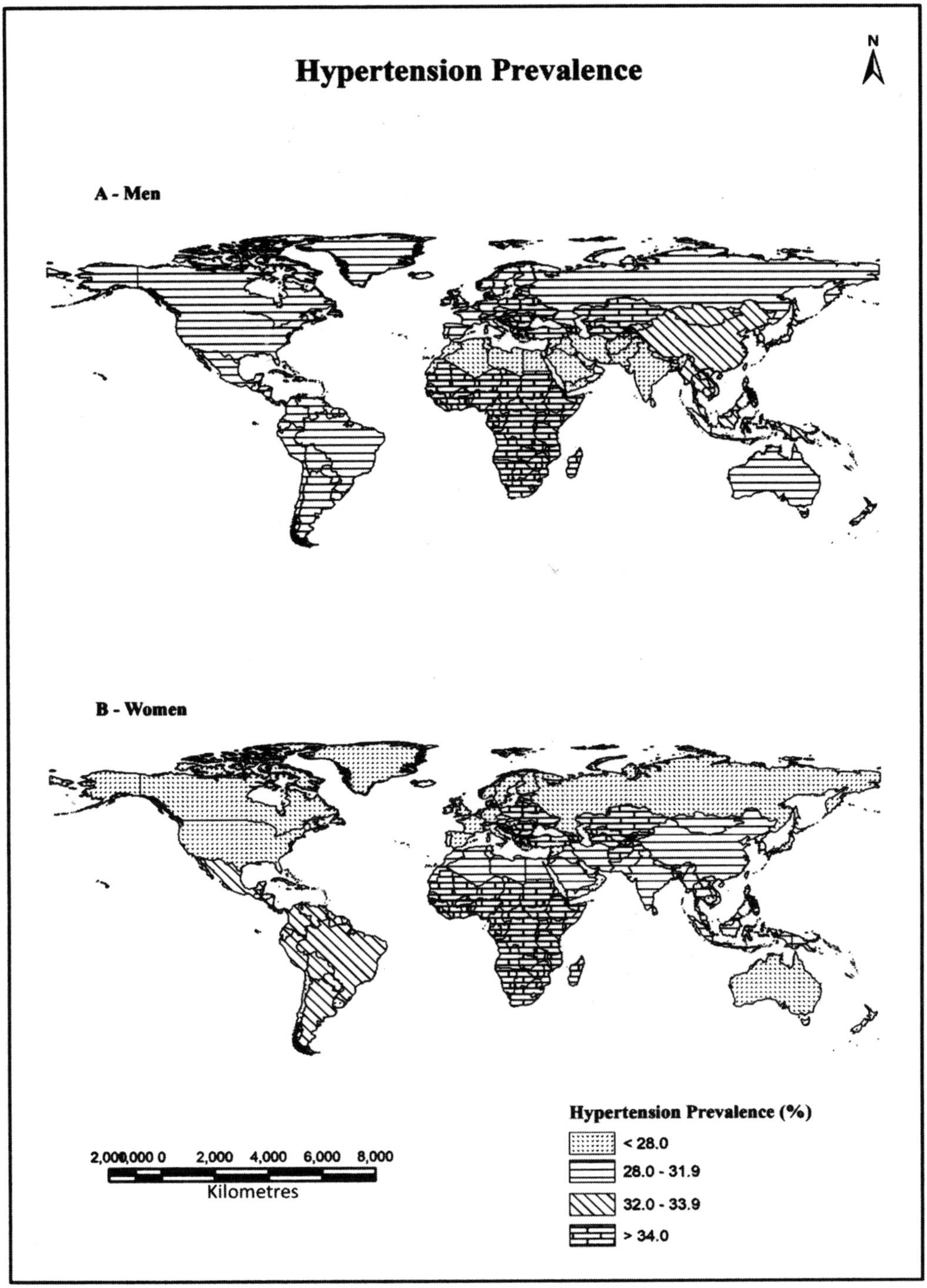

Fig. 5.19: Hypertension Prevalence in World.

Source: Adopted from Mills, K.T., Stefanescu, A. & He, J. The global epidemiology of hypertension. *Nat Rev Nephrol* 16, 223-237 (2020). https://doi.org/10.1038/s41581-019-0244-2

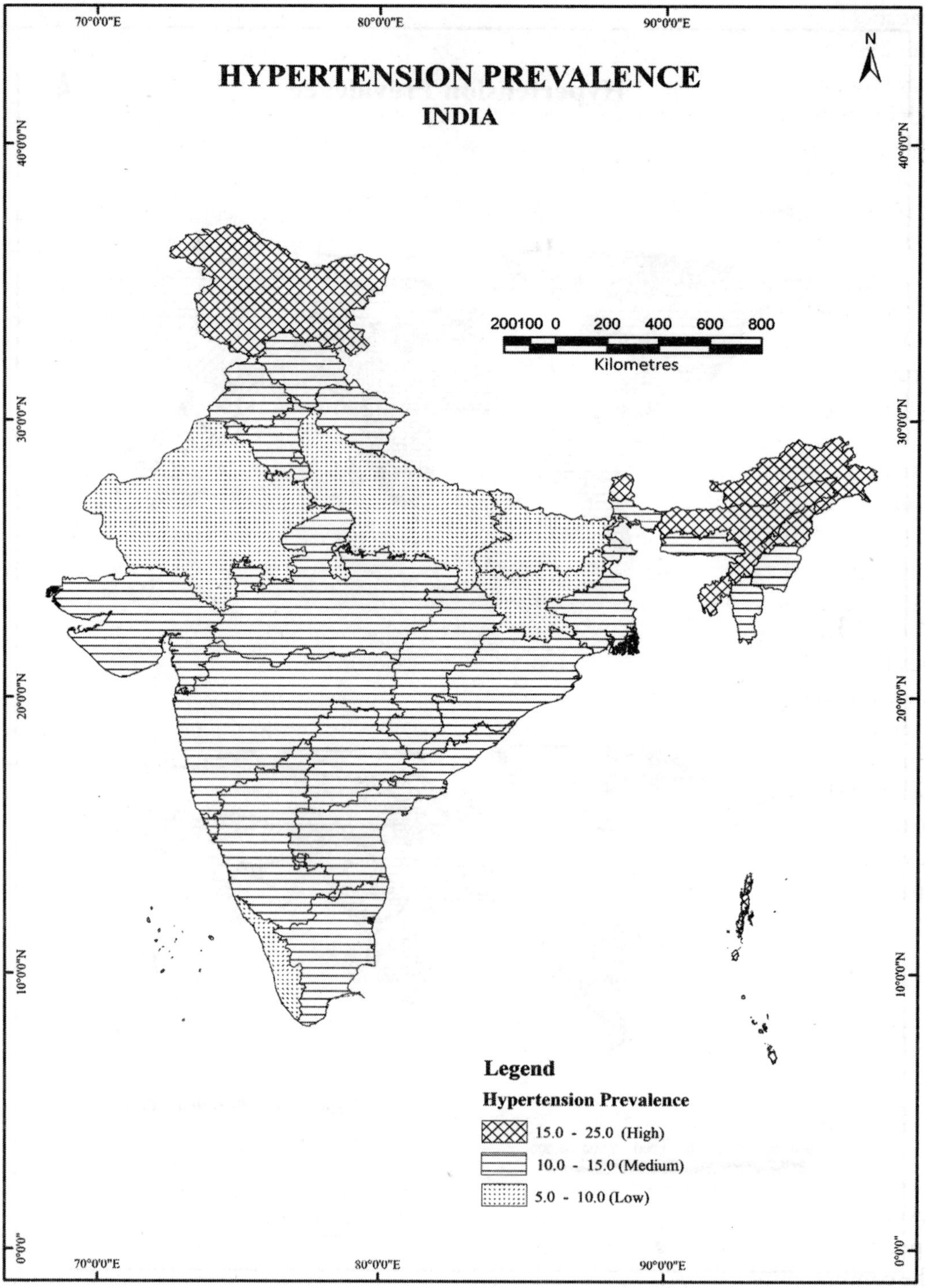

Fig. 5.20: Hypertension Prevalence in India (in percentage).

Source: Adopted from Ghosh and Kumar, 2019.

Statistics show that men are more prone to hypertension as compared to women. On a global average, 29.2 per cent of men and 24.8 per cent of women are suffering from hypertension. Croatia, Hungary, Slovenia, Lithuania, and Latvia are the top five countries which are notable for high blood pressure among men; correspondingly Mali, Burkina, Niger, Chad and Somalia are ranked as the top five countries which are notable for high blood pressure among women (*India Today*, 2017).

In India, the age-adjusted prevalence of hypertension was 11.3 per cent (95% CI 11.16% to 11.43%) among persons aged between 15 and 49 and was four percentage points higher among males 13.8 per cent (95% CI 13.46% to 14.19%) than among females 10.9 per cent (95% CI 10.79% to 11.06%). Persons in the urban location (12.5%, 95% CI 12.25% to 12.80%) had a marginally higher prevalence than persons in rural location (10.6%, 95% CI 10.50% to 10.78%). The proportion of population suffering from hypertension varied greatly between states, with a prevalence of 8.2 per cent (95% CI 7.58% to 8.85%) in Kerala to 20.3 per cent (95% CI 18.81% to 21.77%) in Sikkim. Advancing age, obesity/overweight, male sex, socio-economic status and consumption of alcohol were found to be the major predictors of hypertension (Ghosh and Kumar, 2019) (Fig. 5.20).

According to a survey published in *India Today* on 17th May, 2017, in India, people in urban areas are greater victims of hypertension (33-40%), as compared to villages (12-17%). The global men-women ratio also replicates in the Indian scenario, with 23.5 per cent of men and 22.60 per cent of women, above the age of 25, falling prey to the silent killer.

Prevalence of Metabolic Syndrome [a state of central obesity, high blood pressure, insulin resistance and dyslipidaemia, i.e. Dyslipidemia is an abnormal amount of lipids (e.g. triglycerides, cholesterol and/or fat phospholipids) in the blood] has reached epidemic proportions in India in recent years. Reported prevalence of MS in some regions of the country ranges from 23.2 to 41.1 per cent (Deepa *et al.*, 2007). Many of the participants of the study by Ray *et al.* would have had metabolic syndrome because of the high prevalence of pre-hypertension, overweight/obesity and adverse lipid profiles in their study cohort. The high CVD risk of this apparently healthy adult population has important implications that should alarm the public health authorities of the country (Pappachan, 2011).

5.4 Management of Lifestyle Diseases

The World Health Assembly adopted a resolution in the year 2000 on the prevention and control of chronic diseases. It called on its Member States to develop national policy frameworks, taking into account healthy public policies as well as fiscal and taxation measures towards healthy and unhealthy goods and services. The resolution also asked to establish programmes for the prevention and control of chronic diseases; assess and monitor mortality and the proportion of sickness in an area due to chronic diseases; promote effective secondary and tertiary prevention; and develop guidelines for cost-effective screening, diagnosis, and treatment of chronic diseases, with special emphasis in developing countries.

The combination of four healthy lifestyle factors—maintaining a healthy weight, exercising regularly, following a healthy diet, and not smoking—seem to be associated with as much as an 80 per cent reduction in the risk of developing the most common and deadly chronic diseases. This reinforces the current public health recommendations for the observance of healthy lifestyle habits, and because the roots of these habits often originate during the formative stages of life, it is especially important to start early in teaching important lessons concerning healthy living.

According to WHO and WebMD report consuming less than one table spoon salt a day and reducing intake of junk food can help to solve the problem of hypertension and cardiovascular diseases. Consuming more of green leafy vegetables and fruits helps to maintain metabolic balance in the body. Moreover, home cooked food with less of sugar, salt and oil can also help to resolve the health issues. One hour exercise physical like brisk walk, swimming, cycling, aerobics, yoga can also act as a stimulus towards improvement of health and managing lifestyle diseases.

National Centre for Chronic Disease Prevention and Health Promotion (NCCDPHP) points out that chronic diseases are mainly caused by risk behaviours like alcohol consumption, smoking, poor nutrition, physically inactive etc.

According to a study by Yangkoo Han *et al.*, Monitoring a person's lifestyle over a long period of time can be helpful for the following purposes:

- **Early identification of the lifestyle:** A person is generally at risk of a lifestyle disease when he/she lives his/her life in a certain style. Moreover, initial signs and symptoms of such diseases appear in people with irregular life patterns. By long term activity monitoring, it would be possible to identify such styles (e.g. irregular and unhealthy) and determine the risk of the disease before the actual disease appears.
- **Prevention of lifestyle diseases:** It is important to identify lifestyle diseases at the very first place. Noticing your regular body functioning and setting a body alarm of something unusual can help to identify the problem. Before that we should monitor our lifestyle because prevention is better than cure. A person can assess his/her lifestyle and become aware of any irregular patterns through monitoring daily activity patterns.
- **Management of lifestyle diseases:** A person who has a lifestyle disease should make changes to assure a healthy lifestyle. For example, there is no cure for type 2 diabetes, but it can be effectively controlled by maintaining normal blood-glucose levels. This can be achieved through weight control by following a nutritious and balanced diet, along with regular and stringent exercise (Han *et al.,* 2012).

We have learnt, lifestyle diseases are a category of diseases that are caused primarily by the way we lead our lives. They include diabetes, heart disease, stroke, and some forms of cancer. Here are some ways to prevent lifestyle diseases supported by data.

5.4.1 *Healthy Diet*

A healthy diet rich in fruits, vegetables, whole grains, and lean proteins can help prevent lifestyle diseases. According to the World Health Organization, an estimated 19 per cent of all deaths worldwide are attributable to low fruit and vegetable intake. Studies have shown that a diet rich in fruits and vegetables, whole grains and lean proteins can reduce the risk of heart diseases and diabetes by up to 70 per cent. According to UNICEF, one of the things that can be done to reduce the risk of developing NCDs is to eat a nutritious diet, ensuring to include enough vegetables and fruits. The more processed foods are in your diet, the farther away they are from their natural state and are more likely to contain added ingredients that in the long run may be harmful to your health (www.unicef.org). According to World Cancer Research Fund International, consuming predominantly plant-based diets reduces the risk of developing obesity, diabetes, cardiovascular diseases, and some forms of cancer. Plant-based diets are high in vegetables and fruits, wholegrains, pulses, nuts and seeds, and have only modest amounts of meat and dairy. These diets help to achieve and maintain a healthy weight, reduce blood pressure, and are also rich in sources of dietary fibre (which protects against colorectal cancer) (www.wcrf.org).

5.4.2 *Regular Exercise*

Regular exercise can reduce the risk of obesity, heart disease, and Type 2 diabetes. The World Health Organization recommends that adults should do at least 150 minutes of moderate-intensity physical activity per week. According to the World Health Organization, the first indicator of health is physical activity at the community level (Sadrollahi *et al.*, 2016). The risk of many chronic diseases such as cancer, cardiovascular condition, and diabetes (type 2) reduce through regular physical activity (Warburton, 2006). To promote active and healthier societies, WHO launched a programme in June 2018 with the title of "More active people for a healthier world." This programme's primary plan is to create more active and healthier societies by improving spaces and places for physical activity. The improved spaces and areas for physical activity will provide more opportunities for every age group to do dance, sport, walking, cycling, and play (Healy, 2007).

5.4.3 *Avoid Tobacco and Alcohol*

Tobacco use is one of the major risk factors for non-communicable diseases like cancer, cardiovascular diseases, and respiratory diseases. According to WHO, tobacco use is the leading cause of preventable death worldwide, with about 8 million deaths annually. Alcohol is also linked to cancer and liver disease. It is important for family and schools to impart the knowledge of harmful effects of consuming alcohol and smoking in early stages of life. Parents and teachers should not hesitate talking to students on any such thing. Governments should take initiatives, form Acts and carry out various campaigns to address the issue of smoking and alcohol. For example, the Government of India has adopted the national tobacco-control legislation, namely "The Cigarettes and other Tobacco Products (Prohibition of Advertisement and Regulation of Trade and Commerce, Production, Supply and Distribution) Act, 2003", WHO-Framework Convention on Tobacco Control (WHO-FCTC) in February 2004. Further, the Ministry of Health and Family Welfare, Government of India launched the National Tobacco Control Programme (NTCP) in 2007-08 in 42 districts of 21 States/Union Territories of the country, in order to facilitate the effective implementation of the Tobacco Control Law, to bring about greater awareness about the harmful effects of tobacco as well as to fulfil the obligations under the WHO-FCTC. Under Copta Act, 2008, certain safeguards have been introduced through the Prohibition on Smoking at Public Place Rules, 2008, such as that smoking area or space shall not be established at the entrance or exit of the hotel, restaurant and the airport etc. All such initiatives can help to halt the growth of non-communicable diseases.

5.4.4 *Manage Stress*

Chronic stress can lead to health problems like high blood pressure, heart disease, and depression. Learning stress management techniques like mindfulness and meditation can help manage stress and reduce the risk of lifestyle diseases. By managing stress, individuals are more likely to adopt and maintain healthy behaviours, such as regular exercise, proper nutrition, and adequate sleep, which can lower the risk of NCDs. Adopting stress management techniques like meditation, deep breathing exercises, and mindfulness can help reduce stress hormones, boost immune function, and improve overall health. Stress management techniques, like regular exercise, deep breathing, and relaxation exercises, can help lower blood pressure, reduce heart rate, and improve overall cardiovascular health.

5.4.5 *Adequate Sleep*

Sleep is essential for good health. Lack of sleep can lead to an increased risk of obesity, diabetes, and heart disease. The American Academy of Sleep Medicine recommends that adults should have 7-9 hours of sleep per night. Insufficient and/or mistimed sleep is also a major risk factor for obesity and NCDs such as CVD and T2DM. Several prospective cohort studies indicate that both short and long sleep are associated with higher mortality rates and increased risk for CVD (Chien, 2010). US National Health Interview Survey data indicate that relative to sleeping 7-8 h per night, self-reported short (≤6 h) and long sleep (>9 h) duration are independently associated with increased obesity, T2DM, hypertension, and CVD (Buxton, OM *et al.*, 2010).

Hence, adopting a healthy lifestyle including a healthy diet, regular exercise, avoiding tobacco and alcohol, managing stress and getting adequate sleep can play a significant role in preventing lifestyle diseases.

REFERENCES

Afshil *et al.,* and GBD (2017, 2019). Health effects of dietary risks in 195 countries, 1990-2017: a systematic analysis for the Global Burden of Disease Study 2017, in www.thelancet.com volume 393, issue 10184, pp. 1958-1972, doi: https: //doi.org/10.1016/S0140-6736(19)30041-8

Ahirwar, R., Mondal, P.R. (2018 Sep. 21). Prevalence of obesity in India: A systematic review. *Diabetes Metab Syndr.* 2019 Jan-Feb; 13(1): 318-321. doi: 10.1016/j.dsx.2018.08.032. Epub. PMID: 30641719

Ahmed, A.M., Ahmed, N.H. (2005 May). History of disorders of thyroid dysfunction. *East Mediterr Health J.,* 11(3): 459-69. PMID: 16602467

Ahmed, A.M. (2002 Apr.). History of diabetes mellitus. *Saudi Med J.,* 23(4): 373-8. PMID: 11953758

Anand, P., Kunnumakkara, A.B., Sundaram, C., Harikumar, K.B., Tharakan, S.T., Lai, O.S., Sung, B., Aggarwal, B.B. (2008 Sep.). Cancer is a preventable disease that requires major lifestyle changes. *Pharm Res.,* 25(9): 2097-116. doi: 10.1007/s11095-008-9661-9. Epub 2008 July 15. Erratum in: *Pharm Res.,* 2008 Sep; 25(9): 2200. Kunnumakara, Ajaikumar, B. [corrected to Kunnumakkara, Ajaikumar, B.]. PMID: 18626751; PMCID: PMC2515569

Baig, M. *et al.,* (2015). Prevalence of obesity and hypertension among University students and their knowledge and attitude towards risk factors of Cardiovascular Disease (CVD) in Jeddah, Saudi Arabia, *Pakistan Journal of Medical Sciences quarterly.* ncbi.nlm.nih.gov, 31(4), pp. 816-820.

Brannon, L. & Feist, J. (2007). *Health Psychology: An Introduction to Behaviour and Health,* 6th Edition, United States of America, Thomspon Wadsworth Publisher.

Bray, G.A. (1996). "Health hazards of obesity", Endocrinology and metabolism clinics of North America. *Elsevier,* 25(4), pp. 907-919.

Burgos, R., Bretón, I., Cereda, E., Desport, J.C., Dziewas, R., Genton, L. (2018 Sep.). ESPEN guideline clinical nutrition in neurology. *Clin Nutr.,* 354-96. https: //doi.org/10.1016/j.clnu.2017.09.003.

Buxton, O.M. *et al.,* (2010). Sleep restriction for 1 week reduces insulin sensitivity in healthy men. *Diabetes,* 59: 2126-2133. doi: 10.2337/db09-0699.

Carmichael, A.R. (2006). Obesity as a risk factor for development and poor prognosis for breast cancer. *BJOG: An International Journal of Obstetrics and Gynaecology,* 113(10): 1160Y1166.

Chien, K.L., *et al.* (2010). Habitual sleep duration and insomnia and the risk of cardiovascular events and all-cause death: report from a community-based cohort. *Sleep.*, 33: 177-184. doi: 10.1093/sleep/33.2.177.

Crino, M., Sacks, G., Vandevijvere, S., Swinburn, B., Neal, B. (2015, March). The Influence on Population Weight Gain and Obesity of the Macronutrient Composition and Energy Density of the Food Supply. *Curr Obes Rep.*, 4(1): 1-10. doi: 10.1007/s13679-014-0134-7. PMID: 26627085

Deepa, M., Farooq, S., Datta, M., Deepa, R., Mohan, V. (2007). Prevalence of metabolic syndrome using WHO, ATP III and IDF definitions in Asian Indians : the Chennai Urban Rural Epidemiology Study (CURES-34), *Diabetes Metab Res Rev.*, 23: 127-34.

Deswal, R., Narwal, V., Dang, A., Pundir, C.S. (2020), The prevalence of polycystic ovary syndrome: a brief systematic review. *J Hum Reprod Sci.*, 13: 261-71. 10.4103/jhrs.JHRS_95_18

Donaldson, K., Beswick, P.S. (1996). Free radical activity associated with the surface of the particles: a unifying factor in determining biological activity. *Toxicol Lett*, 88: 293-8.

Drewnowski, A. & Popkin, B.M. (1997). The nutrition transition: trends in the global diet. *Nutr. Rev.*, 55(2): 31-43.

Ehrmann, D.A. (2005). Polycystic ovary syndrome. *N Engl J Med.*, 352: 1223-36. 10.1056/NEJMra041536

El-Bassel, N., Shaw, S.A., Dasgupta, A., Strathdee, S.A. (2014). Drug use as a driver of HIV risks: re-emerging and emerging issues. *Curr Opin HIV AIDS,* 9(2): 150-155. doi: 10.1097/COH.0000000000000035

Ezzati, M., Lopez, A.D. (2003). Estimates of global mortality attributable to smoking in 2000. *Lancet,* 362: 847-852. 10.1016/S0140-6736(03)14338-3

Franceschi, S., Talamini, R., Barra, S., *et al.* (1990). Smoking and drinking in relation to cancers of the oral cavity, pharynx, larynx, and esophagus in Northern Italy. *Cancer Research,* 50: 6502-6507. PMID: 2208109

Ghosh, S., Kumar, M., (2019). Prevalence and associated risk factors of hypertension among persons aged 15-49 in India: a cross-sectional study, *BMJ Open,* 9: e029714. doi: 10.1136/bmjopen-2019-029714

Han, Yongkoo, Manhyung Han, Sungyoung Lee, A.M. Jehad Sarkar, and Young-Koo Lee (2012). "A Framework for Supervising Lifestyle Diseases Using Long-Term Activity Monitoring", *Sensors,*12, No. 5: 5363-5379. https: //doi.org/10.3390/s120505363

Healy, G.N., Wijndaele, K., Dunstan, D.W. *et al.* (2007). Objectively measured sedentary time, physical activity, and metabolic risk: the Australian diabetes, obesity and lifestyle study (AusDiab). *Diabetes Care.* 31(2): 369-371. doi: 10.2337/dc07-1795

Howe, H.L., Wingo, P.A., Thun, M.J. *et al.* (2001). Annual report to the nation on the status of cancer (1973 through 1998), featuring cancers with recent increasing trends. *Journal of the National Cancer Institute* 93: 824-842, 11390532

http: //timesofindia.indiatimes.com/articleshow/89838065.cms?utm_source=contentofinterest&utm_medium=text&utm_campaign=cppst

http: //timesofindia.indiatimes.com/articleshow/90617150.cms?utm_source=contentofinterest&utm_medium=text&utm_campaign=cppst

https: //www.thehindu.com/news/national/cancer-cases-in-india

Institute for Health Metrics and Evaluation (2011).*The Challenge Ahead: Progress in Breast and Cervical Cancer. Institute of Health Metrics and Evaluation.* [Last accessed on 2016 Jan. 21]. Available from: http: //www.healthmetricsandevaluation.org/publications/policyreport/challenge-ahead-progress-and-setbacksbreastand-cervical-cancer

International Diabetes Federation. *IDF Diabetes Atlas.* (9th ed.) Brussels, Belgium: International Diabetes Federation, 2019.

Jabeen, A., Yamini, V., Rahman Amberina, A. *et al.* (August 12, 2022). Polycystic Ovarian Syndrome: Prevalence, Predisposing Factors, and Awareness Among Adolescent and Young Girls of South India. *Cureus,* 14(8): e27943. doi: 10.7759/cureus.27943

Jain, T., Negris, O., Brown, D. *et al.* (2021). Characterization of polycystic ovary syndrome among Flo app users around the world. *Reprod Biol Endocrinol,* 19, 36. https: //doi.org/10.1186/s12958-021-00719-y

Klevens, R.M., Hu, D.J., Jiles, R., Holmberg, S.D. (2012). Evolving epidemiology of Hepatitis C virus in the United States. *Clin Infect Dis Off Publ Infect Dis Soc Am.,* 55 Suppl 1: S3-S9. doi: 10.1093/cid/cis393

Kobyliska , M., Katarzyna A., Agnieszka, D., and Katarzyna K. (2022). Malnutrition in Obesity: Is It Possible? *Obes Facts,* 15 (1): 19-25. https: //doi.org/10.1159/000519503

Monteiro, C.A., Benicio, M.H.D.A., Iunes, R., Gouveia, N.C., Taddei, J.A.C. & Cardoso, M.A.A. (1992). Nutritional status of Brazilian children: trends from 1975 to 1989. *Bull. WHO,* 70(5): 657-666.

Negri, E., La Vecchia, C., Franceschi, S. *et al.* (1993). Attributable risk for oral cancer in Northern Italy. *Cancer Epidemiology, Biomarkers, and Prevention,* 2: 189-193, PMID: 8318870

NIDA (2022, March 22). Addiction and Health. Retrieved from https: //nida.nih.gov/publications/drugs-brains-behaviour-science-addiction/addiction-health on 2023.

Owen, N. Healy, G.N. Mathew, C.E. & Dunstan, D.W. (2010). *Too Much Sitting: The Population Health Science of Sedentary Behaviour.* Vol. 38(3), pp. 105-113.

Padrão, P., Lunet, N., Santos, A.C. *et al.* (2007). Smoking, alcohol, and dietary choices: evidence from the Portuguese National Health Survey. *BMC Public Health,* 7, 138. https: //doi.org/10.1186/1471-2458-7-138

Pappachan, M.J. (2011 Aug.) Increasing prevalence of lifestyle diseases: high time for action. *Indian J. Med Res.,* 134(2): 143-5. PMID: 21911964; PMCID: PMC3181012

Perappadan, B.S. (2023). Explained | Why is India rethinking its anaemia policy? Why are anaemia estimates being shifted from the National Family Health Survey to Diet and Biomarkers Survey? *The Hindu,* June 04, 2023, 02:18 am | Updated 12: 20 pm IST retrieved from https: //www.thehindu.com/

Popkin, B.M. (1993). Nutrition patterns and transitions. *Pop. Dev. Rev.,* 19: 138-157.

Pradeepa, R., Mohan, V. (2021 Nov.). Epidemiology of type 2 diabetes in India. *Indian J Ophthalmol.,* 69(11): 2932-2938. doi: 10.4103/ijo.IJO_1627_21. PMID: 34708726; PMCID: PMC8725109.

Rasquin Leon, L.I., Anastasopoulou, C., Mayrin, J.V., *Polycystic ovarian disease.* StatPearls [Internet]. StatPearls Publishing, Treasure Island, FL.

Sadrollahi, A., Hosseinian, M., Alavi, N.M. *et al.* (2016). Physical activity patterns in the elderly Kashan population. *Iran Red Crescent Med J.,* 18(6). [PMC free article] [PubMed] [Google Scholar].

Steyn, K., Damasceno, A. (2006). Lifestyle and Related Risk Factors for Chronic Diseases. In Jamison, D.T., Feachem, R.G., Makgoba, M.W. *et al.,* (editors). *Disease and Mortality in Sub-Saharan Africa.* 2nd edition. Washington (DC): The International Bank for Reconstruction and Development/The World Bank; Chapter 18. Available from: https: //www.ncbi.nlm.nih.gov/books/NBK2290

Tabish, S.A. (2017). Lifestyle Diseases: Consequences, Characteristics, Causes and Control. *J. Cardiol Curr Res,* 9(3): 00326. DOI: 10.15406/jccr.2017.09.0032

Tao, Z., Shi, A., Zhao, J. (2015). Epidemiological perspectives of diabetes. *Cell Biochem Biophys,* 73: 181-5.

The untapped potential of the thyroid axis (thelancet.com) retrieved from https: //www.thelancet.com/action/showPdf?pii=S2213-8587%2813%2970166-9

Warburton, D.E. (2006). Health benefits of physical activity: the evidence. *Can Med Assoc J.,* 174(6): 801-809. doi: 10.1503/cmaj.051351

Warren, T.Y. *et al.* (2010). Sedentary behaviours increase risk of cardiovascular disease mortality in men, *Medicine and science in sports and exercise,* 42(5), pp. 879-885.

Washington State Institute for Public Policy. (2017). *Benefit cost results.* Retrieved from http: //www.wsipp.wa.gov/BenefitCost?topicId=. Accessed on June 14, 2018.

WHO (1998). *Obesity: preventing and managing the global epidemic.* Working Group on Obesity. Geneva, World Health Organization.

Xing, Y.F., Xu, Y.H., Shi, M.H., Lian, Y. (2016). The impact of PM2.5 on the human respiratory system. *J Thorac Dis.,* Jan., 8(1): E69-74.

Zobel, E.H., Hansen, T.W., Rossing, P., von Scholten, B.J. (2016 Dec.). Global Changes in Food Supply and the Obesity Epidemic. *Current Obesity Reports*, 5(4): 449-455. doi: 10.1007/s13679-016-0233-8. PMID: 27696237

Zheng, T., Boyle, P., Zhang, B., *et al.* (2004). Tobacco use and risk of oral cancer. In: Boycle, P., Gray, N., Henningfield, J., Seffrin, J., and Zatonski, W. (eds.). *Tobacco: Science, Policy and Public Health.* Oxford: Oxford University Press, pp. 399-432.

Zheng, T.Z., Boycle, P., Hu, H.F. *et al.* (1990). Tobacco smoking, alcohol consumption, and risk of oral cancer: A case-control study in Beijing, People's Republic of China. *Cancer Causes and Control,* 1: 173-179, PMID: 2102288

Chapter

6

Mental Health

"Mana evam Manushyanam Karanam Bandhamokshayoh."
(Human's captivity or freedom is dependent on the state of his mind. From this it follows that whether a human is healthy or unhealthy depends on himself. Illness is the result not only of our actions but also of our thoughts.)

6.1 Concept and Definition

During the Renaissance, philosophers such as René Descartes and John Locke laid the groundwork for understanding the mind and mental health. Descartes (1596-1650) advocated for the separation of the mind and body, while Locke (1632-1704) emphasized the role of empiricism and the influence of societal factors on mental well-being. Sigmund Freud (1856-1939), the founder of psychoanalysis, revolutionized our understanding of the unconscious mind and its impact on mental health. Freud's theories emphasized the importance of childhood experiences and the role of the unconscious in shaping behaviour and disorders. In 1893, Isaac Ray, a founder of the American Psychiatric Association, provided a definition of the term mental hygiene as "the art of preserving the mind against all incidents and influences calculated to deteriorate its qualities, impair its energies, or derange its movements. The humanistic movement, of 20th Centuery, led by Carl Rogers and Abraham Maslow, focused on promoting self-actualization and the importance of empathy and unconditional positive regard in therapeutic relationships.The focus of various definitions has changed over period of time. From absence of illness to holistic approach to health has made to relook into the definition of mental health too.

1. **The absence of mental illness:** One of the earliest definitions of mental health focused on the absence of mental illness. This approach saw mental health as the opposite of mental disorder and defined mental health as the absence of symptoms of mental illness. This definition is criticized for being too narrow and for failing to account for the positive aspects of mental well-being.
2. **Positive mental health:** This definition emphasized the positive aspects of mental health. It viewed mental health as the presence of positive emotions, the ability to cope with

stressors, and the ability to lead a fulfilling life. This definition sought to move beyond the concept of mental illness and focused on building resilience and promoting well-being.

3. **The World Health Organization (WHO) definition:** The WHO defines mental health as a state of well-being in which a person can realize their potential, cope with normal life stressors, work productively, and contribute to their community. This definition acknowledges the role of a person's environment, social conditions, and individual characteristics in shaping their mental state.

4. **Recovery-oriented perspective:** This definition of mental health views it as an ongoing process of recovery from mental illness. It emphasizes the importance of hope, empowerment, and resilience in helping individuals with mental health conditions to achieve their full potential and improve their quality of life.

C.E.A. Winslow, professor of Public Health at Yale, was also concerned to include mental hygiene in public health education. He described mental hygiene in 1933 as "an organized community response to a recognized community need; and it lays its prime emphasis on the detection and the control of those incipient maladjustments with which the physician *qua* physician never comes into contact, unless specific community machinery and far-flung educational facilities are provided for the purpose" (Winslow, 1938). The first International Congress on Mental Hygiene was convened in 1933. Included in the purpose statement there was the idea that it was necessary to determine "how best to care for and treat the mentally sick, to prevent mental illness, and to conserve mental health" (in National Committee for Mental Hygiene, The Mental Hygiene Movement).

According to Centre for Disease Control and Prevention, mental health includes our emotional, psychological, and social well-being. It affects how we think, feel, and act. It also helps determine how we handle stress, relate to others, and make healthy choices. Mental health is all about how people think, feel, and behave. Mental health specialists can help people with depression, anxiety, bipolar disorder, addiction, and other conditions that affect their thoughts, feelings, and behaviours (*Medical News Today*, www.medicalnewstoday.com).

Keyes (2006, 2014) identifies three components of mental health: emotional well-being, psychological well-being and social well-being.

(a) ***Emotional well-being:*** It includes happiness, interest in life, and satisfaction;
(b) ***Psychological well-being:*** It includes liking most parts of one's own personality, being good at managing the responsibilities of daily life, having good relationships with others, and being satisfied with one's own life; and
(c) ***Social well-being:*** It refers to positive functioning and involves having something to contribute to society (social contribution), feeling part of a community (social integration), believing that society is becoming a better place for all people (social actualization), and that the way society works makes sense to them (social coherence).

Mental health is a dynamic state of internal equilibrium which enables individuals to use their abilities in harmony with universal values of society. Basic cognitive and social skills; ability to recognize, express and modulate one's own emotions, as well as empathize with others; flexibility and ability to cope with adverse life events and function in social roles; and harmonious relationship between body and mind represent important components of mental health which contribute, to varying degrees, to the state of internal equilibrium (Galderisi, 2015).

The concept of "*dynamic state of internal equilibrium*" is meant to reflect the fact that different life epochs require changes in the achieved equilibrium: adolescent crises, marriage, becoming a parent or retirement are good examples of life epochs requiring an active search for a new mental equilibrium. Basic cognitive and social skills are regarded as an important component of mental health in the light of their impact on all aspects of everyday life (Artero, 2001). Cognitive skills include the ability to pay attention, remember and organize information, solve problems, and make decisions; social skills involve the ability to use one's own repertoire of verbal/non-verbal abilities to communicate and interact with others. The inclusion of a harmonious relationship between body and mind is based on the concept that mind, brain, organism and environment are heavily interconnected, and the overall experience of being in the world cannot be separated from the way in which one's body feels in its environment (Fuchs, T. Schlimme, 2009).

Mental health definitions have evolved over time, moving from narrow conceptions that focused solely on the absence of mental illness to more holistic perspectives that emphasize well-being, resilience, and recovery. These definitions recognize that mental health is a complex and multifaceted concept that involves a range of social, emotional, and psychological factors and that it can be influenced by both individual and environmental factors. Like physical health, mental health is not fixed. Mental health exists on a continuum, or range: from positive, healthy functioning at one end through to severe symptoms of mental health conditions at the other (www.un.org).

In the field of geography, the conceptualization of mental health and its study within the context of health geography has evolved over time. One influential scholar who pioneered the incorporation of mental health into geographical research is Susan Smith. Susan Smith, a geographer from the United Kingdom, played a crucial role in raising awareness about the significance of mental health in geography. Her work focused on understanding the spatial dimensions of mental health, exploring how place and environment influence mental well-being. Smith's research contributed to the emergence of a subfield known as "geographies of mental health", which examines the social, economic, and physical factors that shape mental health outcomes at various scales. This subfield recognizes that mental health is not solely an individual or biological issue but is also intricately connected to social and environmental factors. Geographical research on mental health continues to evolve, addressing emerging challenges such as the impacts of urbanization, globalization, climate change, and the COVID-19 pandemic on mental health. As an interdisciplinary field, it draws on theories and methodologies from geography, psychology, sociology, public health, and urban planning to deepen our understanding of the geographical dimensions of mental health and contribute to the development of more effective policies and interventions.

6.2 Significance of Mental Health

Positive mental health is crucial in today's world, as it profoundly influences every aspect of our lives. Mental health can impact our thoughts, actions, and interactions. It empowers us to navigate challenges, build meaningful relationships, and make informed decisions (talkspace.

com). Negative mental health leads to downfall in career, ambitions, day-to-day work and physical fitness. It poses challenge to self-growth and development.

6.2.1 *Productivity and Performance*

Poor mental health, manifesting most often as depression, anxiety, or burnout, can severely decrease motivation and production while increasing stress, leading to it can have serious consequences for a person and their relationships. Other mental health disorders, like ADHD, can interfere with focus and attention and make it much harder to get things done (www.psychologytoday.com). Globally, an estimated 12 billion working days are lost every year due to depression and anxiety at a cost of US$ 1 trillion per year in lost productivity (www.who.int).

Mental health problems have an impact on employers and businesses directly through increased absenteeism, negative impact on productivity and profits, as well as an increase in costs to deal with the issue (European Network for Workplace Health Promotion, 2010). Data from different countries around the world indicate that mental health problems are a cause of a number of employees dropping out of work. In the Netherlands, around 58 per cent of the work-related disabilities are related to mental health (Grundemann *et al.,* 1991). Good mental health positively affects productivity and performance at work. When individuals are mentally healthy, they tend to be more focused, motivated, and engaged, leading to increased productivity levels. This, in turn, contributes to higher economic output and growth. A healthy population is an economically productive population and it is in the benefit of companies to safeguard public health (Rajgopal, 2010).

6.2.2 *Absenteeism at Workplace*

Mental health issues like anxiety, depression, and stress can lead to increased absenteeism from work. By promoting mental well-being and providing support, organizations can help reduce absenteeism rates, minimize disruption to workflow, and avoid additional costs associated with finding replacements or reduced output. In the UK, it is estimated that around 30-40 per cent of the sickness absence is attributable to some form of mental illness (O'Leary, 1993). Workplaces that promote good mental health and support individuals with mental illnesses are more likely to reduce absenteeism (i.e. decreased number of days away from work) and presenteeism (i.e. diminished productivity while at work), and thus increase worker productivity (Hamberg-van Reenen *et al.,* 2012). The workplace policies that provide employees with access to evidence-based care result in reduced absenteeism, disability and lost productivity (Burton *et al.,* 2008). Thereore, for companies and organizations it is important that workers' laws should be promoting welfare and taking care of their needs so that workers attend their workplaces happily and reduce absenteesim. Healthy workplace environments that prioritize mental health tend to have better employee retention rates. By creating supportive and inclusive cultures that address mental health concerns, organizations can retain skilled employees, reduce turnover costs, and maintain the knowledge and expertise critical for long-term economic growth.

6.2.3 *Innovation and Creativity*

The world is run by creative and innovative minds. Mental well-being is closely linked to creativity, innovation, and problem-solving abilities. According to Milan Rajkovic, CEO at

Otto IT, creativity is a fundamental element of innovation, as it involves generating new and unique ideas, perspectives, and approaches to solving problems or addressing challenges. Mental health plays a critical role in fostering creativity by providing employees with the cognitive, emotional, and psychological resources necessary to think innovatively. When employees are mentally healthy, they are better able to access their creative capacities, such as divergent thinking, curiosity, and imagination. They are also more likely to engage in exploratory thinking, take risks, and challenge the *status quo*, which are essential elements of the innovation process (www.linkedin.com).

Stress and anxiety stall creativity and innovation. When we are in stress we are unable to think creatively. The ability to think out of box or to envision something that does not exist, to build up strategies etc, one need healthy and stressfree mind. When individuals are in a positive mental state, they are more likely to think creatively, come up with innovative ideas, and contribute to the growth and development of their organizations and industries. For example, parents nurture their children with values, love and care. Creativity of parenthood lies in strategies and creating a contented and successful human being. But, if parents are mentally engrossed in managing their stress they cannot be able to envision their goal clearly. Their job is full of innovations and creativity everyday. An unhealthy parent can have rarely a healthy child. Similarly, if an adverstising firm hire an employee who always remain in stress, the person will not be able to create an interesting advertisement or marketing strategy for his/her company.

6.2.4 *Economic Burden*

Mental health issues impose a significant economic burden on society through healthcare costs, lost productivity, and decreased quality of life. By investing in mental health support and prevention programmes, societies can reduce the economic burden associated with mental health issues, allowing resources to be allocated more efficiently towards economic growth and development. Society also bears many of the costs of mental health disorders through public disability programmes that pay for income support for those who cannot work. According to a report by CEA, people with psychiatric disabilities were the largest contributor to growth in Social Security Disability Insurance (SSDI) rolls in the early 2000s. As of 2020, 18 per cent of SSDI beneficiaries, or 1.4 million individuals in current payment status, suffered from depression, bipolar, or psychotic disorders. Overall, the mental disorder category accounted for 29 per cent of beneficiaries in 2020, or 2.4 million people—a share larger than beneficiaries who cannot work due to injuries, cancer, or diseases of the circulatory and nervous system, combined. While these supports are important and necessary, too many people fall through the cracks and do not receive the treatment that could both improve their livelihoods and reduce their reliance on disability insurance (CEA, 2022). Based on data from 2010, the global direct and indirect economic costs of mental disorders were estimated at US$2.5 trillion. Importantly, the indirect costs (US$1.7 trillion) are much higher than the direct costs (US$0.8 trillion), which contrasts with other key disease groups, such as cardiovascular diseases and cancer. For the EU, a region with highly developed healthcare systems, the direct and indirect costs were estimated at €798 billion in 2010 (Gustavsson *et al.*, 2010). Therefore, to ensure that direct or indirect cost of any mental illness should not impact economic growth, the organizations or state needs to develop mental harmony in society by various possible means.

6.2.5 *Relationships and Social Harmony*

Mental health influences an individual's relationships and social interactions. The dynamic stability that we try to preserve in our relationships and social interactions is known as sociostasis. Achieving a harmonic state in which individual behaviours, expectations, and group standards are in line with one another in a way that encourages general social stability and cohesion is at the heart of sociostasis. Kleinman (1999) describes the clustering of mental and social health problems in "broken communities" in shanty towns and slums and among vulnerable and marginal migrant populations: civil violence, domestic violence, suicide, substance abuse, depression, and post traumatic disorder cluster and coalesce (Kleinman, 1999). In order to build up social harmony in society, it is important to develop social well-being. Good mental health allows individuals to establish and maintain healthy, meaningful connections with others. Conversely, poor mental health can strain relationships, leading to conflicts and isolation. Nurturing mental health promotes positive social dynamics and fosters a sense of belonging within communities.

6.2.6 *Sense of Fulfilment and Achievement of Self-esteem and Personal Well-being*

Mental health is crucial for individual well-being and quality of life. When individuals have good mental health, they experience greater happiness, satisfaction, and fulfilment in their personal lives. Positive mental health allows individuals to effectively cope with stress, maintain healthy relationships, and achieve their goals. Good mental health leads to build confidence and helps to perform better at school, workplace and sectors of society. It also helps you to develop a feeling of fulfilment and contentment (Refer Fig. 6.1).

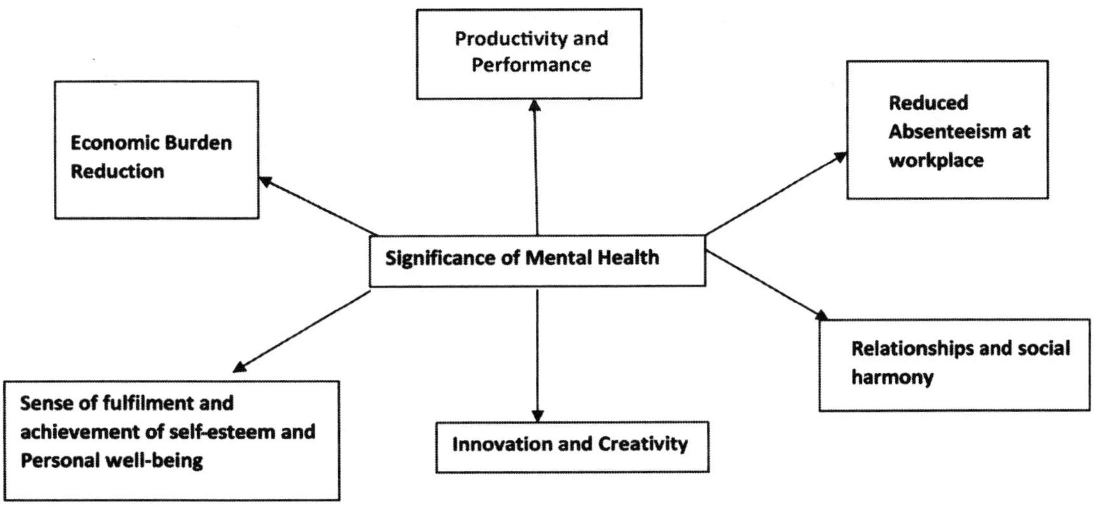

Fig. 6.1: Significance of Mental Health.

6.3 Type of Mental Health Challenges

World Health Organization identifies mainly 8 mental health disorders: Fig. 6.2 shows that 63 per cent of disorders are related to substance, alcohol and smoking or drugs. Anxiety is very common, around 17 per cent of total mental disorders are anxiety disorders and 15 per cent are depression cases.

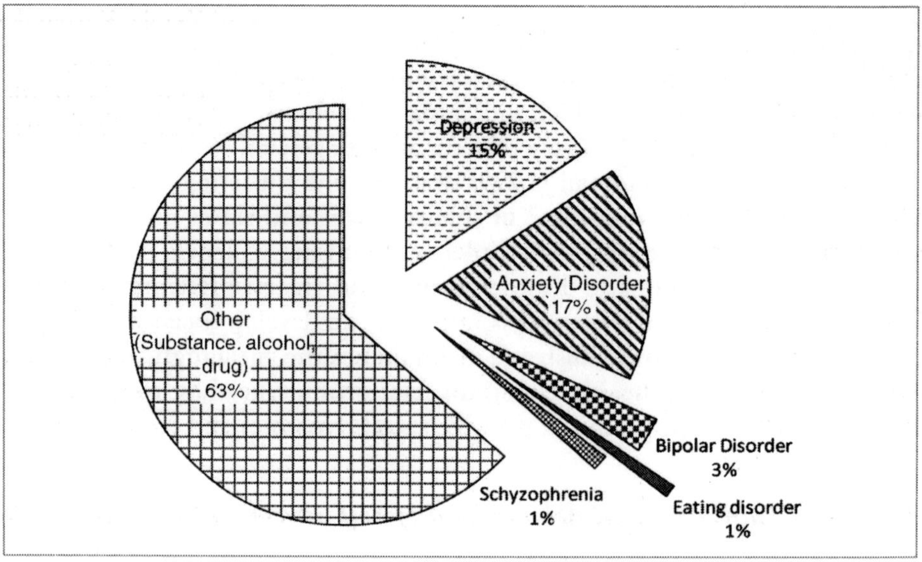

Fig. 6.2: Type of Mental Health Challenges in the World, 2017.

Source: Dattani *et al.,* 2021.

6.3.1 *Anxiety*

The word 'anxiety' is derived from the Latin "anxietas" (to choke, throttle, trouble, and upset) and encompasses behavioural, effective and cognitive responses to the perception of danger. Anxiety is a normal human emotion. In moderation, anxiety stimulates an anticipatory and adaptive response to challenging or stressful events. In excess, anxiety destabilizes the individual and dysfunctional state results (Trivedi, 2010). There are several different kinds of anxiety disorders, such as generalised anxiety disorder (characterised by excessive worry), panic disorder (characterised by panic attacks), social anxiety disorder (characterised by excessive fear and worry in social situations), separation anxiety disorder (characterised by excessive fear or anxiety about separation from those individuals to whom the person has a deep emotional bond), and others. Childhood, adolescence, or adulthood traumatic experiences are frequently the start of anxiety disorders. Being subjected to stress and trauma when you are very young is probably going to have a significant effect. Experiences like physical and emotional abuse, losing a parent, racism etc. can significantly impact human brain and leads to depression. It might cause you to sweat, feel restless and tense, and have a rapid heartbeat. It can be a normal reaction to stress. For example, you might feel anxious when faced with a difficult problem at work, before taking a test, or before making an important decision. It can help you to cope. The anxiety may give you a boost of energy or help you focus.

But for people with anxiety disorders, the fear is not temporary and can be overwhelming. It is estimated that 264 million adults around the globe have anxiety (World Health Organization, 2017). Of these adults, 179 million are female (63%) and 105 million are male (37%) (Our World in Data, 2018). The prevalence of all mental disorders increased by 50 per cent worldwide from 416 million to 615 million between 1990 and 2013 (World Health Organization, 2016).

In 2017, 44·9 million people had anxiety disorders in India. The prevalence varied 1·4 times across the states, with the high prevalence observed in the states of Kerala, Karnataka, Telangana, Tamil Nadu, Himachal Pradesh, and Maharashtra all lie in the high SDI state group; and Andhra Pradesh, Manipur, and West Bengal in the middle SDI state group (The burden of mental disorders across the states of India: the Global Burden of Disease Study 1990-2017, December 20, 2019).

Table 6.1: Type of anxiety disorders

Type of Anxiety disorder	Meaning
Generalized anxiety disorder	It involves persistent and excessive worry that interferes with daily activities. This ongoing worry and tension may be accompanied by physical symptoms, such as restlessness, feeling on edge or easily fatigued, difficulty concentrating, muscle tension or problems in sleeping.
Panic disorder	The core symptom of panic disorder is recurrent panic attacks, an overwhelming combination of physical and psychological distress. During an attack, several of these symptoms occur in combination like palpitations, pounding heart or rapid heart rate, sweating, trembling or shaking, feeling of shortness of breath or smothering sensations, chest pain etc.
Phobias	A specific phobia is excessive and persistent fear of a specific object, situation or activity that is generally not harmful. Patients know their fear is excessive, but they cannot overcome it. These fears cause such distress that some people go to extreme lengths to avoid what they fear. Examples are public speaking, fear of flying or fear of spiders.
Social Anxiety Disorder	A person with social anxiety disorder has significant anxiety and discomfort about being embarrassed, humiliated, rejected or looked down on in social interactions. People with this disorder will try to avoid the situation or endure it with great anxiety. Common examples are extreme fear of public speaking, meeting new people or eating/drinking in public.
Separation Anxiety Disorder	A person with separation anxiety disorder is excessively fearful or anxious about separation from those with whom he or she is attached. The feeling is beyond what is appropriate for the person's age, persists (at least four weeks in children and six months in adults) and causes problems in functioning. A person with separation anxiety disorder may be persistently worried about losing the person closest to him or her, may be reluctant or refuse to go out or sleep away from home or without that person, or may experience nightmares about separation.
Selective Mutism	Children with selective mutism do not speak in some social situations where they are expected to speak, such as school, even though they speak in other situations. They will speak in their home around immediate family members, but often will not speak even in front of others, such as close friends or grandparents.

Source: Compiled by author from www.psychiatry.org

6.3.2 *Depression*

According to American Psychiatrists Association, depression (major depressive disorder) is a common and serious medical illness that negatively affects how you feel, the way you think and how you act. It is mood disorder that causes a persistent feeling of sadness and loss of interest. Also called major depressive disorder or clinical depression, it affects how you feel, think and behave and can lead to a variety of emotional and physical problems (www.mayoclinic.org). Feelings of sadness, tearfulness, emptiness or hopelessness; angry outbursts, irritability or frustration, even over small matters; loss of interest or pleasure in most or all normal activities, such as sex, hobbies or sports; sleep disturbances, including insomnia or sleeping too much; tiredness and lack of energy, so even small tasks take extra effort; reduced appetite and weight loss or increased cravings for food and weight gain; anxiety, agitation or restlessness; slowed thinking, speaking or body movements; feelings of worthlessness or guilt, fixating on past failures or self-blame; trouble thinking, concentrating, making decisions and remembering things; frequent or recurrent thoughts of death, suicidal thoughts, suicide attempts or suicide; unexplained physical problems, such as back pain or headaches (www.mayoclinic.org). According to WHO, globally, an estimated 5 per cent of adults suffer from depression. Approximately, 280 million people in the world have depression.

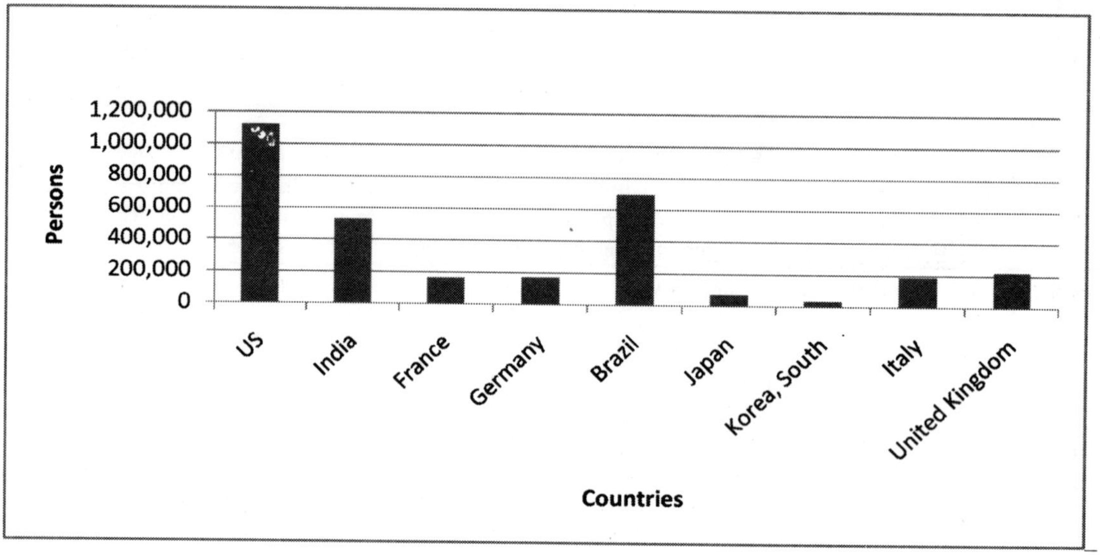

Fig. 6.3: Deaths due to depression, 2023.

Source: WHO, CDC, ECDC, NHC, mohfw.gov.in and DXY and local media reports.

More women are affected by depression than men. Depression is about 50 per cent more common among women than among men. Worldwide, more than 10 per cent of pregnant women and women who have just given birth experience depression (Woody *et al.*, 2017). More than 7,00,000 people die due to suicide every year. Suicide is the fourth leading cause of death in 15-29-year-olds. In a 2021 UNICEF survey, around 14 per cent of 15 to 24-year-olds in India reported frequently feeling depressed or disinterested. The World Health Organization's 2015 report suggested that 4.5 per cent of the Indian population, or approximately 5,66,75,969 people, were affected by depressive disorders (mindvoyage.in). In world, USA has the highest deaths due to depression followed by Brazil, India, Russia, Mexico, UK, Peru and Italy. Depression cases are highest in USA, i.e., more than 10 million.

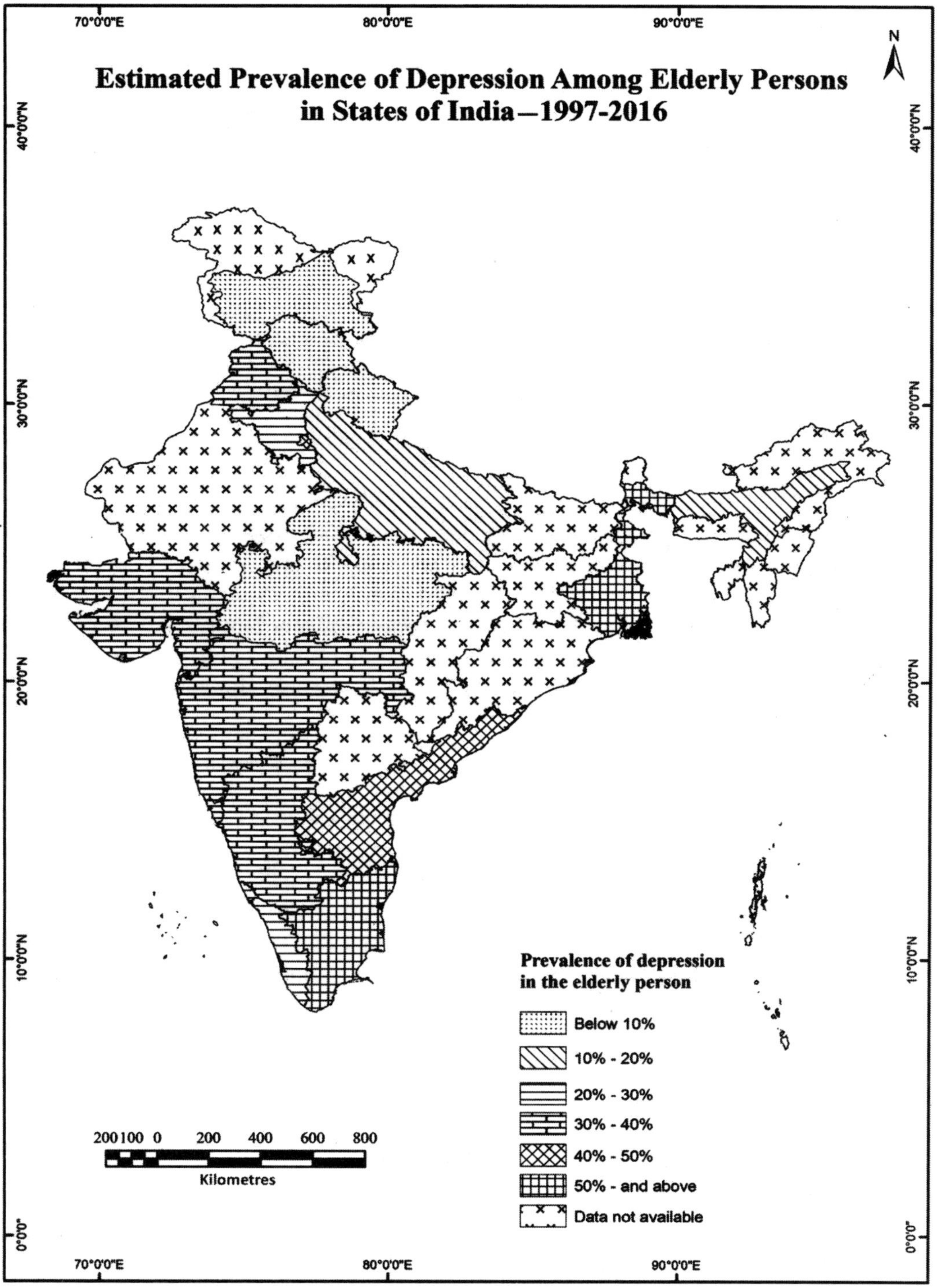

Fig. 6.4: Prevalence of Depression in the elderly persons.

Table 6.2: Depression cases in India

States	Depression cases	Deaths due to depression
Maharashtra	81,68,584	1,48,547
Kerala	69,04,252	71,909
Karnataka	40,87,933	40,353
Tamil Nadu	36,10,352	38,077
Andhra Pradesh	23,40,659	14,733
Uttar Pradesh	21,44,881	23,699
West Bengal	21,24,472	21,547
Delhi	2,04,053	26,654

Last Updated: 18 May 2023 at 9:42 AM.
Sources: WHO, CDC, ECDC, NHC, mohfw.gov.in and DXY and local media reports.

In India, Maharashtra has highest cases and deaths linked to depression. Cases are also high in Kerala, Karnataka, Tamil Nadu etc. Depression deaths are high in states of Kerala, Karnataka, Tamil Nadu, Delhi respectively. Elderly population in India suffer from depression. According to a study, depression in elderly people are more than 40 per cent in Tamil Nadu, Andhra Pradesh and West Bengal. Depression among elderly is prevalent in Gujarat, Maharashtra, Karnataka and Punjab, where 30-40 per cent of elderly suffer from depression. Comparatively, low depression cases are reported in states of Himachal Pradesh, Uttrakhand and Jammu and Madhya Pradesh (Fig. 6.4). Among elderly people, chronic diseases, restricted mobility, bereavement, elderly abuse, isolation, and loss of income are major risk factors for depression, in addition to common risk factors in all age groups (Fiske, Wetherell and Gatz, 2009).

6.3.3 *Bipolar Disorder*

According to WHO, people with bipolar disorder experience alternating depressive episodes with periods of manic symptoms. During a depressive episode, the person experiences depressed mood (feeling sad, irritable, empty) or a loss of pleasure or interest in activities, for most of the day, nearly everyday. According to Mayo Clinic, Bipolar disorder, formerly called manic depression, is a mental health condition that causes extreme mood swings that include emotional highs (mania or hypomania) and lows (depression). Symptoms can cause unpredictable changes in mood and behaviour, resulting in significant distress and difficulty in life.

- *Bipolar I disorder:* You've had at least one manic episode that may be preceded or followed by hypomanic or major depressive episodes. In some cases, mania may trigger a break from reality (psychosis).
- *Bipolar II disorder:* You have had at least one major depressive episode and at least one hypomanic episode, but you have never had a manic episode.
- *Cyclothymic disorder:* You have had at least two years—or one year in children and teenagers—of many periods of hypomania symptoms and periods of depressive symptoms (though less severe than major depression).
- *Other types:* These include, for example, bipolar and related disorders induced by certain drugs or alcohol or due to a medical condition, such as Cushing's disease, multiple sclerosis or stroke (www.mayoclinic.org).

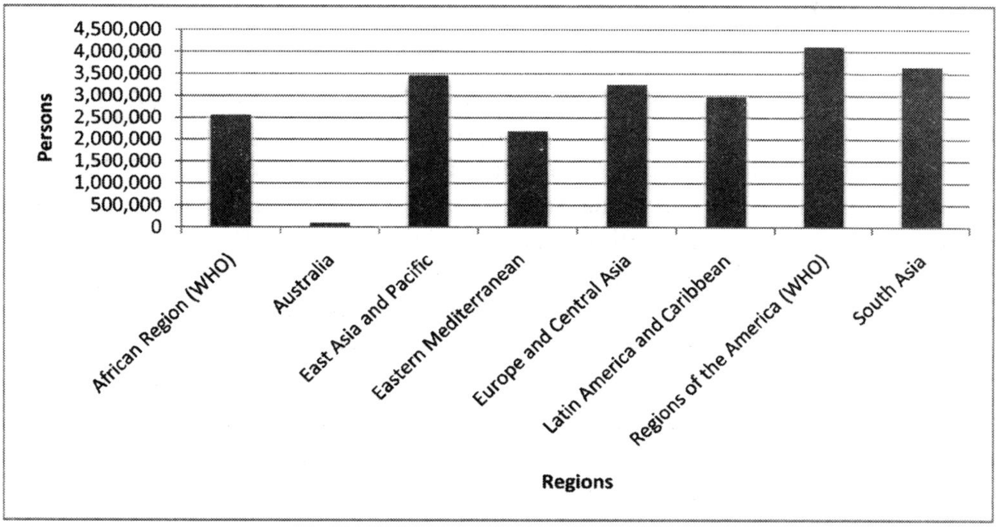

Fig. 6.5: Number of People with Bi-Polar Disorder, 2019.

Source: Global Burden of Disease Collaborative Network. Global Burden of Disease Study 2019 (GBD, 2019) Results. Seattle, United States: Institute for Health Metrics and Evaluation (IHME), 2021. Institute for Health Metrics and Evaluation, Global Burden of Disease (2019).

It can be seen from Fig. 6.5, Regions of America have the highest bipolar cases in the world. This is followed by South Asia, East Asia and Pacific, Latin America and Caribbean, Affican Region and Australia respectively.

According to a report published in *Times of India*, The National Mental Health Survey of India 2016, states that one out of 150 suffer from bipolar disorder in India and around 70 per cent of them remain untreated. The bipolar disorder is less reported and diagnosed. In India state of Goa has the highest number of cases followed by Kerela, Sikkim and Himachal Pradesh (Fig. 6.6).

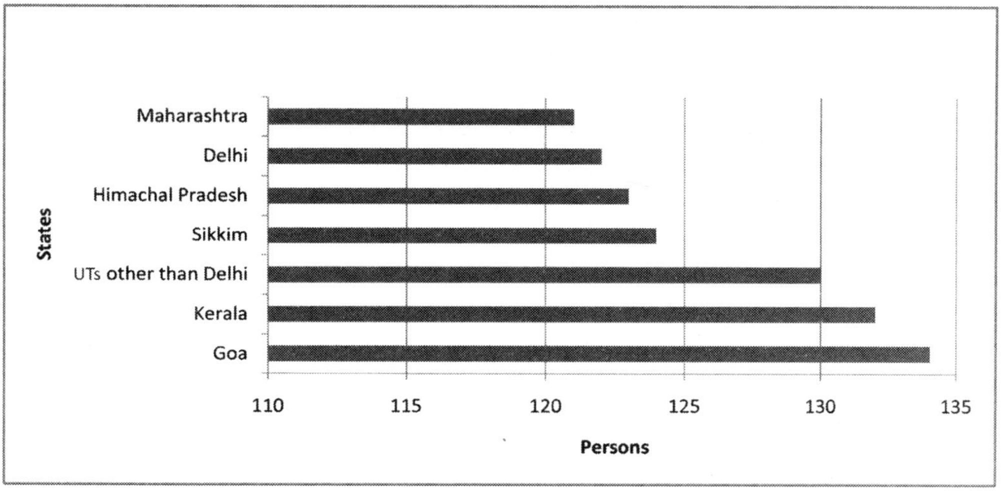

Fig. 6.6: DALYs relative to bipolar disorder across Indian states in 2017, by SDI (per 1,00,000 inhabitants).
Source: www.statista.com

6.3.4 *Post Traumatic Stress Disorder*

According to American Psychiatrists Association, Post Traumatic Stress Disorder (PTSD) is a psychiatric disorder that may occur in people who have experienced or witnessed a traumatic event, series of events or set of circumstances. An individual may experience this as emotionally or physically harmful or life-threatening and may affect mental, physical, social, and/or spiritual well-being. Examples include natural disasters, serious accidents, terrorist acts, war/combat, rape/sexual assault, historical trauma, intimate partner violence and bullying (www.psychiatry.org). According to the National Centre for PTSD, about 6 of every 10 men (or 60%) and 5 of every 10 women (or 50%) experience at least one trauma in their lives. Canada has highest rates of PTSD in their lifetime. Almost 20 per cent of American experience trauma after disastrous events.

A recent meta-analysis on infectious disease outbreaks showed that about three out of ten who survived other coronavirus infections experienced PTSD symptoms during the outbreak (Salehi, 2021). More specifically, up-to-date evidence on COVID-19 shows a PTSD prevalence from 9.5 per cent to 30.2 per cent after hospitalization (Serra *et al.*, 2022). Post-earthquake PTSD is generally attributed to high levels of chronic stress due to uncertainty about the immediate future in terms of material, social, and family possessions (Martínez, 2016). This condition is exacerbated by the presence of unfavourable characteristics. For example, a systematic review based on studies from Peru, Taiwan, Turkey, China, Greece, Haiti, Pakistan, Italy, Iran, and Japan has shown that low family income is an important predictor of PTSD (Dai *et al.*, 2016).

6.3.5 *Schizophrenia*

According to WHO, Schizophrenia is characterised by significant impairments in the way reality is perceived and changes in behaviour related to:

- *Persistent delusions*: the person has fixed beliefs that something is true, despite evidence to the contrary;
- *Persistent hallucinations*: the person may hear, smell, see, touch, or feel things that are not there;
- *Experiences of influence, control or passivity*: the experience that one's feelings, impulses, actions, or thoughts are not generated by oneself, are being placed in one's mind or withdrawn from one's mind by others, or that one's thoughts are being broadcast to others;
- *Disorganized thinking*, which is often observed as jumbled or irrelevant speech;
- *Highly disorganised behaviour*, e.g. the person does things that appear bizarre or purposeless, or the person has unpredictable or inappropriate emotional responses that interfere with their ability to organise their behaviour;
- "*Negative symptoms*" such as very limited speech, restricted experience and expression of emotions, inability to experience interest or pleasure, and social withdrawal; and/or
- *Extreme agitation or slowing of movements*, maintenance of unusual postures (WHO, www.who.int/news).

In 2000, the World Health Organization found the prevalence and incidence of schizophrenia to be roughly similar around the world, with age-standardized prevalence per 1,00,000 ranging from 343 in Africa to 544 in Japan and Oceania for men and from 378 in Africa to 527 in South-eastern Europe for women (Global burden of schizophrenia in the year, 2000).

However, the impact of schizophrenia tends to be highest in Oceania, the Middle East, and East Asia, while the nations of Australia, Japan, the United States, and most of Europe typically have low impact. Despite relative geographical proximity, the DALY rate of schizophrenia in Indonesia is nearly double that of Australia (the nations with the highest and lowest respective DALY rates). Discrepancies between DALY rates and prevalence may arise from differences in availability of medical treatment: years lived with mental disorders carry significantly higher DALY values when unmedicated than when medicated (Global burden of schizophrenia in the year, 2000).

In 2010, there were approximately 3,97,200 hospitalizations for schizophrenia in the United States. About 88,600 (22.3%) were readmitted within 30 days (Elixhauser A. Steiner, 2013).

In India, where about 1.1 billion people reside, the prevalence of schizophrenia is about 3/1000 individuals (Gururaj, Girish & Isaac, 2005). It is more common in men, and in terms of age of onset, men tend to be younger by an average of about five years than women when they develop schizophrenia. In 2017, the highest DALY rates attributed to schizophrenia was seen in Goa, categorized as a high SDI state with 210. DALYs or disability adjusted life years is a metric used to quantify the overall disease burden which is the number of years that are lost as a result of ill health, disability, or premature death. Furthermore, Arunachal Pradesh, a medium SDI state recorded a DALY rate of 177. By contrast, the lowest DALY rate relative to schizophrenia was seen in Bihar, which is a low SDI state with 133 (www.statista.com).

6.3.6 *Eating Disorder*

Eating disorders are behavioural conditions characterized by severe and persistent disturbance in eating behaviours and associated distressing thoughts and emotions. They can be very serious conditions affecting physical, psychological and social function. Types of eating disorders include anorexia nervosa, bulimia nervosa, binge eating disorder, avoidant restrictive food intake disorder, other specified feeding and eating disorder, pica and rumination disorder (www.psychiatry.org). Eating disorders often co-occur with other psychiatric disorders most commonly, mood and anxiety disorders, obsessive-compulsive disorder, and alcohol and substance use disorders.

Eating disorders affect at least 9 per cent of the global population. 9 per cent of the US population suffers from eating disorders. The percentage accounts for 28.8 million Americans. Of all the countries in Asia, Japan records the highest rates of eating disorders. Additionally, Singapore, Hong Kong, South Korea, and Taiwan have led Asians to high rates of eating disorders. The highest prevalence rate for eating disorders in Europe occurs in Austria, having 1.55 per cent in 2012 (www.crossrivertherapy.co).

In 2017, the highest DALY rates attributed to eating disorders was seen in Goa, categorized as a high SDI state with 54. DALYs or disability adjusted life years is a metric used to quantify the overall disease burden which is the number of years that are lost as a result of ill health, disability, or premature death. Furthermore, in Haryana, a medium SDI state recorded a DALY rate of 43. By contrast, the lowest DALY rate relative to eating disorders was seen in Bihar, which is a low SDI state with 26 (www.statista.com).

6.3.7 *Disruptive Behaviour and Dissocial Disorders*

Disruptive behaviour disorders (DBD) can seriously impact a child's daily life. Children with disruptive behaviour disoıders show ongoing patterns of uncooperative and defiant behaviour. The most common types of disruptive behaviour disorders include an other or unspecified disruptive, impulse-control, and conduct disorder (previously known as disruptive behaviour disorder), oppositional defiant disorder (ODD) and conduct disorder (CD) (www.nationwidechildrens.org). Problematic behaviours and issues with self-control associated with these disorders are typically first observed in childhood and can persist into adulthood. In general, disruptive, impulse-control, and conduct disorders tend to be more common in males than females (/www.psychiatry.org). Youth with disruptive behaviour disorders experience difficulties with their parents, peers, and teachers, and are at risk for academic underachievement. Furthermore, for many youth, these difficulties persist into adolescence and adulthood, presenting additional risk for substance use, suicide, and incarceration (Frick *et al.*, 2010; Loeber *et al.*, 2000a, b).

According to Institute of Health Metrics and Evaluation, Global Health, 40 million people, including children and adolescents, were living with conduct-dissocial disorder in 2019. As per Mathew *et al.,* in their article Psychosocial interventions for disruptive behavioural problems in children living in low- and middle-income countries: study protocol of a systematic review, oppositional defiant disorder (ODD) and conduct disorder (CD) have an estimated worldwide prevalence of 3.3 per cent and 3.2 per cent, respectively (Canino *et al.,* 2010). The sizeable burden of behavioural problems over the lifespan is suggested by their early age of onset (Kesseler *et al.*, 2007), stability over time and increased risk of onset of other psychiatric disorders throughout childhood, adolescence and adulthood, including conduct disorder (for ODD) (Cohen and Flory, 1998), depression and substance abuse (Boyle, 1991). Disruptive behavioural problems are associated with low school achievement, school dropout (Tramotina, 2001) and suicide (Nock *et al.,* 2008). Long-term follow-up studies have demonstrated that childhood behavioural problems are associated with later lower educational achievement, increased delinquency and increased risk of later serious, violent and chronic criminal offending (Loeber and Farrington, 2000).

There is paucity of data especially with reference to spatio temporal data. The researches are also limited and focused only on small scale like a school or college etc.

6.3.8 *Neuro-developmental Disorders*

According to American Psychiatric Association, "Developmental disorders" were included for the first time in *DSM-III,* for the category that comprised autistic disorder. "Neurodevelopmental disorders (NDDs) is a disorder usually first diagnosed in infancy, childhood, or adolescence." In *ICD11,* the latest revision of the International Classification of Diseases published by the WHO, NDDs gained even more prominence by becoming an integral part of the title of the chapter on psychiatry: "Mental, behavioural or neurodevelopmental disorders." NDDs are defined as a group of conditions with onset in the developmental period, inducing deficits that produce impairments of functioning. NDDs comprise intellectual disability (ID); Communication Disorders; Autism Spectrum Disorder (ASD); Attention-Deficit/Hyperactivity Disorder (ADHD); Neurodevelopmental Motor Disorders, including Tic Disorders; and Specific Learning

Disorders (Morris and Crocq, 2020). Autism Spectrum Disorder (ASD) and attention deficit and hyperactivity disorder (ADHD) are the two most common neurodevelopmental disorders observed in childhood (Scandurra, 2019). 'Autism' is defined by characteristics of abnormal functioning in all three areas of social interaction, communication, and restricted, repetitive behaviour. Globally, around 62 million people were estimated to have autistic spectrum disorder in 2016. Just under 50 million of these cases were in males. Of the 62 million with autistic spectrum disorder, around 18 million had Autism, and 44 million had Asperger syndrome and other spectrum disorders (ourworldindata.org). According to Centres for Disease Control and Prevention (CDC) 2016, about 6.1 million children in the United States (9.4%) between ages 2 and 17 are estimated to have ever been diagnosed with attention deficit hyperactivity disorder (ADHD or ADD). The worldwide prevalence of adult ADHD is estimated at 2.8 per cent, according to a 2016 study (www.additudemag.com). According to CDC, in USA in 2003, 7.8 per cent of children were ever diagnosed with ADHD which increased to 9.5 per cent in 2007 and 11 per cent in 2011.

In India, according to the 2011 Census, more than 6 million children below the age of nine are afflicted by all kinds of disabilities. The census divides disabilities into eight categories—seeing, hearing, speech, movement, mental retardation, mental illness, multiple disabilities and others—and probably underestimates number of children suffering from NDDs. The new study published in *PLoS Medicine* projects that more than 23 million children below nine years have NDDs alone. Almost one in eight children aged 2-9 years living in India may have at least one neurodevelopmental disorder (NDD), according to prevalence estimates published this week in *PLoS Medicine* (www.eurekalert.org). Due to paucity of data the proper spatiotemporal analysis isn't possible.

6.4 Mental Health Management

Maintaining good mental health varies from person to person and depends on a variety of factors, such as genetics, upbringing, lifestyle, and life events. However, there are some general strategies that can help people manage their mental health and improve their overall well-being.

1. **Practice self-care:** Take care of yourself physically and emotionally by exercising regularly, eating a healthy diet, getting enough sleep, and participating in activities you enjoy. Self-care practices can help reduce stress and promote positive emotions.
2. **Develop a support system:** Build and maintain positive relationships with family, friends, and other people who are supportive and empathetic. Spending time with others who share similar interests can provide a sense of belonging and reduce feelings of isolation.
3. **Seek therapy or counselling:** It is okay to ask for help. If you are struggling with mental health problems, like depression, anxiety, or addiction, seeking professional help can be a game-changer. Speaking to a therapist can help you get clarity, understand your emotions, and learn how to cope with difficult situations.
4. **Practice mindfulness:** Engage in mindfulness practices, such as meditation, deep breathing, yoga or journaling, to help reduce stress and manage negative emotions. Mindfulness practices can also help you improve your focus and concentration, which can enhance your overall well-being.

5. **Keep a positive outlook:** Practice positive self-talk, embrace your strengths and weaknesses, and cultivate an attitude of gratitude. Cultivating a positive mindset can help you cope with difficult situations and maintain a positive outlook on life.
6. **Engage in hobbies and creative pursuits:** Participating in creative activities like painting, music, writing, or gardening can provide a sense of purpose and joy. Hobbies can also be a healthy outlet for emotions and a way to recharge your mental batteries.

Check WHO website for help: https://apps.who.int/iris/bitstream/handle/10665/331901/9789240003910-eng.pdf

Managing mental health requires a multifaceted approach that involves taking care of oneself physically and emotionally, building a support system, seeking professional help when necessary, practicing mindfulness, cultivating a positive mindset, and engaging in hobbies and creative pursuits that bring joy and purpose. By incorporating these strategies into your daily routine, you can maintain good mental health and improve your overall well-being.

REFERENCES

Artero, S., Touchon, J., Ritchie, K. (2001). Disability and mild cognitive impairment: a longitudinal population-based study. *Int J Geriatr Psychiatry*, 16: 1092-7.

Ayuso-Mateos, J.L. "Global burden of schizophrenia in the year 2000" (PDF). World Health Organization.

Burton, W.N., Schultz, A.B., Chen, C., Edington, D.W. (2008). The association of worker productivity and mental health: a review of the literature. *Int J Workplace Health Manag*, 1(2): 78-94.

Canino, G., Polanczyk, G., Bauermeister, J.J. *et al.*. (2010). Does the prevalence of CD and ODD vary across cultures? *Soc Psychiatry Psychiatr Epidemiol*, 45: 695-704. 10.1007/s00127-010-0242-y

Cohen, P., Flory, M. (1998). Issues in the disruptive behaviour disorders: attention deficit disorder without hyperactivity and the differential validity of oppositional defiant and conduct disorders. *DSM-IV Sourcebook*, 4: 455-63.

Dai, W., Chen, L., Lai, Z., Li, Y., Wang, J., Liu, A. (2016). The Incidence of Post-Traumatic Stress Disorder among Survivors after Earthquakes: A Systematic Review and Meta-Analysis. *BMC Psychiatry*, 16: 188. doi: 10.1186/s12888-016-0891-9.

Dariush, D. Farhud (2015). Impact of Lifestyle on Health in Iran. *J Public Health*, Vol. 44, No.11, Nov., pp. 1442-1444.

Einvik, G., Dammen, T., Ghanima, W., Heir T., Stavem, K. (2021). Prevalence and Risk Factors for Post-Traumatic Stress in Hospitalized and Non-Hospitalized COVID-19 Patients. *Int. J. Environ. Res. Public Health*, 18: 2079. doi: 10.3390/ijerph18042079. [PMC free article] [PubMed] [CrossRef] [Google Scholar].

Elixhauser, A., Steiner, C. (2010). *Readmissions to U.S. Hospitals by Diagnosis*, HCUP Statistical Brief #153. Agency for Healthcare Research and Quality. April 2013.

European Network for Workplace Health Promotion. *Newsletter* 09/2010. //www.enwhp.org/fileadmin/downloads/8th_Initiative/MentalHealth_Broschuere_businesscase.pdf

Fiske, A., Wetherell, J.L., Gatz, M. (2009). Depression in older adults. *Annu Rev Clin Psychol*, 5: 363-89.

Fuchs, T., Schlimme, J.E. Embodiment and psychopathology: a phenomenological perspective. *Curr Opin Psychiatry*, 22: 570-75.

Galderisi, S., Heinz, A., Kastrup, M., Beezhold, J., Sartorius, N. (2015 June). Towards a new definition of mental health. *World Psychiatry*, 14(2): 231-3. doi: 10.1002/wps.20231. PMID: 26043341; PMCID: PMC4471980

Global Cancer Facts and Figures, 4th edition, 2018, American Cancer Society, retrieved from https: //www.cancer.org/content/dam/cancer-org/research/cancer-facts-and-statistics/global-cancer-facts-and-figures/global-cancer-facts-and-figures-4th-edition.pdf

Grundemann, R.W., Nijboer, D., Schellart, A.J. (1991). Den Haag: Ministry of Social Affairs and Employment; 1991. The work relatedness of drop-out from work for medical reasons.

Gururaj, G., Girish, N., Isaac, M.K. (2005). *NCMH Background papers—Burden of disease in India.* New Delhi: Ministry of Health & Family Welfare, Mental, neurological and substance abuse disorders: Strategies towards a systems approach.

Gustavsson, A., Svensson, M., Jacobi, F., Allgulander, C., Alonso, J., Beghi, E., Dodel, R., Ekman, M., Faravelli, C., Fratiglioni, L. *et al.* (2011). Cost of disorders of the brain in Europe 2010. *Eur Neuropsychopharmacol* 21: 718-779.

Hamberg-van Reenen, H.H., Proper, K.I., van den Berg, M. (2012). Worksite mental health interventions: a systematic review of economic evaluations. *Occup Environ Med.,* 69: 837-45.

Institute of Health Metrics and Evaluation. Global Health Data Exchange (GHDx), (https: //vizhub.healthdata.org/gbd-results/, accessed 14 May, 2022)

Janiri, D., Carfì, A., Kotzalidis, G.D., Bernabei, R., Landi, F., Sani, G. (2021). Posttraumatic Stress Disorder in Patients After Severe COVID-19 Infection. *JAMA Psychiatry,* 78: 567. doi: 10.1001/jamapsychiatry.2021.01.09.

Kessler, R.C., Angermeyer, M., Anthony, J.C. *et al.* (2007). Lifetime prevalence and age-of-onset distributions of mental disorders in the World Health Organization's World Mental Health Survey Initiative. *World Psychiatry,* 6: 168.

Keyes, C.L. (2006). Mental health in adolescence: is America's youth flourishing? *Am J Orthopsychiatry,* 76: 395-402.

Keyes, C.L.M. (2014). Mental health as a complete state: how the salutogenic perspective completes the picture. In: Bauer, G.F., Hämmig, O., editors. *Bridging occupational, organizational and public health.* Dordrecht: Springer, pp. 179-92.

Kleinman, A. (1999). Social violence: research questions on local experiences and global responses. *Archives of General Psychiatry,* 56: 978-79.

Loeber, R., Farrington, D.P. (2000). Young children who commit crime: Epidemiology, developmental origins, risk factors, early interventions, and policy implications. *Dev Psychopathol,* 12: 737-62. 10.1017/S0954579400004107

Martínez, X.D., Bastías, C.M., Aravena, M.A.M., López, R.C., Castillo, S.M., Mena, J.O., Díaz, R.M. (2016). Síntomas del trastorno por estrés postraumático en la comuna chilena de Cobquecura, 2010. *Rev. Cuba. De Salud Pública,* 42: 284-293.

Morris-Rosendahl, D.J., Crocq, M.A. (2020 March). Neurodevelopmental disorders—the history and future of a diagnostic concept. *Dialogues Clin Neurosci,* 22(1): 65-72. doi: 10.31887/DCNS.2020.22.1/macrocq

Nock, M.K., Borges, G., Bromet, E.J. *et al.* (2008). Cross-national prevalence and risk factors for suicidal ideation, plans and attempts. *Br J Psychiatry,* 192: 98-105. 10.1192/bjp.bp.107.040113

O'Leary, L. (1993). Mental Health at work. In *Occup Health Rev.,* 45: 23-26.

Pal, D., Sahu, D.P., Maji, S., Taywade, M. (2022, Aug. 16). Prevalence of Anxiety Disorder in Adolescents in India: A Systematic Review and Meta-Analysis. *Cureus,* 14(8): e28084. doi: 10.7759/cureus.28084. PMID: 36127986

Pardini, D., Frick, P.J. (2013). Multiple developmental pathways to conduct disorder: current conceptualizations and clinical implications. *J Can Acad Child Adolesc Psychiatry.*

Rajgopal, T. (2010 Sep.). Mental well-being at the workplace. *Indian J Occup Environ Med.,* 14(3): 63-5. doi: 10.4103/0019-5278.75691. PMID: 21461156; PMCID: PMC3062016

Reducing the Economic Burden of Unmet Mental Health Needs, 2022, CEA, retrieved from www.whitehouse.gov/cea.

Salehi, M., Amanat, M., Mohammadi, M., Salmanian, M., Rezaei, N., Saghazadeh, A., Garakani, A. (2021). The prevalence of post-traumatic stress disorder related symptoms in Coronavirus outbreaks: A systematic-review and meta-analysis. *J. Affect. Disord,* 282: 527-538. doi: 10.1016/j.jad.2020.12.188. [PMC free article] [PubMed] [CrossRef] [Google Scholar].

Saloni Dattani, Hannah Ritchie and Max Roser (2021). "Mental Health". Published online at OurWorldInData.org. Retrieved from: 'https: //ourworldindata.org/mental-health'

Scandurra, V., Emberti Gialloreti, L., Barbanera, F., Scordo, M.R., Pierini, A., Canitano, R. (2019, Sep. 4). Neurodevelopmental Disorders and Adaptive Functions: A Study of Children With Autism Spectrum Disorders (ASD) and/or Attention Deficit and Hyperactivity Disorder (ADHD). *Front Psychiatry,* 10: 673. doi: 10.3389/fpsyt.2019.00673.

Serra, R., Borrazzo, C., Vassalini, P., Di Nicolantonio, C., Koukopoulos, A.E., Tosato, C., Cherubini, F., Alessandri, F., Ceccarelli, G., Mastroianni, C.M., D'Ettorre, G., Tarsitani, L. (2022, July 11). Post-Traumatic Stress Disorder Trajectories the Year after COVID-19 Hospitalization. *Int J Environ Res Public Health,* 19(14): 8452. doi: 10.3390/ijerph19148452

Tarsitani, L., Vassalini, P., Koukopoulos, A., Borrazzo, C., Alessi, F., Di Nicolantonio, C., Serra, R., Alessandri, F., Ceccarelli, G., Mastroianni, C.M. *et al.* (2021). Post-traumatic Stress Disorder Among COVID-19 Survivors at 3-Month Follow-up After Hospital Discharge. *J. Gen. Intern Med.,* 36: 1702-1707. doi: 10.1007/s11606-021-06731-7. [PMC free article] [PubMed] [CrossRef] [Google Scholar].

The burden of mental disorders across the states of India: the Global Burden of Disease Study 1990-2017, December 20, 2019, volume 7, issue 2, pp. 148-161, February 2020, DOI: HTTPS: //DOI.ORG/10.1016/S2215-0366(19)30475-4

Tramontina, S., Martins, S., Michalowski, M.B. *et al.*. (2001). School drop-out and conduct disorder in Brazilian elementary school students. *Can J Psychiatry,* 46: 941-47.

Trivedi, J.K., Gupta, P.K. (2010 Jan.). An overview of Indian research in anxiety disorders. *Indian J Psychiatry.* 52 (Suppl. 1): S210-8. doi: 10.4103/0019-5545.69234. PMID: 21836680; PMCID: PMC3146193

Winslow, C.A.E. (1938). *The mental hygiene movement and its founder,* in National Committee on Mental Hygiene, The Mental Hygiene Movement, Garden City, NY, Country Life Press, pp. 303-17.

Woody, C.A., Ferrari, A.J., Siskind, D.J., Whiteford, H.A., Harris, M.G. (2017). A systematic review and meta-regression of the prevalence and incidence of perinatal depression. *J Affect Disord,* 219: 86-92.

Ziglio, E., Currie, C., Rasmussen, V.B. (2004). The WHO cross-national study of health behaviour in school aged children from 35 countries: findings from 2001-2002. *J School Health,* 74 (6): 204-206. [PubMed] [Google Scholar] [Ref list].

Chapter

7

Healthcare Policies, Programmes and Institutions

Globally, health is one of the most important areas of concern. Health concerns are not just limited to individuals or states; they have wider impacts and need to be tackled by formulating global strategies. Global health concern caters to the health issues that transcend national borders and have an impact on people across the globe. These health issues include infectious diseases such as Zika, Ebola, and COVID-19, non-communicable diseases (NCDs) such as cancer, heart diseases and diabetes, as well as other health related challenges such as food and nutrition insecurity, violence, and climate change. All global initiatives pinpoints to the relevance of equity and universal access in a substantial way. Several international health initiatives in the form of campaigns, programmes etc. designed and implemented by international organizations are followed by various countries. The global agendas are guiding principles for national policies and required local actions. For example United Nations Conference on Environment and Development held in 1992, also known as Agenda 21, took an initiative of formulating targets for world and various countries to achieve goal of sustainable development. The section 1 of Agenda 21 focused on socio-economic development directed towards combating poverty, especially in developing countries, changing consumption patterns, promoting health, achieving a more sustainable population, and sustainable settlement in decision making. For example, the North African countries are signatories but little to no adoption on the local-government level is formally done. In fact, countries in sub-Saharan Africa and North Africa generally have poorly documented Agenda 21 status reports. By contrast, South Africa's participation in Agenda 21 mirrors that of modern Europe, with 21 city members of ICLEI (Local governments for Sustainability) and support of Agenda 21 by national-level government.

7.1 The Significance of Global Health Organizations, Policies and Programmes

The question arises why we need global agendas or global health parameters? As mentioned earlier health concerns are not just individual specific rather they are universal, so the formulation of agendas at global level sets guideline principles for policymakers at national and state levels. The significance of Global initiatives are:

7.1.1 *Emergence of Pandemics and Infectious Diseases*

An outbreak of an infectious disease in one part of the world can quickly spread to other regions, eventually becoming a pandemic. This can have severe and widespread repercussions, including loss of life, social and economic disruption, and a significant burden on healthcare systems. Global health policies can play a crucial role in responding to pandemics and mitigating their impact on communities around the world. Effective communication and coordination between countries and international organizations is essential for containing the spread of pandemics. The World Health Organization (WHO) plays a critical role in coordinating the global response to pandemics and sharing information on best practices and guidelines. For example, during the COVID-19 pandemic, the WHO organized regular briefings and shared information on the spread of the virus, prevention measures, and treatment options. Global health policies can also help mobilize resources and funding to support countries in responding to pandemics. The World Bank, for instance, has created a Pandemic Emergency Financing Facility that provides funds to countries affected by pandemics. The facility provides rapid funding to support countries in responding to pandemics and provides a financial safety net for communities in need. Global health policies can facilitate the development and distribution of vaccines and treatments for pandemics. For example, the COVAX initiative is a global effort to ensure equitable access to COVID-19 vaccines, particularly for low- and middle-income countries. The initiative brings together governments, organizations, and manufacturers to accelerate the development, production, and equitable access to COVID-19 vaccines.

7.1.2 *Economic Impact*

Poor health can worsen poverty, low productivity, and an increased financial burden on healthcare systems. Global Health policies can have short-term and long-term economic impacts which can be both positive as well as negative. During pandemics, many countries implement travel bans and restrictions to prevent the spread of the virus. These restrictions can have a significant economic impact, particularly on the tourism industry. For example, during the 2002-2004 SARS outbreak, the Chinese government imposed travel restrictions, leading to a 55 per cent decrease in international tourism in China and a significant loss of revenue for the tourism industry. During pandemics, businesses may have to shut down or reduce their operations due to health and safety concerns. This can have a significant economic impact, particularly on small and medium-sized enterprises. For example, during the 2014 Ebola outbreak in West Africa, many businesses in affected countries had to shut down, leading to a decrease in economic activity and loss of jobs. The governments may need to invest significant resources to respond to the outbreak. This can lead to increased healthcare costs and additional expenses for the government. For example, during the COVID-19 pandemic, many governments had to invest in additional resources such as personal protective equipment, testing, and contact tracing, leading to increased healthcare expenditures. Pandemics can disrupt global supply chains and lead to a decrease in international trade. For example, during the COVID-19 pandemic, many countries implemented trade restrictions on medical equipment and supplies, leading to shortages and delays in the availability of critical goods. So it can effect inter-regional trade and commerce; inflation and food prices and availability of various items worldwide.

Therefore, embracing global health can prevent the spread of diseases and the occurrence of other health complications that can harm people's health and the economy. While the economic impact of pandemics is significant, it is important to prioritize public health and safety measures to prevent the spread of the virus and protect populations.

7.1.3 *Health Equity*

Health equities are the differences in health outcomes between different groups of people, caused by factors such as socio-economic status, race, and gender. Global health aims to promote health equity by addressing the health needs of marginalized and disadvantageous populations, including low-income communities, and reducing health disparities between low-, middle-, and high-income countries around the world. It can affect poor, handicapped, migrants and children in a serious manner. Poor can become poorer and people might not have accessibility and affordability of health services. One example of how a global health crisis can impact health equities is the Ebola outbreak that occurred in West Africa in 2014. The outbreak disproportionately affected low-income communities, where access to healthcare and information was limited. These communities also lacked basic resources such as clean water, which made it difficult to practice good hygiene and prevent the spread of the disease. The outbreak led to a significant number of deaths and had a long-lasting impact on the affected communities' economy and social well-being. Another example is the ongoing COVID-19 pandemic, which has highlighted health inequities around the world. The pandemic has disproportionately affected low-income and marginalized communities, who may have limited access to healthcare, live in overcrowded conditions, and work in essential jobs that expose them to higher risk of infection. In addition, the pandemic has exacerbated existing health inequities based on race and ethnicity too.

7.1.4 *The Impact of Climate Change on Health*

The impact of climate change on the planet can lead to various health hazards, including natural disasters, and the spread of diseases that can be spread from animals to human beings. Global health policies focused on mitigating climate change can help reduce the incidence of climate-sensitive health outcomes such as respiratory illness, skin cancer, and heat stress. Policies aimed at reducing greenhouse gas emissions, renewable energy, and sustainable transportation can help mitigate climate change and prevent its harmful effects on human health. For example, the Paris Agreement, which aims to limit global warming to below 2 degrees Celsius, will help decrease the incidence of heat-related deaths, respiratory illness, and infectious diseases that thrive in warmer temperatures. Global health policies focused on preparedness and response to climate change can help mitigate the impact of extreme weather events such as hurricanes, floods, and droughts. These policies can help decrease the loss of life, restore food and water security, and promote disaster resilience. For example, the Sendai Framework for Disaster Risk Reduction provides an integrated approach to reducing disaster risk and supporting resilient societies.

7.2 Global Health Organizations and Committees

7.2.1 *World Health Organization (WHO)*

The WHO was established on April 7, 1948 and this day is regarded as World Health Day. WHO is a specialized agency of the United Nations that is responsible for international public health. Its role is to coordinate and direct international health programmes, provide technical support and assistance to countries, promote health research and standards, and develop policies and strategies to combat global health issues, some of the key contributions of WHO include the eradication of smallpox, polio, and Guinea worm disease and the advancement of universal health coverage. The goal of WHO is to ensure that a billion more people have universal health coverage, to protect a billion more people from health emergencies, and provide a further billion people with better health and well-being. The World Health Organization (WHO) plays a critical role in meeting global health challenges by coordinating the global response to health threats and providing guidance on best practices and policies. The main objective of WHO is "the attainment of highest level of Health for all". The key responsibilities of WHO are:

1. **Epidemic and pandemic response:** WHO's role in responding to epidemics and pandemics is critical to preventing their spread and mitigating their impact. For example, during the COVID-19 pandemic, WHO played an important role in coordinating the global response, providing guidance on public health measures, and coordinating global efforts to develop and distribute vaccines.
2. **Health education and promotion:** WHO plays an important role in educating the public about health issues and promoting healthy behaviours. For example, WHO campaigns have raised awareness of key health issues such as tobacco use, mental health, and communicable diseases.
3. **Disease eradication:** WHO has played a key role in eradicating diseases such as smallpox and polio through vaccination campaigns and public health initiatives. For example, in 2019, WHO announced the eradication of wild polio virus in Africa, a milestone achievement in public health.
4. **Global health policy and regulation:** WHO is responsible for the development of global health policies and the regulation of health products and services. For example, WHO's Framework Convention on Tobacco Control (FCTC) is a global treaty that has helped reduce tobacco use and its related health consequences around the world. In addition, WHO regulates the use of pharmaceuticals and medical devices through the prequalification programme. A recent example of WHO's role in meeting global health challenges is the COVID-19 pandemic. WHO has provided guidance on public health measures, such as wearing masks and social distancing, and has coordinated global efforts to develop and distribute vaccines. In addition, WHO has worked to raise awareness of the pandemic and promote healthy behaviours.
5. **During emergencies:** WHO prepares for emergencies by identifying, mitigating and managing risks. It prevents emergencies and support development of tools necessary during outbreaks. WHO also detect and respond to acute health emergencies by support delivery of essential health services in fragile settings.

The World Health Organization consists of 3 Principal organs:

(a) The World Health Assembly: akin to a Parliament,
(b) The Executive Board: akin to a Cabinet, and
(c) The Secretariat.

WHO has 191 member states. It divides world into six regions namely: Africa, The Americas, Eastern Mediterranean, Europe, South East Asia, Western Pacific.

7.2.2 *United Nations Children's Fund (UNICEF)*

UNICEF was established in 1946 with the aim of promoting children's rights, health, education, and equality. Its focus is on providing healthcare services, education, nutrition, water, and sanitation to mothers and children in low- and middle-income countries. It also provides emergency assistance during humanitarian crises such as natural disasters and wars. UNICEF plays following roles related to health challenges and emergencies:

1. **Emergency response:** UNICEF is frequently involved in emergency response efforts during natural disasters and conflict situations. For example, UNICEF was involved in the response to the Ebola outbreak in West Africa, where it provided essential medical supplies and equipment, and supported hand-washing and sanitation programmes to prevent the spread of the disease.
2. **Immunization:** UNICEF plays a critical role in promoting immunization campaigns to protect children against preventable diseases such as measles, polio, and rubella. For example, in 2020, UNICEF delivered more than 2 billion vaccine doses to 110 countries, despite the challenges posed by the COVID-19 pandemic.
3. **Nutrition:** UNICEF promotes nutrition programmes to support children's health and growth and prevent malnutrition. For example, UNICEF supports programmes that promote breastfeeding, provide nutritional supplements, and ensure access to safe drinking water and sanitation.
4. **Education:** UNICEF promotes education programmes that help improve children's health and well-being. For example, UNICEF supports programmes that promote school attendance, provide educational materials, and prioritize the needs of children in conflict-affected areas.
5. **Advocacy and policy:** UNICEF advocates for policies that support the health and well-being of children and families around the world. For example, UNICEF played a critical role in advocating for the inclusion of childhood immunizations as part of the Sustainable Development Goals.

7.2.3 *Food and Agricultural Organization (FAO)*

FAO is an agency of United Nations which was established in 1945 and has its headquarters in Rome. The main objective of FAO is raising food production and ensuring adequate food availability in the face of increasing population. The goal is to achieve food security for all and make sure that people have regular access to enough high-quality food to lead active, healthy lives. The FAO is also linked to World Food Programme (WFP). In 1960, FAO launched Freedom from Hunger Campaign. Since 1994, FAO has been focussing on food security.

7.2.4 *The Global Fund to Fight AIDS, Tuberculosis and Malaria*

The Global Fund was founded in 2002 and is an international financing institution that aims to mobilize and provide resources to combat HIV/AIDS, tuberculosis, and malaria. It partners with countries, communities, and the private sector to fund prevention, treatment, and care programmes, and also supports health system strengthening to ensure sustainability.

7.2.5 *Doctors without Borders*

It is also known as Médecins Sans Frontières (MSF) was established in 1971 and is an international medical humanitarian organization that provides emergency medical care and aid to people affected by conflict, epidemics, and disasters in over 70 countries. MSF operates independently and provides medical assistance based solely on the needs of the population at hand. MSF has played a crucial role in tackling global health issues:

1. **Ebola outbreak in West Africa (2014-2016):** MSF played a critical role in responding to the Ebola outbreak in West Africa, providing medical care, setting up isolation centres, and training local health workers. MSF was one of the first organizations to respond to the outbreak, and their timely intervention saved countless lives.
2. **Refugee crisis in Syria and neighbouring countries:** MSF has been providing essential medical assistance to refugees fleeing the conflict in Syria since the outbreak of the war. MSF operates medical facilities in Syria and neighbouring countries that provide treatment for those affected by the conflict, including war wounds and other conditions.
3. **HIV/AIDS epidemic:** MSF has been active in responding to the HIV/AIDS epidemic since the 1990s. MSF provides HIV testing and treatment in countries affected by the epidemic, trains local health workers, and advocates for policies that support access to essential medicines.
4. **Natural disasters:** MSF has responded to many natural disasters, including earthquakes, cyclones, and floods, providing essential medical assistance to those affected. For example, in 2010, MSF responded to the earthquake in Haiti, setting up medical facilities and providing treatment and surgery for those injured.

7.2.6 *International Committee of Red Cross*

It is a Non-Governmental Organization formulated in 1863 with an aim of ensuring protection and assistance for victims of armed conflict and strife. It takes action in response to emergencies. The first Geneva Convention was held in 1864. Now it has branches all over the world. Its objectives are provision of amenities for soldiers. It also organizes disaster relief services in times of disasters. They also maintain blood banks, maternity welfare services and child welfare services for emergencies.

These global health organizations have made significant contributions to improving health outcomes worldwide, and their works have been instrumental in fighting different health challenges globally.

7.3 International Health Policies and Programmes

International and national health policies help to ensure a consistent and standardized approach to healthcare across the globe or within a specific country. These policies provide guidance for healthcare providers and institutions to deliver quality care to individuals and communities. International health policies include:

7.3.1 *International Health Regulations*

The IHR are an instrument of international law that is legally-binding on 196 countries, including the 194 WHO Member States. IHR create rights and obligations for countries, including the requirement to report public health events. The Regulations also outline the criteria to determine whether or not a particular event constitutes a "public health emergency of international concern". IHR helps all the countries to formulate their own regulations to manage communicable diseases. It was adopted in 1969 by WHO and revised in 2005. Here is a chronological order of significant events related to the International Health Regulations.

In 1851, the International Sanitary Regulations were established at the International Sanitary Conference to prevent the spread of cholera in Europe. It focused on six quarantinable diseases; cholera, plague, relapsing fever, smallpox, typhoid and yellow fever. In 1969, the ISR were revised and renamed the 'International Health Regulations' (Collins, 2010). A Public Health Emergency of International Concern, or PHEIC, is defined in the IHR (2005) as, "an extraordinary event which is determined to constitute a public health risk to other States through the international spread of disease and to potentially require a coordinated international response" (WHO, 2019). This definition implies a situation, that is, serious, sudden, unusual or unexpected; carries implications for public health beyond the affected State's national border; and may require immediate international action. In 2003, the IHR was revised, with an increased focus on transparency and capacity-building in developing countries, following the outbreak of severe acute respiratory syndrome (SARS). In 2005, the World Health Assembly adopted the revised IHR, which required all countries to strengthen their public health systems and report certain infectious disease outbreaks to WHO within 24 hours. In 2009, the IHR were put to the test when the H1N1 influenza pandemic spread across the globe. The IHR allowed countries to implement effective information sharing channels and establish measures to ensure public health safety.

In 2014, the Ebola virus outbreak in West Africa demonstrated the importance of the IHR and the urgent need for global cooperation. The IHR enabled countries to establish control measures and limit the spread of the virus. In 2020, the COVID-19 pandemic highlighted the limitations of the IHR and the need for further strengthening of global public health systems to prevent and respond to future pandemics.

7.3.2 *Universal Health Coverage*

This standard aims to ensure that all individuals and communities have access to the essential health services they need without experiencing financial hardship. It covers the full continuum of essential health services, from health promotion to prevention, treatment, rehabilitation and palliative care (WHO). The SDG 3.8 target aims to "achieve universal health coverage (UHC), including financial risk protection, access to quality essential healthcare services, and access to safe, effective, quality, and affordable essential medicines and vaccines for all." Though the UHC is the target for all countries still many people across the globe suffer because of accessibility or affordability of health services. The poor and downtrodden are the most effective ones. According to WHO, almost 90 million people are impoverished by health expenses every year. It was in 2019, the UHC got the momentum. UHC focuses upon maternal deaths, child mortality, High fertility, adolescent fertility, mental, neurological and substance disorder.

7.3.3 *Primary Health Care*

This standard promotes the provision of comprehensive, community-based health services that are accessible, affordable, and culturally appropriate. *"PHC is a whole-of-society approach to health that aims at ensuring the highest possible level of health and well-being and their equitable distribution by focusing on people's needs and as early as possible along the continuum from health promotion and disease prevention to treatment, rehabilitation and palliative care, and as close as feasible to people's everyday environment" (www.who.int).* According to WHO, scaling up primary healthcare (PHC) interventions across low- and middle-income countries could save 60 million lives and increase average life expectancy by 3.7 years by 2030. Solidarity, equity and participation are rooted commitment in PHC. It is the most effective and efficient approach to ensure global healthcare.

7.3.4 *Disease Prevention and Control*

This standard aims to prevent and control the spread of communicable and non-communicable diseases, and to ensure that appropriate treatments are available and accessible. Primary prevention refers to actions aimed at avoiding the manifestation of a disease (this may include actions to improve health through changing the impact of social and economic determinants on health; the provision of information on behavioural and medical health risks, alongside consultation and measures to decrease them at the personal and community level; nutritional and food supplementation; oral and dental hygiene education; and clinical preventive services such as immunization and vaccination of children, adults and the elderly, as well as vaccination or post-exposure prophylaxis for people exposed to a communicable disease) (www.emro.who.int). Health promotion is the process of empowering people to increase control over their health and its determinants through health literacy efforts and multisectoral action to increase healthy behaviours. This process includes activities for the community-at-large or for populations at increased risk of negative health outcomes. Health promotion usually addresses behavioural risk factors such as tobacco use, obesity, diet and physical inactivity, as well as the areas of mental health, injury prevention, drug abuse control, alcohol control, health behaviour related to HIV, and sexual health (www.emro.who.int).

7.3.5 *Health System Resilience*

This standard is concerned with ensuring that health systems are able to withstand and respond to crises, such as natural disasters, disease outbreaks, or other emergencies. It is significant at the global level as it ensures that health systems can provide essential health services to people around the world, even during emergencies. The significance of health system resilience at the global level during past can be understood through various examples:

1. **COVID-19 pandemic:** Health system resilience has been critical in responding to the COVID-19 pandemic. Health systems that have been able to quickly adapt and respond to the pandemic have been better able to provide essential health services to those affected by the virus. For example, health systems that were able to quickly set up testing and contact tracing systems, provide personal protective equipment to healthcare workers, and increase hospital capacity were better equipped to respond to the pandemic.
2. **Natural disasters:** Health system resilience is crucial in responding to natural disasters such as earthquakes, hurricanes, and floods. Health systems that are able to quickly respond to natural disasters and provide essential health services to those affected are better able to mitigate the impact of the disaster. For example, in the aftermath of the 2010 earthquake in Haiti, health system resilience was critical in providing essential health services to those affected by the disaster.
3. **Epidemics and pandemics:** Health system resilience is critical in responding to epidemics and pandemics such as Ebola, Zika, and COVID-19. Health systems that are able to adapt and respond to epidemics and pandemics are better able to provide essential health services to those affected by the disease and contain the spread of the disease. For example, health systems in countries such as South Korea and Taiwan, that were able to quickly respond to the COVID-19 pandemic, were able to provide essential health services to those affected by the virus while also containing the spread of the disease.

7.4 Health Care System of USA

There are several countries with strong and efficient healthcare systems that are often looked up to as models for other countries, one of it is USA. The healthcare system in the United States is a complex, multi-layered system involving multiple public and private entities. Some of the components and policies of the healthcare system in the United States are:

7.4.1 *Health Insurance*

The majority of Americans receive health insurance through their employer. The Affordable Care Act (ACA), also known as Obamacare, requires most employers to provide health insurance to their employees, and it established a health insurance exchange where individuals can purchase insurance plans. The Medicaid programme provides health insurance for low-income individuals, and the Medicare programme provides health insurance for individuals over 65 and those with disabilities. According to the US Census Bureau, the percentage of people without health insurance decreased from 16 per cent in 2010 to 8.6 per cent in 2019. In addition, the ACA requires insurers to cover pre-existing conditions and allows children to stay on their parents' insurance until the age of 26. The ACA also included an expansion of Medicaid, the government health insurance programme for low-income individuals. As of 2020, 38 states and Washington, DC., have expanded Medicaid, providing coverage to millions of previously uninsured Americans.

7.4.2 *Public Health Agencies*

The United States has several public health agencies, including the Centres for Disease Control and Prevention (CDC), the National Institutes of Health (NIH), and the Food and Drug

Administration (FDA). These agencies are responsible for regulating and monitoring health issues such as infectious diseases, drug safety, and food safety. Selected few public health agencies in the United States are:

(i) **Centres for Disease Control and Prevention (CDC):** The CDC is responsible for monitoring and preventing the spread of infectious diseases, such as COVID-19, and promoting overall health and wellness. The CDC has been instrumental in the US response to the COVID-19 pandemic, providing guidance on public health measures such as mask-wearing and vaccination, conducting research, and coordinating with state and local public health departments.

(ii) **National Institute of Health (NIH):** The NIH is a federal agency responsible for conducting and supporting medical research. The NIH has made significant contributions to the development of vaccines, treatments, and therapies for a range of diseases, including cancer, HIV/AIDS, and COVID-19.

(iii) **Food and Drug Administration (FDA):** The FDA is responsible for regulating food, drugs, medical devices, and other products to ensure their safety and efficacy. The FDA has been involved in the approval and regulation of vaccines and therapies for COVID-19 and other diseases.

(iv) **Substance Abuse and Mental Health Services Administration (SAMHSA):** SAMHSA is responsible for promoting the prevention and treatment of mental and substance use disorders. SAMHSA has been instrumental in improving access to mental health and substance use disorder treatment services and promoting prevention strategies to reduce the incidence of these conditions.

(v) **Environmental Protection Agency (EPA):** The EPA is responsible for protecting human health and the environment. The EPA has been involved in efforts to reduce pollution and promote clean air and water, which have been linked to improved health outcomes.

7.4.3 *Health Policy*

Health policy in the United States is heavily influenced by politics and public opinion. For example, the ACA was a controversial policy, and there have been ongoing debates about the role of government in healthcare and the best way to provide universal coverage. The healthcare policy in the United States has undergone multiple changes and reforms over time. Some of the significant policies that have shaped the healthcare system in the United States are Social Security Act of 1935 that established the Social Security system and included provisions to create programmes to support public health, including maternal and child health services and disease prevention; medicare and Medicaid Programmes that were created to provide health insurance for low-income individuals, the elderly, and those with disabilities; Health Maintenance Organization Act of 1973, an Act that encouraged the formation of health maintenance organizations (HMOs) as an alternative to fee-for-service healthcare. HMOs emphasized preventive care and coordinated care to improve the quality of care provided to patients. Health Insurance Portability and Accountability Act (HIPAA) of 1996 established national standards for the protection of personal health information and provided individuals with the right to access their medical records. Another Act was Patient Protection and Affordable Care Act (ACA) of

2010. This law, also known as Obamacare, was a comprehensive reform of the healthcare system that included provisions to expand access to health insurance, improve quality, and control healthcare costs. The ACA required most Americans to obtain health insurance, established health insurance exchanges where individuals can purchase insurance plans, and expanded Medicaid to provide health insurance for low-income individuals. 21st Century Cures Act of 2016 provides funding for medical research, including research on precision medicine and cancer, and included provisions to promote patient access to medical information and improve mental health policies.

The Mental Health Parity and Addiction Equity Act of 2008 is a federal law that requires health insurance companies to provide equal coverage for mental health and substance use disorder treatment as they do for physical illnesses. Prior to the law, many health insurance policies provided limited or no coverage for mental health and substance use disorder treatment, leading to higher out-of-pocket costs and limited access to care. Canada has a universal healthcare system that provides coverage for all legal residents and citizens. The government regulates the prices of medical services and medications, which makes healthcare more affordable for everyone.

7.5 Health Care System of India

The Constitution of India outlines "Public Health, Sanitation, Hospitals and Dispensaries" as a state subject, while "Population Control and Family Planning", "adulteration of foodstuff", control of infectious and contagious diseases across state boundaries and issues governing medical profession are placed under the Concurrent List where both the Central Government and the State Governments have jurisdiction. Hospitals attached to port facilities for quarantine or seamen's hospitals are exclusively under the jurisdiction of the Central Government. Policy formulation and regulation on health insurance is largely under the jurisdiction of the Central Government, social health insurance (SHI) is in the Concurrent List, paving the way for state-level policy formulation (Mahal, 2020).

The Parliament of India endorsed the first India's National Health Policy in 1983. The draft of the Indian National Health Policy deals with health as a fundamental right, the expenses of health, health as an integral part of national development, the health movement, the role of indigenous systems, priority in healthcare, and the infrastructure of healthcare delivery. The principles outlined in the policy focus on improvement of living conditions, health education and the health movement, preventive and promotive health, coverage of the felt needs of the people, primary healthcare, continuing medical education, pharmaceuticals, medical education curriculum, biomedical engineering, legislation, coordination, health insurance, and nationalization. In order for this policy to be implemented, proper strategy and planning needs to be carried out after identifying short-term and long-tern goals (IMA, 1979). The health policy was revised in 2002 and latest in 2017. It is to note as the disease pattern, occurrence and types have changes in last two to three decades; the policy needs to be revised as per the requirements. The context is changed from previous policies to 2017 health policy, i.e.:

1. There is growing burden on account of non-communicable diseases and some infectious diseases.
2. The emergence of a robust healthcare industry estimated to be growing at double digit.
3. Change is the growing incidences of catastrophic expenditure due to healthcare costs,

which are presently estimated to be one of the major contributors to poverty.

4. A rising economic growth enables enhanced fiscal capacity. Therefore, a new health policy responsive to these contextual changes is required.

7.5.1 *Some Prominent Healthcare Agencies in India*

There are several health agencies in India that play a significant role in promoting and maintaining the health and well-being of the population. Some of the most important health agencies in India are as follows:

1. **Ministry of Health and Family Welfare:** The Ministry of Health and Family Welfare is the primary body responsible for formulating and implementing policies related to healthcare in India. It is responsible for planning, implementing, and evaluating national health programmes, as well as coordinating with state governments and other stakeholders.
2. **National Health Authority:** The National Health Authority is an autonomous body responsible for implementing the flagship Pradhan Mantri Jan Arogya Yojana (PM-JAY) scheme, which aims to provide health insurance cover to the poorest of the poor in India. The agency is also responsible for setting standards for healthcare providers in the country.

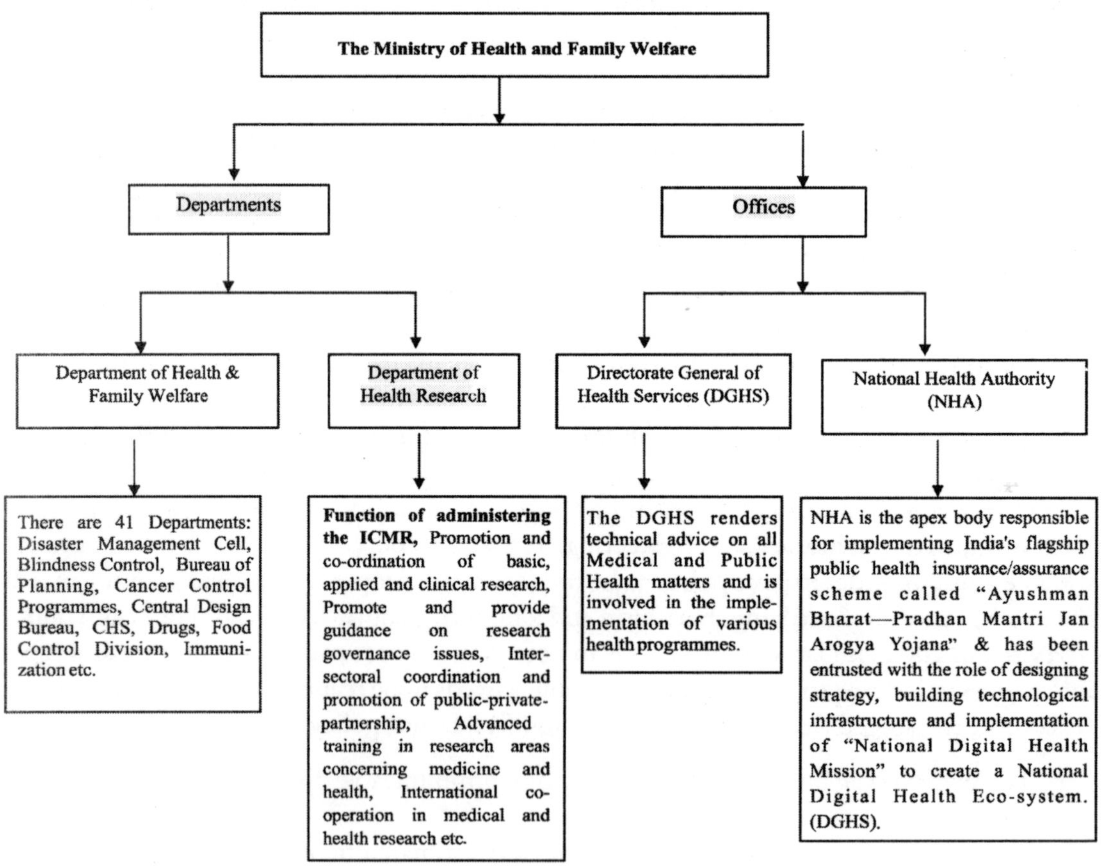

Fig. 7.1: Healthcare System of India.

3. **Indian Council of Medical Research:** The Indian Council of Medical Research is a premier research institution in India that conducts research on various health issues, including infectious diseases, non-communicable diseases, and medical technologies. The agency is also responsible for coordinating and promoting biomedical research in the country.
4. **Central Drugs Standard Control Organization:** The Central Drugs Standard Control Organization is responsible for regulating the import, manufacture, distribution, and sale of drugs and cosmetics in India. The agency is responsible for ensuring that drugs and cosmetics are safe and effective, and that they meet the standards prescribed by law.
5. **National Centre for Disease Control:** The National Centre for Disease Control is responsible for the prevention and control of communicable diseases in India. The agency works closely with state governments and other stakeholders to identify and respond to disease outbreaks and epidemics.

7.5.2 *Prominent Health Schemes and Programmes*

7.5.2.1 *National Health Mission (NHM)*

The NHM envisages achievement of universal access to equitable, affordable and quality healthcare services that are accountable and responsive to people's needs. National Rural Health Mission (NRHM) seeks to provide quality healthcare to the rural population, especially the vulnerable groups. The key policy objectives of National Health Mission are:

1. **Universal Health Coverage:** The policy aims to achieve universal health coverage through a comprehensive and integrative approach that includes prevention, promotion, and healthcare services.
2. **Health in All Policies:** The policy recognizes that health is influenced by a wide range of determinants, and calls for a coordinated approach that integrates health into all policies that affect the health and well-being of the population.
3. **Focus on Primary Healthcare:** The policy prioritizes the strengthening of primary healthcare services, including community engagement, health promotion, and preventive and curative services.
4. **Quality of Care:** The policy emphasizes the importance of ensuring quality of care across all levels of the healthcare system, and encourages the adoption of a patient-centred approach that values the dignity and rights of patients.
5. **Health System Resilience:** The policy aims to build a resilient health system that is able to respond to emergencies and disasters, and that is able to adapt to changing health needs and challenges.
6. **Partnerships and Convergence:** The policy recognizes the importance of partnerships and convergence across sectors, and calls for the engagement of all stakeholders in the health system, including the private sector, civil society, and communities.

7.5.2.2 *Chronological Order of Other Health Policies and Programmes*

1. **Family Planning Programme (1952):** This programme was launched to control population growth and improve maternal and child health. The programme focused on providing family planning services and reproductive health education to couples. It is currently being repositioned to not only achieve population stabilization goals but also promote reproductive health and reduce maternal, infant & child mortality and morbidity.
2. **National Malaria Eradication Programme (1958):** This programme was launched to control the spread of malaria in India. The programme involved spraying insecticides, distribution of mosquito nets, and providing treatment to patients. The programme has gone through several phases of implementation, with the current phase running from 2017-2022. However, despite these efforts, malaria remains a significant public health challenge in India, with an estimated 5.6 million cases and 870 deaths reported in 2019. Some of the reasons for this include drug resistance, insecticide resistance, and inadequate funding. To further strengthen the NMEP, the Indian government has taken several steps, such as increasing funding for malaria control, leveraging technology for better surveillance and monitoring, and collaborating with international partners to address the problem. There is also a renewed focus on community engagement and awareness-raising activities, especially in high-burden states. The programme has been effective in reducing the burden of malaria in India.
3. **Smallpox Eradication Programme (1962):** This programme was launched to eradicate smallpox from India. It was a massive vaccination campaign that covered the entire population of the country. India was declared smallpox-free in 1975. According to a report published by Michigan University, the challenge of vaccinating such huge population was humongous. In 1977, the islands were also being scrutinised for smallpox. The International Commission finally certified that India was free of smallpox. Two years later, in December 1979, the Global Commission for the Certification of Smallpox Eradication declared that smallpox had been eradicated from the planet.
4. **National Tuberculosis Control Programme (1962):** The National Tuberculosis (TB) Programme in India was launched in 1962, with the aim of reducing morbidity, mortality, and transmission of TB in the country. The programme's current phase, the Revised National TB Control Programme (RNTCP), was launched in 1997 and has undergone several upgrades since then. The RNTCP's key strategies include early detection and diagnosis of TB cases, standardized treatment with directly observed therapy, short-course (DOTS), and infection control measures. The programme has made significant progress in reducing the burden of TB in India over the years. According to the World Health Organization (WHO), India has the highest burden of TB cases, accounting for 27 per cent of the global burden. However, the RNTCP has achieved some significant milestones, such as reaching the WHO's benchmark of 85 per cent treatment success rate for all TB cases, reducing TB deaths by 19 per cent from 2015 to 2019, and achieving a 16 per cent decline in incidence rate during the same period. Moreover, the Government of India has taken several steps to strengthen the RNTCP, such as increasing funding, expanding diagnostic services, promoting community engagement, and adopting innovative digital

technologies for monitoring and surveillance. For instance, the use of mobile apps and web-based portals has enabled the programme to increase the efficiency of reporting and tracking TB cases across the country.

5. **Pulse Polio Programme (1995):** The Pulse Polio Immunization (PPI) programme in India was launched in 1995 with the aim of eradicating polio from the country. It was a massive public health initiative that involved administering oral polio vaccine (OPV) drops to children under the age of five years in a phased manner, at regular intervals. The pulse polio programme had several waves, each involving multiple rounds of vaccine administration.

   The PPI programme was instrumental in controlling and eventually eradicating polio from India. According to the World Health Organization (WHO), India was once considered among the world's largest endemic reservoirs of polio virus, with thousands of cases reported every year. However, thanks to the PPI, India was officially declared free of polio in 2014, after no new cases were reported for three consecutive years. The PPI programme's success can be attributed to various strategies, including high-level political commitment, intensive communication campaigns, community mobilization, and innovative operational approaches. For instance, the programme utilized a large network of trained healthcare workers, volunteers, and social workers to reach out to remote and marginalized communities. Moreover, the PPI programme had a strong monitoring and evaluation system, which enabled timely identification and correction of gaps in implementation. The programme's success also helped strengthen the overall immunization infrastructure in India, leading to better coverage and outcomes for other vaccines.

6. **National Rural Health Mission (2005):** The National Rural Health Mission (NRHM) in India was launched in April 2005 with the aim of improving overall healthcare delivery in rural areas by providing accessible, affordable, and quality healthcare to every person. The mission had six key goals, including reducing child mortality, maternal mortality, and the burden of diseases such as tuberculosis, malaria, and HIV/AIDS.

   Over the years, the NRHM has achieved some significant milestones. For instance, the NRHM was instrumental in enhancing the health infrastructure in rural areas through the construction of new health facilities, renovation of old ones, and the expansion of health workforce, including the establishment of a community health worker programme. The NRHM also made significant progress towards improving maternal and child health. For instance, the Maternal Mortality Ratio (MMR) in India declined from 301 deaths per 1,00,000 live births in 2001-03 to 130 deaths per 1,00,000 live births in 2014-16. Similarly, the Infant Mortality Rate (IMR) declined from 58 per 1000 live births in 2005 to 32 per 1000 live births in 2018. NRHM played a crucial role in ramping up health financing in India by increasing the budget allocation towards health and promoting innovative financing models, such as risk pooling schemes. The NRHM also leveraged technology to improve healthcare delivery in rural areas by establishing a robust health information system, telemedicine services, and deploying mobile health vans.

   However, the NRHM also faced several challenges in terms of implementation, including inadequate funding, shortage of human resources, and poor governance. Moreover, the programme was affected by the COVID-19 pandemic, leading to disruptions in healthcare services delivery and infrastructure development. National Tobacco Control Programme (NTCP), launched in 2007, the NTCP is a national programme aimed at preventing and controlling the consumption of tobacco. It aims to create awareness about the harmful effects of tobacco, to enforce tobacco control laws, to provide tobacco cessation services, and to facilitate research on tobacco control.

7. **Rashtriya Swasthya Biına Yojana (2008):** The Rashtriya Swasthya Bima Yojana (RSBY) is a health insurance scheme launched by the Government of India in 2008, aimed at providing health coverage to the below poverty line families in the country. The scheme aimed to make quality healthcare accessible to everyone, regardless of their socio-economic status. Under the RSBY, beneficiaries are provided with smart cards containing their insurance details. The scheme covers inpatient hospitalization expenses up to Rs. 30,000 per annum per family, including pre-existing diseases. Along with hospitalization charges, the scheme also covers transportation costs, pre- and post-hospitalization expenses, and other medical expenses. The RSBY has achieved some significant milestones, particularly in the area of financial protection of vulnerable populations. The scheme has significantly reduced the financial burden and out-of-pocket expenditure on healthcare for poor households. According to a study conducted by the World Bank in 2012, households that enrolled in the RSBY spent 29 per cent less on healthcare than those who were not enrolled.

   Moreover, the RSBY has also led to increased access to healthcare services, particularly in remote and under-served areas. The scheme has provided an incentive for private hospitals to deliver healthcare services to the poor, as more than 50 per cent of the hospitals empanelled under the RSBY are private. According to the Ministry of Health and Family Welfare, more than 4 crore BPL families have been covered under the scheme since its launch. However, the RSBY has also faced some challenges in terms of implementation, including inefficiencies in the smart card system, inadequate awareness among beneficiaries, and low coverage among certain population groups.
8. **Mission Indradhanush (2014):** Launched in 2014, Mission Indradhanush is a national programme that aims to increase the coverage of immunization in India by targeting unvaccinated or partially vaccinated children. The programme aims to achieve full immunization coverage for all children by 2020. Priority would be to further improve immunization coverage with quality and safety, improve vaccine security as per National Vaccine Policy 2011 and introduction of newer vaccines based on epidemiological considerations.
9. **Mental Health Policy (2014):** This policy takes into consideration the provisions of the National Mental Health Policy 2014 with simultaneous action on the following fronts: (1) Increase creation of specialists through public financing and develop special rules to give preference to those willing to work in public systems, (2) Create network of community members to provide psycho-social support to strengthen mental health services at primary level facilities, and (3) Leverage digital technology in a context where access to qualified psychiatrists is difficult (NHP, 2017).

10. **Ayushman Bharat Yojana (2018):** This programme, also known as PMJAY (Pradhan Mantri Jan Aarogya Yojana), was launched to provide health insurance coverage to low-income households. The programme aims to provide financial protection to vulnerable populations by providing health insurance coverage for medical and hospitalization expenses. The scheme provides free-of-cost insurance coverage of up to Rs. 5 lakh per family per year for secondary and tertiary healthcare. Ayushman Bharat Yojana has provided much-needed financial protection to millions of families in India and has helped them manage the costs of expensive treatment. Ayushman Bharat Yojana has resulted in improved access to healthcare services for many people living in rural and remote areas of the country. The scheme has also created incentives for private hospitals to provide healthcare services to the poor, with more than 22,000 hospitals empanelled under the scheme. The scheme has encouraged the digitization of health records, making it easier to track medical history, and ensuring better coordination across healthcare providers. The scheme has started showing results in terms of improved healthcare outcomes. The National Health Authority (NHA), which runs the Ayushman Bharat scheme, reported over 1.26 crore hospitalizations and more than one crore beneficiaries treated under the scheme. The scheme has also helped in reducing out-of-pocket expenditures, resulting in better primary care and long-term health outcomes. Ayushman Bharat Yojana has led to the creation of a robust public health infrastructure across the country. This infrastructure includes dedicated healthcare centres and hospitals providing cashless healthcare services to beneficiaries.
11. **Jan Aushadhi:** Jan Aushadhi is a generic medicine programme launched by the Government of India to provide affordable and quality medicines to the masses. Under this programme, generic medicines are made available in specialized Jan Aushadhi Kendras (JAKs) across country. The medicines at up to 90 per cent discount on the branded medicines' market price are made available at various government shops. The Jan Aushadhi programme has achieved significant success in making quality medicines accessible to the masses at an affordable price. Jan Aushadhi provides essential medicines at significantly lower prices, making a significant difference in the lives of those who face financial stress due to high medical costs. In the capital city of Delhi, there are more than 100 Jan Aushadhi Kendras across the city, making essential medicines accessible to the masses. These Kendras help to overcome the challenges of accessing affordable medicines in remote and underserved areas, thus increasing outreach. The medicines sold under the programme go through strict quality checks and are procured from reputed public and private pharma companies. It ensures that these Kendras maintain quality measures as prescribed by the Food and Drug Administration. Jan Aushadhi has been successful in reducing the out-of-pocket expenditure of patients on medicines significantly, thereby alleviating the financial burden on families. The programme has expanded its product range to include various essential medicines, such as children's medicines, diabetic medicines, and more.

Affordable medicines provided under Jan Aushadhi have helped many households in Delhi, and particularly among the poor and underprivileged, to manage life-threatening illnesses that were previously beyond their financial capability.

In addition to the above-mentioned programmes, every Indian state has implemented its own health programmes to cater to the specific healthcare needs of their citizens. For instance, the Tamil Nadu government has implemented the Tamil Nadu Health System Reform Programme (TNHSRP), which aims to provide universal healthcare for the population. Similarly, in Maharashtra, the Rajiv Gandhi Jeevandayee Arogya Yojana programme provides free quality medical care to the poor and vulnerable population. While progress has been made to improve healthcare access, there remains a need to address the high burden of communicable and non-communicable diseases and to provide higher quality healthcare services to all citizens.

7.6 New Delhi Healthcare Initiatives (A Case Study)

The Government of Delhi has implemented several health schemes and programmes aimed at providing accessible and affordable healthcare to its citizens. Some of the major health policies and programmes of the Delhi government that are appreciated worldwide are as under:

7.6.1 *Mohalla Clinics (2015)*

The Mohalla Clinic is a primary healthcare delivery system established by the Delhi government in 2015, with the aim of providing accessible and affordable healthcare services to residents in urban slums and low-income communities. Under this initiative, primary healthcare clinics are set-up in various neighbourhoods to provide free health check-ups, diagnostic tests, and medical consultations. The Mohalla Clinic approach has achieved significant success in improving access to primary healthcare services in Delhi. The major contributions are:

1. **Access to Basic Healthcare:** The Mohalla Clinics have provided basic healthcare access to millions of citizens living in Delhi's urban slums and low-income neighbourhoods, who were previously deprived of medical services or could not afford them.
2. **Timely Diagnosis and Treatment:** The Mohalla Clinics provide free laboratory and diagnostic services like blood tests, urine tests, and X-rays, ensuring timely diagnosis and treatment of various illnesses. The clinics also provide prescription medicine for common ailments like fever, cough, cold, and flu.
3. **Improved Community Participation:** The community has been actively participating and contributing towards the success of Mohalla Clinics. The community has been helping in identifying potential beneficiaries, spreading awareness about the availability of services in their neighbourhood, and providing feedback to improve the quality of services provided.
4. **Cost-Effective Health Services:** Mohalla Clinics offer cost-effective healthcare delivery as the clinics are located within walking distance to the poor and marginalized and the services provided are free of cost.
5. **Reduction in Hospitalization Cost:** Mohalla Clinics have reduced the financial burden on families by providing affordable primary healthcare services. Ashoka University in a report revealed that the Mohalla Clinics have reduced the cost of hospitalization by approximately 50 per cent.

The Mohalla Clinics have been recognized nationally and internationally for their contribution towards improving primary healthcare delivery. Harvard University has done a case study on Mohalla Clinics and World Health Organization (WHO) has appreciated the contribution of Mohalla Clinics to healthcare services in Delhi,

7.6.2 *Health Information Management System (HIMS) (2019)*

The Health Information Management System (HIMS) 2019 is an e-governance initiative launched by the Delhi government in 2019. The system aims to create a comprehensive digital platform that enables the government to store, access, and share healthcare data from across all public healthcare facilities in Delhi. The HIMS 2019 is a cloud-based platform designed to ease the burden of manual record-keeping and to provide real-time data sharing to improve the effectiveness of health policies in Delhi. The system allows the government to monitor the healthcare status of citizens, and to take timely action in response to emerging health issues. The HIMS 2019 system is designed to integrate healthcare data from various public health facilities in Delhi, including hospitals, clinics, and dispensaries. The system enables healthcare providers to manage electronic medical records of patients, including their medical histories, treatment plans, and diagnostic test results. The system processes and analyses healthcare data in real-time, enabling the government to identify disease trends and risk factors quickly and take timely preventive measures. HIMS 2019 provides a dashboard display, which presents detailed healthcare data in a user-friendly manner to policymakers and healthcare professionals, enabling them to make well-informed decisions. The system's health analytics tools draw actionable insights from health data and provide valuable insights about health service utilization and performance, medication compliance, and patient treatment outcomes. The HIMS 2019 system has a mobile application to enable healthcare providers to access patient data anytime, anywhere and improve their overall efficiency.

The HIMS 2019 system has been successful in improving the efficiency of healthcare delivery in Delhi, particularly during the COVID-19 pandemic. The system enabled the government to monitor the number of COVID-19 cases, track hospitalizations, and ensure suitable treatment. The HIMS system helped improve the responsiveness of medical facilities and minimized the response time in Delhi during the crisis.

7.6.3 *Delhi Arogya Kosh (2017)*

Launched in 2017, the Delhi Arogya Kosh is a health scheme that provides assistance to economically disadvantaged patients seeking medical treatment in private hospitals. This scheme provides financial support in the form of cashless hospitalization up to Rs. 10 lakhs, ensuring that patients have access to quality medical care. The fund was set up to provide financial assistance to deserving patients who wish to access expensive medical treatment but cannot afford to do so. The Arogya Kosh initiative has achieved significant success in its objective of providing financial assistance to patients who need expensive medical treatments. Arogya Kosh provides financial assistance to patients from low-income groups who are unable to afford costly medical treatment like cancer treatment, heart surgeries, organ transplants, or other life-saving surgeries. The initiative helps reduce the financial burden on patients by covering a portion of their medical expenses, including medical tests, therapies, surgeries etc. Through Arogya Kosh, patients have access to an easy and transparent system of receiving financial assistance. The application process is hassle-free, and the money is transferred directly to the hospital's account, reducing the administrative burden on patients' families. Arogya Kosh leverages new-age technology tools, including machine learning, artificial intelligence, and blockchain, to fast-track the application process and ensure transparency.

7.6.4 *Delhi Health Bill (2021)*

In a recent move, the Delhi government has introduced the Delhi Health Bill, which seeks to establish a regulatory framework and streamline healthcare delivery in Delhi. This Bill aims to make healthcare services more accessible and affordable to all citizens of Delhi. The Delhi Health Bill is a legislation passed by the Delhi Legislative Assembly in March 2021, with the aim of improving the health infrastructure and systems in Delhi. The Bill aims to create a state-funded corporation to manage and govern all Delhi Government health facilities. The corporation will be responsible for budget plans, effective delivery of health services, and the creation of a Delhi Health Information Management System. The Bill aims to establish Universal Health Care in the National Capital Territory of Delhi, providing free healthcare services to every citizen. The HIMS will be an e-governance initiative aimed at providing policymakers with access to real-time data from public health facilities. The HIMS will enable the government to make well-informed decisions based on the data received. The Bill proposes to establish a Delhi Health Tribunal, which will hear disputes relating to health services and determine appropriate remedies. The Bill envisages increasing public-private partnership in healthcare through innovative financing mechanisms to encourage private players to participate in providing health services. The Bill proposes to set up a Delhi Arogya Kosh to support patients who need expensive medical treatments. The Bill promotes the importance of preventive healthcare by integrating Yoga, Ayurveda, and other traditional medical practices in its healthcare system. Delhi government has implemented various health policies and programmes to improve healthcare access and affordability in the state. The programmes outlined above strive to provide quality healthcare services to all citizens, irrespective of their socio-economic background. However, there is still a long way to go in addressing the gaps in healthcare delivery and ensuring that all citizens have access to quality healthcare services.

7.7 Merits and Demerits of Indian Health Care System

The Indian Healthcare System, like any other healthcare system around the world, has its merits and demerits. India has one of the largest healthcare systems in the world but the inequitable distribution of healthcare facilities especially in urban and rural areas is the major challenge of Indian system. Below are some of the advantages and disadvantages of the Indian Healthcare System:

7.7.1 *Merits*

1. **Widespread accessibility:** The Indian healthcare system provides accessibility to healthcare facilities for all individuals regardless of their socio-economic background. The government provides free or low-cost medical care to the poor and marginalized population. Furthermore, telemedicine technology and mobile healthcare clinics have made healthcare facilities accessible to rural areas. Number of hospitals in India has increased from 11,174 in 1991 to 18,218 in 2000. Moreover, under Ayushman Bharat

Scheme, i.e., government-led health insurance fund that provides healthcare to millions of individuals who cannot even afford primary healthcare costs. The Pradhan Mantri Jan Arogya Yojana (PM-JAY), also known as Ayushman Bharat, aims to provide health insurance coverage to around 500 million vulnerable citizens. As of June 2021, more than 29 million hospitalizations have been covered under PM-JAY, offering financial protection to those in need.The Indian government has taken proactive measures to improve primary healthcare accessibility, resulting in increased coverage across rural and urban areas. For instance, the National Health Mission (NHM) has played a pivotal role in establishing and strengthening primary healthcare centres (PHCs) and sub-centres across the country. According to 2020 data, India has approximately 25,308 PHCs, catering to the healthcare needs of millions.

2. **Cost-effectiveness:** Compared to other healthcare systems around the world, healthcare services in India are affordable due to lower treatment costs and low physician fees. The cost of surgery in India is about one-tenth of that in the US or Western Europe. The healthcare sector in India is expected to grow to reach a size of $50 billion by 2025, while the global medical tourism market is estimated to be worth about $72 billion. "India's share in medical tourism is expected to be around 10 billion dollars by 2023. The country is also world's largest supplier of generic drugs" (www.livemint.com/).
3. **Alternative healthcare options:** India is known for its alternative healthcare options such as Ayurveda, Yoga, and Homoeopathy, which provide holistic treatment options and drug-free therapies. The growth of allopathic medicine rests upon higher funding and resources for research, development and in marketing. Still nearly 70 per cent of India's rural population relies on traditional medicine for their basic care. The Ayurveda, Yoga, naturopathy, Unani, Siddha, and Homoeopathy make up India's system of alternative medicine (AYUSH) and alternative medicine sector in India is anticipated to grow at a CAGR of 8.6 per cent during the forecast period of 2022-27. Ayurveda, yoga, naturopathy, Unani, Siddha, and Homoeopathy make up India's system of alternative medicine (AYUSH). India is regarded as the centre of alternative medicine, including Unani, Ayurveda, Siddha, and Homoeopathy, due to the wealth of old scientific knowledge here (Bahl, 2022).
4. **Thriving Telemedicine Revolution:** India has witnessed a significant rise in telemedicine initiatives, especially in recent years. With the advent of digital technology, telemedicine has become a transformative solution, bridging the gap between healthcare providers and patients in remote areas. For example, eSanjeevani, a national telemedicine initiative, provided over 9.3 million teleconsultations as of June 2021. This has allowed patients to receive expert medical advice from specialists without the need for physical travel, thereby increasing accessibility and reducing healthcare costs.
5. **Competitive Pharmaceutical Industry:** India's pharmaceutical industry is globally recognized for its vast production and affordability, making it a merit of the Indian healthcare system. It is known as the "Pharmacy of the World" due to its ability to manufacture and export high-quality generic medications at affordable prices. The Indian pharmaceutical industry caters not only to domestic needs but also supplies affordable medicines to developing nations worldwide. This merits commendation, as it significantly

contributes to making healthcare more accessible and affordable, both within India and globally.

6. **Skilled medical professionals:** India is known for the quality of its medical professionals, who are highly skilled and well-trained in their respective fields. As of 2021, the Indian healthcare sector employs a total of 4.7 million people. The sector has generated 2.7 million additional jobs in India between 2017-22. It generates over 5,00,000 new jobs per year.

7.7.2 *Demerits*

1. **Limited expenditure on Healthcare infrastructure:** The Indian healthcare system faces several infrastructure challenges, including a shortage of medical facilities, equipment, and trained healthcare workers. Rural areas and remote regions lack adequate healthcare facilities and are underserved by healthcare professionals. It is believed that overall expenditure on Healthcare is responsible for deteriorating condition of the system. India's public expenditure on healthcare is only 2.1 per cent of GDP in 2021-22 while Japan, Canada and France spend about 10 per cent of their GDP on public healthcare.
2. **Lack of health insurance coverage and high out-of-pocket expenditure:** Despite the launch of the Ayushman Bharat Yojana, millions of Indians are still not covered by health insurance. Private healthcare is very expensive and unaffordable for much of the population. One of the significant demerits of the Indian healthcare system is the lack of universal healthcare coverage. According to the National Sample Survey 75th Round, only about 12 per cent of the rural population and 18 per cent of the urban population were covered under any health insurance scheme in 2017-18. This leaves a large portion of the population vulnerable to high out-of-pocket healthcare expenditures. The lack of comprehensive healthcare coverage often leads to financial burdens, making healthcare services unaffordable for many. Individuals and families are forced to bear the brunt of medical expenses, pushing them into poverty or crippling them financially.

   Therefore, India's healthcare system heavily relies on out-of-pocket expenditures, which contributes to the financial burden on individuals. As per a study published in *The Lancet*, an estimated 70 per cent of healthcare expenses in India are paid out-of-pocket, significantly higher than the global average of 18 per cent. High out-of-pocket expenditures deter individuals from seeking timely medical care, leading to delayed diagnoses and treatment, potentially worsening health conditions. This burden especially affects marginalized communities and lower-income groups, deepening healthcare inequalities within the country.
3. **Inadequate and Inequitable healthcare services:** A major demerit is the insufficient healthcare infrastructure, particularly in rural areas. According to the National Health Profile 2020, India has a shortage of 24 per cent of sub-centres, 18 per cent of primary health centres (PHCs), and 16 per cent of community health centres (CHCs). This inadequacy limits access to basic healthcare services for a significant portion of the population, especially those in remote and underserved regions. Inequitable distribution of healthcare services and facilities based on socio-demographic circumstances creates vast inequalities in healthcare access and outcomes. In rural areas, the primary healthcare

centres are often understaffed, lack necessary equipment, medicines, and diagnostic facilities. This compromises the quality of healthcare services provided and leads to a suboptimal patient experience.

4. **Lack of healthcare professionals:** Despite the presence of skilled medical professionals, many healthcare facilities in India lack the necessary infrastructure and resources to deliver adequate care. India suffers from a chronic shortage of skilled medical professionals, which has only been intensified by the pandemic. The recommended ratio of medical service providers to people by the WHO is 1:1000. India's ratio stands at a mere 1:10,189 (104% short), posing a desperate need for more healthcare professionals (shapecharity.org). India faces a significant shortage of healthcare professionals, including doctors, nurses, and paramedics. The doctor-patient ratio in India stands at approximately 1:1,404, significantly below the World Health Organization's recommended ratio of 1:1,000. Similarly, the nurse-patient ratio is estimated at 1:614, compared to the desired ratio of 1:300. This shortage of healthcare professionals puts immense strain on the existing workforce, leading to longer wait times, decreased patient-doctor interaction time, and compromised healthcare quality. It also results in overburdened hospitals where doctors are forced to handle an excessive number of patients, compromising their ability to provide personalized care.
5. **Lack of medical research:** Medical research in the country needs to be focused on drugs and vaccines for tropical diseases which are normally neglected by international pharmaceutical companies on account of their limited profitability potential. The National Health Policy 2002 suggests to allocate more funds to boost medical research in this direction (www.economicsdiscussion.net). India has neglected biomedical engineering, which is responsible for medical advancements and technology. According to the 2017 ET report, the ICMR, which employs over 800 scientists across 32 institutions nationwide, is unable to name even one new intervention, such as a new medication, vaccine, diagnostic tool, or treatment technique that has been produced by its many researchers over the past two years. In India, there are 64 stand alone PG institutes and 596 medical colleges. However, only a small number of these universities have committed resources to research or integrated research into their medical curricula. In a report in *The Economic Times* in 2017, it was revealed that in a span of 2 years, 685 research papers were published by the ICMR scientists whereas All India Institute of Medical Sciences (AIIMS) published more than 1100 research papers in a year. Also, an extensive research paper on the state of research in India revealed many reasons for the sorry state of medical research in the country, which is alarming given we have more than 6,00,000 medical graduates per year (www.healthcareexecutive.in).

The Indian healthcare system has made significant progress in improving healthcare accessibility and affordability. However, it still faces significant challenges such as inadequate infrastructure, a shortage of healthcare workers in rural areas, and uneven distribution of healthcare resources, which leads to healthcare inequality and compromises the quality of care. The future of health and healthcare in India holds immense potential for growth and development. With a dynamic and rapidly evolving healthcare landscape, advancements in technology, and various reforms and initiatives, India is poised to make significant progress in improving healthcare access and outcomes. The integration of technology in healthcare, commonly known as digital health, is transforming the sector in India. The rise of mobile technology, telemedicine, artificial intelligence (AI), and health apps are set to revolutionize how healthcare is delivered, accessed, and managed. According to a report by McKinsey, the Indian digital health market is expected to reach $5.5 billion by 2025, driven by increased internet penetration, smartphone usage, and government initiatives. Precision medicine, an emerging approach that customizes healthcare based on an individual's genetic makeup, is gaining traction in India. The field of genomics plays a crucial role in advancing precision medicine and is expected to have a significant impact on diagnostics, treatment, and disease prevention. The future of health and the healthcare system in India is marked by the integration of technology, expansion of health insurance coverage, emphasis on preventive and public health initiatives, precision medicine, and strengthening primary healthcare. Continued efforts, collaboration between public and private sectors, and sustained investment in healthcare infrastructure will be crucial in realizing a future where healthcare is accessible, affordable, and of high quality for all citizens.

REFERENCES

Bahl, A.S. (2022). India's alternative medicine industry grows, boosted by the Covid-19 pandemic in *TOI*, retrieved from timesofindia.indiatimes.com

Collins, E. (2010). "Communication with the Public". In Van-Tam, Jonathan; Sellwood, Chloe (eds.). *Introduction to Pandemic Influenza*. Wallingford, Oxford: CAB International. p. 192. ISBN 978-1-84593-578-8.

https: //main.mohfw.gov.in/

https: //www.icrc.org/en

Mahal, A., Selvaraj., S. *et al.,* (ed.) (2022). *India Health System Review in Health System in Transition*, Vol. 11, No. 1202, WHO Pub.

National health policy: a draft prepared by the Indian Medical Association. *J. Indian Med Assoc.* 1979, Mar 16; 72(6): 144-7. PMID: 512387.

WHO, "What are the International Health Regulations and Emergency Committees? Q&A". www.who.int. World Health Organization. 19 December, 2019.

Index